Nanoparticle-Macrophage Interactions: Implications for Nanosafety and Nanomedicine

Nanoparticle-Macrophage Interactions: Implications for Nanosafety and Nanomedicine

Editors

Olesja Bondarenko
Fernando Torres Andón

MDPI • Basel • Beijing • Wuhan • Barcelona • Belgrade • Manchester • Tokyo • Cluj • Tianjin

Editors
Olesja Bondarenko
National Institute of Chemical Physics and Biophysics,
Tallinn, Estonia

Fernando Torres Andón
Center for Research in Molecular Medicine & Chronic Diseases (CiMUS),
Universidade de Santiago de Compostela,
Santiago de Compostela,
Spain

Editorial Office
MDPI
St. Alban-Anlage 66
4052 Basel, Switzerland

This is a reprint of articles from the Special Issue published online in the open access journal *Nanomaterials* (ISSN 2079-4991) (available at: https://www.mdpi.com/journal/nanomaterials/special_issues/nanomedicine_nanosafety).

For citation purposes, cite each article independently as indicated on the article page online and as indicated below:

LastName, A.A.; LastName, B.B.; LastName, C.C. Article Title. *Journal Name* **Year**, *Volume Number*, Page Range.

ISBN 978-3-0365-4599-8 (Hbk)
ISBN 978-3-0365-4600-1 (PDF)

Contents

About the Editors . . . . **vii**

Fernando Torres Andón and Olesja Bondarenko
Recent Discoveries in Nanoparticle–Macrophage Interactions: In Vitro Models for Nanosafety Testing and Novel Nanomedical Approaches for Immunotherapy
Reprinted from: *Nanomaterials* **2021**, *11*, 2971, doi:10.3390/nano11112971 . . . . **1**

Sandeep Keshavan, Fernando Torres Andón, Audrey Gallud, Wei Chen, Knut Reinert, Lang Tran and Bengt Fadeel
Profiling of Sub-Lethal in Vitro Effects of Multi-Walled Carbon Nanotubes Reveals Changes in Chemokines and Chemokine Receptors
Reprinted from: *Nanomaterials* **2021**, *11*, 883, doi:10.3390/nano11040883 . . . . **5**

Martin Wiemann, Antje Vennemann, Cornel Venzago, Gottlieb-Georg Lindner, Tobias B. Schuster and Nils Krueger
Serum Lowers Bioactivity and Uptake of Synthetic Amorphous Silica by Alveolar Macrophages in a Particle Specific Manner
Reprinted from: *Nanomaterials* **2021**, *11*, 628, doi:10.3390/nano11030628 . . . . **21**

Mai T. Huynh, Carole Mikoryak, Paul Pantano and Rockford Draper
Scavenger Receptor A1 Mediates the Uptake of Carboxylated and Pristine Multi-Walled Carbon Nanotubes Coated with Bovine Serum Albumin
Reprinted from: *Nanomaterials* **2021**, *11*, 539, doi:10.3390/nano11020539 . . . . **39**

Benjamin J. Swartzwelter, Alessandro Verde, Laura Rehak, Mariusz Madej, Victor. F. Puntes, Anna Chiara De Luca, Diana Boraschi and Paola Italiani
Interaction between Macrophages and Nanoparticles: In Vitro 3D Cultures for the Realistic Assessment of Inflammatory Activation and Modulation of Innate Memory
Reprinted from: *Nanomaterials* **2021**, *11*, 207, doi:10.3390/nano11010207 . . . . **63**

Ruhung Wang, Rishabh Lohray, Erik Chow, Pratima Gangupantula, Loren Smith and Rockford Draper
Selective Uptake of Carboxylated Multi-Walled Carbon Nanotubes by Class A Type 1 Scavenger Receptors and Impaired Phagocytosis in Alveolar Macrophages
Reprinted from: *Nanomaterials* **2020**, *10*, 2417, doi:10.3390/nano10122417 . . . . **77**

Helena Rouco, Patricia Diaz-Rodriguez, Diana P. Gaspar, Lídia M. D. Gonçalves, Miguel Cuerva, Carmen Remuñán-López, António J. Almeida and Mariana Landin
Rifabutin-Loaded Nanostructured Lipid Carriers as a Tool in Oral Anti-Mycobacterial Treatment of Crohn's Disease
Reprinted from: *Nanomaterials* **2020**, *10*, 2138, doi:10.3390/nano10112138 . . . . **107**

Edorta Santos-Vizcaino, Aiala Salvador, Claudia Vairo, Manoli Igartua, Rosa Maria Hernandez, Luis Correa, Silvia Villullas and Garazi Gainza
Overcoming the Inflammatory Stage of Non-Healing Wounds: In Vitro Mechanism of Action of Negatively Charged Microspheres (NCMs)
Reprinted from: *Nanomaterials* **2020**, *10*, 1108, doi:10.3390/nano10061108 . . . . **127**

Alba Pensado-López, Juan Fernández-Rey, Pedro Reimunde, José Crecente-Campo, Laura Sánchez and Fernando Torres Andón
Zebrafish Models for the Safety and Therapeutic Testing of Nanoparticles with a Focus on Macrophages
Reprinted from: *Nanomaterials* **2021**, *11*, 1784, doi:10.3390/nano11071784 . . . . **141**

About the Editors

Olesja Bondarenko

Olesja Bondarenko is a senior researcher and team leader at the National Institute of Chemical Physics and Biophysics (Estonia) and a Marie Curie Individual Fellowship-funded postdoctoral researcher at the University of Helsinki (Finland). She co-authored over 30 peer-reviewed publications on the antibacterial and immune effects of nanoparticles, including several highly cited publications. Dr. Bondarenko is also a co-founder of the biotechnological company Nanordica Medical, which focuses on developing advanced antibacterial nanotechnology.

Fernando Torres Andón

Fernando Torres Andón is an AECC Researcher in Nanomedicine for cancer immunotherapy at CiMUS, University of Santiago de Compostela, Spain. He is a pharmacist with a PhD in Molecular Biology, a postdoc in Nanotoxicology with Prof. Bengt Fadeel at Karolinska Institutet, Sweden, and a postdoc in Tumor Immunology with Prof. Paola Allavena at the Humanitas Institute, Italy. His current research at Alonso's lab (CiMUS) is focused on the development and evaluation of new nanostructures for the targeting and reprograming of tumor-associated macrophages into antitumor macrophages with the ability to kill tumor cells, inhibit angiogenesis and promote adaptive immune responses in solid tumors, with the ultimate goal of providing new solutions for patients with cancer.

nanomaterials

Editorial

Recent Discoveries in Nanoparticle–Macrophage Interactions: In Vitro Models for Nanosafety Testing and Novel Nanomedical Approaches for Immunotherapy

Fernando Torres Andón [1,2,*] and Olesja Bondarenko [3,4,*]

1 Center for Research in Molecular Medicine & Chronic Diseases (CiMUS), Universidade de Santiago de Compostela, Campus Vida, 15706 Santiago de Compostela, Spain
2 IRCCS Istituto Clinico Humanitas, Via A. Manzoni 56, Rozzano, 20089 Milan, Italy
3 National Institute of Chemical Physics and Biophysics, Akadeemia tee 23, 12618 Tallinn, Estonia
4 Institute of Biotechnology, HiLIFE, University of Helsinki, Viikinkaari 5d, 00790 Helsinki, Finland
* Correspondence: fernando.torres.andon@usc.es (F.T.A.); olesja.bondarenko@kbfi.ee (O.B.)

Citation: Torres Andón, F.; Bondarenko, O. Recent Discoveries in Nanoparticle–Macrophage Interactions: In Vitro Models for Nanosafety Testing and Novel Nanomedical Approaches for Immunotherapy. *Nanomaterials* **2021**, *11*, 2971. https://doi.org/10.3390/nano11112971

Received: 25 October 2021
Accepted: 29 October 2021
Published: 5 November 2021

Nanoparticles (NPs) offer unique properties for biomedical applications, leading to new nanomedicines. Recent examples of advanced nanoparticle-based nanomedicines are COVID-19 RNA vaccines. Regardless of the delivery route of the NPs into the body (intravenous or subcutaneous injection, oral, intranasal, etc.), NPs inevitably come into contact with immune cells, such as macrophages. Macrophages are phagocytizing cells that determine the fate and the lifetime of NPs in relevant biological fluids or tissues, which has consequences for both nanosafety and nanomedicine.

The aim of this Special Issue is to cover recent advancements in our understanding of NP–macrophage interactions, with a focus on in vitro models for nanosafety and novel nanomedicine approaches that allow the modulation of the immunological profile of macrophages. The current Special Issue compiles nine papers: seven research articles and two review articles. The original articles include studies on the interaction of different nanomaterials, such as multi-walled carbon nanotubes (MWCNTs) [1–3], amorphous silica [4], gold nanoparticles [3,5], lipid carriers [6], and microspheres [7], with macrophages in different scenarios.

Most of the articles in this Special Issue are focused on the toxicological aspects of nanomaterials and in vitro models. Wang et al. found that carboxylated-MWCNTs (cMWCNTs) coated with Pluronic®F-108 (PF108) interacted with the class A scavenger receptor (SR-A1) on the surface of alveolar macrophages, whereas both pristine-MWCNTs (pMWCNTs) and amino-functionalized-MWCNTs coated with PF108 did not. This interaction was crucial for the uptake of cMWCNTs by macrophages resulting in higher toxicity and impaired phagocytic activity for other SR-A1 ligands. Similarly, Huynh et al. [2] coated cMWCNTs and pMWCNTs with bovine serum albumin (BSA) and observed an increased uptake for BSA-cMWCNTs versus BSA-pMWCNTs by RAW264.7 macrophages. The authors hypothesized that SR-A1 can interact with two structural features of BSA-cMWNTs, one inherent to the oxidized nanotubes and the other provided by the BSA corona. In another work, Wiemann et al. studied the interaction of serum-coated synthetic amorphous silica (SAS) NPs with alveolar NR8383 macrophages. While under serum-free conditions, SAS NPs were taken up by macrophages, which resulted in toxicity; these effects were mitigated by the presence of serum [4]. Similar results were previously observed by Gallud et al. [8] with mesoporous silica, where the cytotoxicity of the NPs was mitigated in the presence of serum. These toxicological studies have implications for the nanosafety of biomaterials, but also for the potential application of NPs in medicine.

Depending on the route of administration [9], NPs interact with different proteins and form a protein corona that heavily influences their interaction with macrophages [10]. Thus, studies on the interaction of NPs with proteins and macrophages with different phenotypes are of foremost importance. Upon the interaction and uptake of NPs by macrophages, different outcomes are possible [11]. In this Special Issue, Keshavan et al. [3] published an in vitro study comparing three benchmark nanomaterials (Ag NPs, TiO_2 NPs, and MWCNTs) procured from the nanomaterial repository at the Joint Research Centre of the European Commission. The exposure of sub-lethal concentrations of macrophage-like cell line (THP-1 pretreated with phorbol-12-myristate-13-acetate) to these NPs induced changes in mRNA expression that was mostly related to immune networks such as cytokine and chemokine signaling pathways. Using sub-lethal concentrations of MWCNTs, modest inductions of IL-6 and IL-1β were observed, while CCR2-CCL2 was identified as the most significantly upregulated pathway [3]. This activation of CCL2, also referred to as monocyte chemoattractant protein-1 (MCP-1), may have a role in the granuloma formation in the lungs, pleural or abdominal cavity following exposure to MWCNTs. In previous studies, we also reported on the secretion of IL-1β by hollow carbon spheres [12], or the specific interaction of single-walled carbon nanotubes (SWCNTs) with TLR2 in the absence of protein corona [13]. Of foremost importance, we demonstrate that these types of experiments must be combined with biodegradation studies in order to understand the benefits and limitations of new nanotechnologies, such as carbon nanotubes [14], for their safe application for industrial or medical purposes.

For immunotoxicology studies, in silico and in vitro methods, including cell- and organ-based assays, are encouraged. Mimicking the immune system in vitro is not easy, and important differences have been observed between two- (2D) and three-dimensional (3D) cell cultures. In this Special Issue, Swartzwelter et al. performed a comprehensive comparison of traditional 2D cultures with 3D collagen-matrix models, representing the skin, including human blood monocytes exposed to gold nanoparticles (AuNPs) [5]. Immediate inflammation related to the stimulation of fresh monocytes, and the secondary reaction of monocyte-derived macrophages after previous priming, were evaluated. They observed similar TNF-α and IL-6 responses in 2D and 3D cultures, but notable differences in IL-8 or IL-1Rα, mainly in the recall/memory response of primed cells to a second stimulation, with the 3D cultures showing a clearer cell activation and memory effect in response to AuNPs. Although our knowledge of innate memory is still largely incomplete, it has been demonstrated that its activation is involved in defensive responses or can lead to a pathological exacerbation of secondary reactions. Furthermore, the therapeutic manipulation of this innate memory using different drugs or even NPs was postulated for medical purposes [15]. Thus, the inclusion of macrophages and the allowing of their long-term culture in vitro in these types of 3D models is crucial for the improved testing of new NPs.

As a step forward in the screening of NPs, but still avoiding the use of mammalians, zebrafish models present important ethical and economic advantages. In the review conducted by Pensado-López et al., we learn that zebrafish (Danio rerio) now constitute a well-established model for the toxicological and pharmacological screening of new drugs and nanomaterials, thanks to their rapid embryo development, small size and transparency, and genetic and physiological conservation [16]. Zebrafish with fluorescently labeled macrophages, including disease models that cause and/or are caused by inflammatory disorders (i.e., cancer, autoimmune or infectious diseases) have been developed. The number of publications tracking the interaction between macrophages and NPs using zebrafish has been clearly increasing in recent years, and it is expected that this research will lead to further knowledge about the role of macrophages in the initiation, progression, and remission of diseases over the course of a treatment, but will also contribute to the safe use of NPs and their translation towards the clinic.

In this Special Issue, we also included some manuscripts with a focus on the therapeutic application of nanotechnological approaches. We presented a review on the most recent nano-based drug delivery strategies to manipulate the immune system in the context of osteoarthritis, with a particular focus on those designed to specifically target and reprogram macrophages [17]. In the context of the joint pathology, macrophages with an M1-like pro-inflammatory phenotype induce chronic inflammation and joint destruction, and they have been correlated with the development and progression of the disease, while the M2-like anti-inflammatory macrophages support the recovery of the disease, promoting tissue repair and the resolution of inflammation. Thus, the use of NPs, liposomes, or hybrid nanosystems to locally improve the delivery of anti-inflammatory drugs to macrophages has been investigated. An interesting approach for wound healing was reported by Santos-Vizcaino et al. [7]. They studied the mechanism of action of negatively charged microspheres (NCM) from a commercial formulation to revert the chronic inflammatory state of stagnant wounds, such as diabetic wounds. After toxicity experiments, they demonstrated the internalization of NCMs by macrophages, driving their polarization towards an anti-inflammatory M2-phenotype that favors the wound-healing processes.

With a different therapeutic purpose, Rouco et al. evaluated, in vitro, the activity of rifabutin-loaded lipid-nanocarriers (RFB-NLC) [6]. These RFB-NLCs showed macrophage uptake and selective intracellular release of RFB, thus constituting a promising strategy to improve oral anti-mycobacterial therapy in Crohn's disease. Although in vivo experiments were not performed, the authors hypothesize that the passage and accumulation of NPs in the intestinal inflamed sites, densely infiltrated by macrophages, might be favored by the disruption of the epithelial barrier observed in inflammatory bowel disease patients.

Overall, as Editors of Nanomaterials, we are fully aware that the present Special Issue cannot fully reflect the high number and diversity of studies on nanoparticle–macrophage interactions. Thus, we also encourage the reading of other general reviews on nanotoxicology and nanomedicine [18], and specific reviews on the interaction of NPs with macrophages for the treatment of cancer [10], infectious diseases [19], other inflammatory disorders [15,20] such as the COVID-19-related cytokine storm [21], or strategies to improve the biocompatibility of antibacterial NPs [22].

In summary, we are confident that this Special Issue will contribute to the research interest in the field, providing our readership with a multi-faceted scenario that outlines the importance of macrophage-based in vitro models for nanosafety, and awareness about novel therapeutic approaches, such as the reprogramming of macrophages, using nanomedicines.

Author Contributions: F.T.A. and O.B. contributed equally to the writing, review and editing of the manuscript. All authors have read and agreed to the published version of the manuscript.

Funding: F.T.A. was supported by a grant from the "Asociación Española Contra el Cáncer (AECC)" and the "Oportunious" grant from "Xunta de Galicia" (Spain). O.B. was supported by the grants PUT1015 and COVSG16 from the Estonian Research Council.

Acknowledgments: We are grateful to all the authors for submitting their studies to the present Special Issue and for its successful completion. We deeply acknowledge the Nanomaterials reviewers for enhancing the quality and impact of all submitted papers. We acknowledge Bengt Fadeel, our previous postdoc supervisor at the Karolinska Institute, for the knowledge we have gained in the field of nanoparticle–macrophage interactions. Finally, we sincerely thank Steve Yan and the editorial staff of Nanomaterials for their excellent support during the development and publication of the Special Issue.

Conflicts of Interest: The authors declare no conflict of interest.

References

1. Wang, R.; Lohray, R.; Chow, E.; Gangupantula, P.; Smith, L.; Draper, R. Selective Uptake of Carboxylated Multi-Walled Carbon Nanotubes by Class a Type 1 Scavenger Receptors and Impaired Phagocytosis in Alveolar Macrophages. *Nanomaterials* **2020**, *10*, 2417. [CrossRef]
2. Huynh, M.T.; Mikoryak, C.; Pantano, P.; Draper, R. Scavenger Receptor A1 Mediates the Uptake of Carboxylated and Pristine Multi-Walled Carbon Nanotubes Coated with Bovine Serum Albumin. *Nanomaterials* **2021**, *11*, 539. [CrossRef] [PubMed]
3. Keshavan, S.; Andón, F.T.; Gallud, A.; Chen, W.; Reinert, K.; Tran, L.; Fadeel, B. Profiling of Sub-lethal in Vitro Effects of Multi-walled Carbon Nanotubes Reveals Changes in Chemokines and Chemokine Receptors. *Nanomaterials* **2021**, *11*, 883. [CrossRef] [PubMed]
4. Wiemann, M.; Vennemann, A.; Venzago, C.; Lindner, G.G.; Schuster, T.B.; Krueger, N. Serum Lowers Bioactivity and Uptake of Synthetic Amorphous Silica by Alveolar Macrophages in a Particle Specific Manner. *Nanomaterials* **2021**, *11*, 628. [CrossRef]

5. Swartzwelter, B.J.; Verde, A.; Rehak, L.; Madej, M.; Puntes, V.F.; De Luca, A.C.; Boraschi, D.; Italiani, P. Interaction between Macrophages and Nanoparticles: In Vitro 3d Cultures for the Realistic Assessment of Inflammatory Activation and Modulation of Innate Memory. *Nanomaterials* **2021**, *11*, 207. [CrossRef] [PubMed]
6. Rouco, H.; Diaz-Rodriguez, P.; Gaspar, D.P.; Gonçalves, L.M.D.; Cuerva, M.; Remuñán-López, C.; Almeida, A.J.; Landin, M. Rifabutin-Loaded Nanostructured Lipid Carriers as a Tool in Oral Anti-Mycobacterial Treatment of Crohn's Disease. *Nanomaterials* **2020**, *10*, 2138. [CrossRef] [PubMed]
7. Santos-Vizcaino, E.; Salvador, A.; Vairo, C.; Igartua, M.; Hernandez, R.M.; Correa, L.; Villullas, S.; Gainza, G. Overcoming the Inflammatory Stage of Non-Healing Wounds: In Vitro Mechanism of Action of Negatively Charged Microspheres (NCMS). *Nanomaterials* **2020**, *10*, 1108. [CrossRef]
8. Gallud, A.; Bondarenko, O.; Feliu, N.; Kupferschmidt, N.; Atluri, R.; Garcia-Bennett, A.; Fadeel, B. Macrophage Activation Status Determines the Internalization of Mesoporous Silica Particles of Different Sizes: Exploring the Role of Different Pattern Recognition Receptors. *Biomaterials* **2017**, *121*, 28–40. [CrossRef] [PubMed]
9. Berrecoso, G.; Crecente-Campo, J.; Alonso, M.J. Unveiling the Pitfalls of the Protein Corona of Polymeric Drug Nanocarriers. *Drug Deliv. Transl. Res.* **2020**, *10*, 730–750. [CrossRef]
10. Andón, F.T.; Digifico, E.; Maeda, A.; Erreni, M.; Mantovani, A.; Alonso, M.J.; Allavena, P. Targeting Tumor Associated Macrophages: The New Challenge for Nanomedicine. *Semin. Immunol.* **2017**, *34*, 103–113. [CrossRef]
11. Andón, F.T.; Fadeel, B. Programmed Cell Death: Molecular Mechanisms and Implications for Safety Assessment of Nanomaterials. *Acc. Chem. Res.* **2013**, *46*, 733–742. [CrossRef]
12. Andón, F.T.; Mukherjee, S.P.; Gessner, I.; Wortmann, L.; Xiao, L.; Hultenby, K.; Shvedova, A.A.; Mathur, S.; Fadeel, B. Hollow Carbon Spheres Trigger Inflammasome-Dependent IL-1β Secretion in Macrophages. *Carbon N. Y.* **2017**, *113*, 243–251. [CrossRef]
13. Mukherjee, S.P.; Bondarenko, O.; Kohonen, P.; Andón, F.T.; Brzicová, T.; Gessner, I.; Mathur, S.; Bottini, M.; Calligari, P.; Stella, L.; et al. Macrophage Sensing of Single-Walled Carbon Nanotubes via Toll-like Receptors. *Sci. Rep.* **2018**, *8*, 1115. [CrossRef] [PubMed]
14. Farrera, C.; Andón, F.T.; Feliu, N. Carbon Nanotubes as Optical Sensors in Biomedicine. *ACS Nano* **2017**, *11*, 10637–10643. [CrossRef]
15. Italiani, P.; Della Camera, G.; Boraschi, D. Induction of Innate Immune Memory by Engineered Nanoparticles in Monocytes/Macrophages: From Hypothesis to Reality. *Front. Immunol.* **2020**, *11*, 2324. [CrossRef] [PubMed]
16. Pensado-López, A.; Fernández-Rey, J.; Reimunde, P.; Crecente-Campo, J.; Sánchez, L.; Andón, F.T. Zebrafish Models for the Safety and Therapeutic Testing of Nanoparticles with a Focus on Macrophages. *Nanomaterials* **2021**, *11*, 1784. [CrossRef]
17. Ummarino, A.; Gambaro, F.M.; Kon, E.; Andón, F.T. Therapeutic Manipulation of Macrophages Using Nanotechnological Approaches for the Treatment of Osteoarthritis. *Nanomaterials* **2020**, *10*, 1562. [CrossRef]
18. Bondarenko, O.; Mortimer, M.; Kahru, A.; Feliu, N.; Javed, I.; Kakinen, A.; Lin, S.; Xia, T.; Song, Y.; Davis, T.P.; et al. Nanotoxicology and Nanomedicine: The Yin and Yang of Nano-Bio Interactions for the New Decade. *Nano Today* **2021**, *39*, 101184. [CrossRef]
19. Shivangi; Meena, L.S. A Novel Approach in Treatment of Tuberculosis by Targeting Drugs to Infected Macrophages Using Biodegradable Nanoparticles. *Appl. Biochem. Biotechnol.* **2018**, *185*, 815–821. [CrossRef]
20. Hu, G.; Guo, M.; Xu, J.; Wu, F.; Fan, J.; Huang, Q.; Yang, G.; Lv, Z.; Wang, X.; Jin, Y. Nanoparticles Targeting Macrophages as Potential Clinical Therapeutic Agents Against Cancer and Inflammation. *Front. Immunol.* **2019**, *10*, 1998. [CrossRef]
21. Liu, J.; Wan, M.; Lyon, C.J.; Hu, T.Y. Nanomedicine Therapies Modulating Macrophage Dysfunction: A Potential Strategy to Attenuate Cytokine Storms in Severe Infections. *Theranostics* **2020**, *10*, 9591–9600. [CrossRef] [PubMed]
22. Kubo, A.L.; Vasiliev, G.; Vija, H.; Krishtal, J.; Tõugu, V.; Visnapuu, M.; Kisand, V.; Kahru, A.; Bondarenko, O. Surface carboxylation or PEGylation decreases CuO nanoparticles' cytotoxicity to human cells in vitro without compromising their antibacterial properties. *Arch. Toxicol.* **2020**, *94*, 1561–1573. [CrossRef] [PubMed]

nanomaterials

MDPI

Article

Profiling of Sub-Lethal in Vitro Effects of Multi-Walled Carbon Nanotubes Reveals Changes in Chemokines and Chemokine Receptors

Sandeep Keshavan [1], Fernando Torres Andón [1,2,3], Audrey Gallud [1,4], Wei Chen [5,6], Knut Reinert [7], Lang Tran [8] and Bengt Fadeel [1,*]

1 Institute of Environmental Medicine, Karolinska Institute, 171 77 Stockholm, Sweden; sandeep.keshavan@unifr.ch (S.K.); fernando.torres.andon@usc.es (F.T.A.); audrey.gallud@gmail.com (A.G.)
2 IRCCS Istituto Clinico Humanitas, 20089 Rozzano, Milan, Italy
3 Center for Research in Molecular Medicine & Chronic Diseases, Universidade de Santiago de Compostela, 15782 Santiago de Compostela, Spain
4 Department of Biology and Biological Engineering, Chalmers University of Technology, 412 96 Göteborg, Sweden
5 Max Delbrück Center for Molecular Medicine, 10115 Berlin, Germany; chenw@sustech.edu.cn
6 Department of Biology, Southern University of Science and Technology, Shenzhen 518055, China
7 Department of Computer Science and Mathematics, Freie Universität Berlin, 14195 Berlin, Germany; Knut.Reinert@fu-berlin.de
8 Statistics and Toxicology Section, Institute of Occupational Medicine, Edinburgh EH14 4AP, UK; lang.tran@iom-world.org
* Correspondence: bengt.fadeel@ki.se

Citation: Keshavan, S.; Andón, F.T.; Gallud, A.; Chen, W.; Reinert, K.; Tran, L.; Fadeel, B. Profiling of Sub-Lethal in Vitro Effects of Multi-Walled Carbon Nanotubes Reveals Changes in Chemokines and Chemokine Receptors. *Nanomaterials* **2021**, *11*, 883. https://doi.org/10.3390/nano11040883

Academic Editors: Werner Blau and Angelina Angelova

Received: 11 February 2021
Accepted: 26 March 2021
Published: 30 March 2021

Abstract: Engineered nanomaterials are potentially very useful for a variety of applications, but studies are needed to ascertain whether these materials pose a risk to human health. Here, we studied three benchmark nanomaterials (Ag nanoparticles, TiO_2 nanoparticles, and multi-walled carbon nanotubes, MWCNTs) procured from the nanomaterial repository at the Joint Research Centre of the European Commission. Having established a sub-lethal concentration of these materials using two human cell lines representative of the immune system and the lungs, respectively, we performed RNA sequencing of the macrophage-like cell line after exposure for 6, 12, and 24 h. Downstream analysis of the transcriptomics data revealed significant effects on chemokine signaling pathways. *CCR2* was identified as the most significantly upregulated gene in MWCNT-exposed cells. Using multiplex assays to evaluate cytokine and chemokine secretion, we could show significant effects of MWCNTs on several chemokines, including CCL2, a ligand of CCR2. The results demonstrate the importance of evaluating sub-lethal concentrations of nanomaterials in relevant target cells.

Keywords: multi-walled carbon nanotubes; nanoparticles; chemokines; macrophages; transcriptomics

1. Introduction

Nanotoxicology is a scientific discipline aimed at assessing the potential adverse effects of engineered nanomaterials (NMs) as well as enabling the safe use of NMs [1]. Nanotoxicology research has made great strides in the past ten to fifteen years, and efforts to pin down the mechanism(s) of NM toxicity may ultimately inform regulatory frameworks with the goal of exploiting nanotechnology in a safe and sustainable manner [2]. However, much attention has been focused on the same basic paradigms, including the so-called oxidative stress paradigm [1,2]. This has certainly provided considerable insight into the biological and toxicological effects of NMs, but there may not be a one-size-fits-all mechanism with which to explain NM toxicity in different cells or tissues. The use of global omics-based approaches enables the exploration more broadly of biological mechanisms that influence the toxicity and efficacy of NMs [3]. Considerable progress has been made in the last few years in terms of applying transcriptomics and proteomics coupled with computational analysis to address the NM effects [4].

The nanomaterial repository of the Joint Research Centre (JRC) of the European Commission (EC) provides a collection of exhaustively characterized NMs that have been applied as benchmark materials in a number of projects, including the large, EC-funded FP7-NANOREG project, a pan-European project aimed at a common approach to the regulatory testing of nanomaterials [5]. Hence, in FP7-NANOREG, we performed cytotoxicity screening and cytokine profiling of nineteen NMs using the human monocyte-like THP-1 cell line and obtained evidence that diverse NMs can be grouped based on their pro-inflammatory potential [6]. Similarly, in the EC-funded FP7-MARINA project on hazard assessment and risk management of NMs, a comprehensive study was performed on a panel of metal oxides from the JRC repository [titanium dioxide (TiO_2) (NM103 and NM104), zinc oxide (ZnO) (NM110 and NM111) and silicon dioxide (SiO_2) (NM200 and NM203)] using a range of cellular assays representing different target organs or systems (immune system, respiratory system, gastrointestinal system, reproductive organs, kidney and embryonic tissues) [7]. The results enabled a hazard ranking of the NMs. The study also revealed cell type-specific response to NMs; overall, the most sensitive cells studied were the murine alveolar macrophages (MH-S). In the EC-funded FP7-ENPRA project, which also focused on hazard assessment of NMs, a panel of NMs procured from the JRC repository were investigated using the human hepatoblastoma C3A cell line, and silver (Ag) and ZnO were found to be more potent with respect to cytotoxicity and cytokine secretion, whereas the multi-walled carbon nanotubes (MWCNTs) and TiO_2 displayed less toxicity [8]. The conclusion that the effects of NMs are cell type-dependent was also demonstrated in a study of 23 NMs using a panel of ten different cell lines [9]. In fact, even when assessing NM toxicity towards cells originating from the same organ, the outcome was dependent on the specific cell line used, and its origin (human or mouse), as illustrated by the fact that the three lung epithelium-derived cell lines used differed in terms of oxidative stress [9].

CNTs have received particular attention due to their apparent similarities with other fiber-like materials, although inadequate or limited evidence of carcinogenicity exists for most CNTs [10]. Notwithstanding, in a recent study of seven different CNTs and two carbon nanofibers (CNFs), all the tested materials except one highly aggregated MWCNT sample induced genotoxicity in human bronchial epithelial cells (BEAS-2B) [11]. There was a tendency for CNTs/CNFs with increasing length and diameter to display slightly greater toxicity. Di Cristo et al. [12] performed a comparative study of the toxicity of three benchmark MWCNTs obtained from the JRC repository (NM400, NM401, and NM402) using two murine macrophage cell lines (RAW264.7 and MH-S) and found that long and needle-like NM401, but not short and tangled NM400 or NM402, affected cell viability in a dose-dependent manner in both cell models. For this reason, we selected NM401 as representative MWCNTs for our studies. For comparison, we chose Ag and TiO_2, which have been shown in numerous previous studies to possess high and low toxicity potential, respectively. The three NMs [Ag (NM300K), TiO_2 (NM104), and MWCNTs (NM401)] were tested using two human cell lines, the lung adenocarcinoma cell line A549 (often used as a model of the lung epithelium) and THP-1. Following cytotoxicity screening using established protocols [6], we performed genome-wide transcriptomics analysis by applying RNA sequencing, coupled with pathway analysis [13,14]. The results were then corroborated by cytokine–chemokine profiling.

2. Materials and Methods

2.1. Nanomaterials

The NMs used in this study are classified as representative test materials and include a (random) sample from one industrial production batch. This ensures that the sample has been homogenized and is sub-sampled into vials under reproducible (GLP) conditions, and that the stability of the sub-samples is monitored. Thus, to the extent possible for industrial materials, all the sub-samples should be identical and differences in test results between laboratories for the same endpoint should not be due to differences in the NMs tested [15]. For detailed physicochemical characterization of the selected NMs [Ag (NM300K), TiO_2 (NM104), and MWCNTs (NM401)] performed at the JRC, refer to: Rasmussen et al. [15] and references therein. For the dispersion of the NMs, the SOP developed under the EC-funded NANOGENOTOX joint action was used, as described previously [6]. Briefly, stock dispersions were prepared by pre-wetting the NM powders in 0.5 vol% ethanol followed by dispersion in sterile-filtered 0.05% w/v bovine serum albumin (BSA)-water (Milli-Q® water, Sigma-Aldrich, Stockholm, Sweden). Both the water and the BSA (obtained from Sigma-Aldrich, Stockholm, Sweden) were endotoxin-free. The samples were then dispersed by sonication (16 min at 400 W) before being added to cell cultures.

2.2. Human Cell Lines

Human THP-1 acute monocytic leukemia cells and A549 lung adenocarcinoma cells were obtained from the American Type Culture Collection (ATCC) (Manassas, VA, USA). The cells were mycoplasma tested regularly using MycoAlert® mycoplasma detection kit (Lonza, Basel, Switzerland). THP-1 cells were maintained in RPMI-1640 medium (Sigma-Aldrich, Stockholm, Sweden), supplemented with 10% heat-inactivated fetal bovine serum (FBS), 2 mM L-glutamine, 1 mM Na-pyruvate, 5.0×10^{-5} M β-mercaptoethanol, 100 U/mL penicillin, and 100 mg/mL streptomycin. A549 cells were cultured in DMEM (ThermoFisher, Stockholm, Sweden), supplemented with 10% heat activated FBS, 2 mM L-glutamine, 1 mM Na-pyruvate, 100 U/mL penicillin, and 100 mg/mL streptomycin. To induce differentiation into macrophage-like cells, THP-1 cells were stimulated for 3 days with 150 nM phorbol myristate acetate (PMA) (Sigma-Aldrich, Stockholm, Sweden).

2.3. Endotoxin Testing

NMs were tested for endotoxin contamination using the LAL test (Limulus Amebocyte Lysate Endochrome, Charles River Endosafe, Charleston, SC, USA) according to the manufacturer's instructions. The NMs were all endotoxin-free (<0.5 EU/mL) (data not shown).

2.4. Cell Viability Assay

Cell viability was monitored with the lactate dehydrogenase (LDH) release assay using the CytoTox96® non-radioactive cytotoxicity kit (Promega, Stockholm, Sweden), as previously described [16]. The samples were analyzed using the Tecan Infinite® F200 plate reader operating with Magellan v7.2 software (Männedorf, Switzerland). The percentage of cell viability was calculated based on the ratio between the absorbance of each sample and the negative control sample.

2.5. Transmission Electron Microscopy

Cellular uptake/localization of NMs was monitored by TEM as described [17]. Briefly, cells were fixed in 2% glutaraldehyde in 0.1 M sodium cacodylate buffer containing 0.1 M sucrose and 3 mM $CaCl_2$, pH 7.4. Cells were then washed and post-fixed in 2% osmium tetroxide in 0.07 M sodium cacodylate buffer containing 1.5 mM $CaCl_2$, pH 7.4, at 4 °C for 2 h, dehydrated in ethanol followed by acetone, and embedded in LX-112, an epoxy derivative. Sections were contrasted with uranyl acetate followed by lead citrate and were examined in a Tecnai 12 Spirit Bio TWIN TEM (FEI, Eindhoven, The Netherlands) at 100 kV. Digital images were obtained using a Veleta camera (Olympus, GmbH, Münster, Germany).

2.6. Cytokine and Chemokine Analysis

TNF-α released in the culture medium was measured using an ELISA kit following the instructions provided by the manufacturer (MabTech, Nacka, Sweden). The absorbance of the reaction product was measured using a spectrophotometer (Tecan Infinite® F200, Männedorf, Switzerland) and the results for each sample were calculated using a standard curve of recombinant human TNF-α protein. Lipopolysaccharide (LPS) (100 ng/mL;

Sigma-Aldrich, Stockholm, Sweden) was used as a positive control for TNF-α release. Results are expressed as ng/mL of released cytokine, based on three independent experiments. Furthermore, profiling of cytokines and chemokines released by THP-1 cells was performed by using the U-PLEX chemokine panel 1 (human) (K15047K-1) and the V-PLEX pro-inflammatory panel 1 (human) (K15049D-1), respectively. We employed the Meso Scale Discovery (MSD) (Rockville, MD, USA) multi-plex electrochemiluminescence (ECL) platform to quantify cell supernatant concentrations of the indicated biomarkers, according to the manufacturer's instructions. As a positive control, cells were exposed to 0.1 μg/mL LPS (Sigma-Aldrich, Stockholm, Sweden) for 24 h. The samples were analyzed on the MSD Meso SECTOR® S600 instrument and the data were analyzed using MSD Discovery Workbench® software (v. 4.0) (Rockville, MD, USA). Samples with values below the lower limit of detection (defined as 2.5 S.D. above the background) were excluded from further analysis. The cytokine and chemokine expression data retrieved from the multi-plex assay were further analyzed using hierarchical clustering analysis, as described previously [6]. Complete linkage and Euclidean distances were employed as metrics to draw association dendrograms between cytokines/chemokines and the different treatment conditions. The cluster analysis and the corresponding heatmaps were prepared using R 3.2 [6].

2.7. Western Blotting

For protein detection, cells were harvested and lysed at 4 °C in RIPA buffer [50 mM Tris HCl (pH 7.4), 150 mM NaCl, 1% Triton X-100, 0.25% sodium deoxycholate, 0.1% SDS, 1 mM EDTA] supplemented with protease and phosphatase inhibitors plus 1 mM DTT (Sigma Aldrich, Stockholm, Sweden) as described previously [18]. Thirty μg total protein were loaded into each well of a NuPAGE 4–12% Bis-Tris gradient gel (ThermoFisher, Stockholm, Sweden) and subjected to electrophoresis. The proteins were then transferred to a Hybond low-fluorescent 0.2 μm PVDF membrane (Amersham, Buckinghamshire, UK), blocked for 1 h in Odyssey® Blocking Buffer (PBS) (LI-COR), and stained overnight at 4°C with antibodies against NLRP12 (Abcam, Stockholm, Sweden) and GAPDH (ThermoFisher, Stockholm, Sweden) as loading control. The membranes were then probed with the goat anti-rabbit IgG (H+L) HRP-conjugated antibody (ThermoFisher, Stockholm, Sweden) or the goat anti-mouse IRDye 680RD antibody (LI-COR Biotechnology, Lincoln, NE, USA) and proteins were detected using Clarity™ ECL substrates (BioRad, Hercules, CA, USA) and Super RX-N film (FujiFilm Nordic AB, Stockholm, Sweden), or the LI-COR Odyssey® CLx scanner operating with Odyssey® Image Studio software (LI-COR Biotechnology).

2.8. RNA Sequencing

Total RNA was extracted from cells harvested at 0 h, 6 h, 12 h, and 24 h of exposure to NMs (25 μg/mL) using the TRIZOL reagent (Life Technologies, Stockholm, Sweden) according to the manufacturer's recommendations. Total RNA was quantified by NanoDrop™ (NanoDrop Technologies, ThermoScientific, Stockholm, Sweden) and RNA quality was assessed using the Bioanalyzer 2100 (Agilent Technologies, Santa Clara, CA, USA). Three biological replicates of each sample were submitted for RNA sequencing [19]. In brief, the sequencing was performed using 1 μg total RNA following the Illumina® mRNA-Seq library preparation protocol (Illumina, San Diego, CA, USA). To this end, poly(A) RNA was isolated by two rounds of oligo (dT)25 Dynabeads™ (Invitrogen, Stockholm, Sweden) purification. Then, the chemically fragmented mRNAs were purified by Agencourt RNA-Clean XP SPRI beads (Agencourt-Beckman Coulter, Beverly, MA, USA) and converted to first strand cDNA, followed by second strand cDNA synthesis. The paired-end sequencing library was prepared from purified double stranded cDNA using the NEBNext® DNA Library Prep Kit (Illumina, San Diego, CA, USA). The purified ligated product was PCR amplified and the prepared libraries were quantified and quality-assessed and sequenced on the Illumina® HiSeq 2000 platform (Illumina, San Diego, CA, USA).

2.9. Pathway Analysis

Canonical pathway analysis was done using the Ingenuity Pathway Analysis (IPA) software (content version 24718999) (Ingenuity Systems, Redwood City, CA, USA). The significance of the pathways was estimated through the curated ingenuity knowledge database using a causal analysis approach [20], complemented by hierarchical cluster analysis, as described in Reference [21]. Significant pathways were filtered by *p*-values < 0.001 and activation z-scores > 2 or >2 (data not shown), representing a significant deactivation or activation, respectively. Data were integrated using hierarchical clustering on quantile-normalized data.

2.10. Statistical Analysis

One-way analysis of variance (ANOVA), followed by a Dunnett's or Sidak's multiple comparison test analysis was used for the analysis of statistical significance, and $p <$ 0.05 was considered significant. For nonparametrically distributed data, the two-tailed Mann-Whitney test was used. Statistical tests were performed using GraphPad Prism 8 (San Diego, CA, USA).

3. Results

3.1. Characterization of Benchmark Nanomaterials

The test materials [Ag (NM300K), TiO_2 (NM104), and MWCNTs (NM401)] were obtained from the JRC nanomaterial repository and detailed characterization has been provided by the JRC (refer to Table S1 for an overview and see references therein). The MWCNTs are characterized by their rigid and needle-like appearance (length: 4048 $\pm$ 2371 nm; diameter: 67 $\pm$ 24 nm). The TiO_2 NMs are rutile, with an average diameter of 25 nm and have been extensively studied in the FP7-MARINA project [7]. The Ag NMs were provided in a colloidal suspension with a primary particle size of 15 nm. The latter NMs were studied extensively in the FP7-NANOREG project (see, for instance, Bhattacharya et al. [6]).

3.2. Cytotoxicity Assessment of Nanomaterials

We utilized two human cell lines: the lung cell line A549 and the monocyte-like cell line THP-1. The latter cells were differentiated into macrophage-like cells using PMA [6]. The cells were exposed for 24 h to the three different NMs at concentrations ranging from 1 to 100 μg/mL and cell viability was monitored using the LDH release assay. The TiO_2 NMs were cytotoxic for THP-1 cells only at the highest dose while Ag NMs and MWCNTs triggered a dose-dependent cytotoxicity at doses above 10 and 25 μg/mL, respectively (Figure 1A). In contrast, the NMs were not cytotoxic towards the A549 lung cell line, apart from a minor effect noted for the Ag NMs at high doses (Figure 1B).

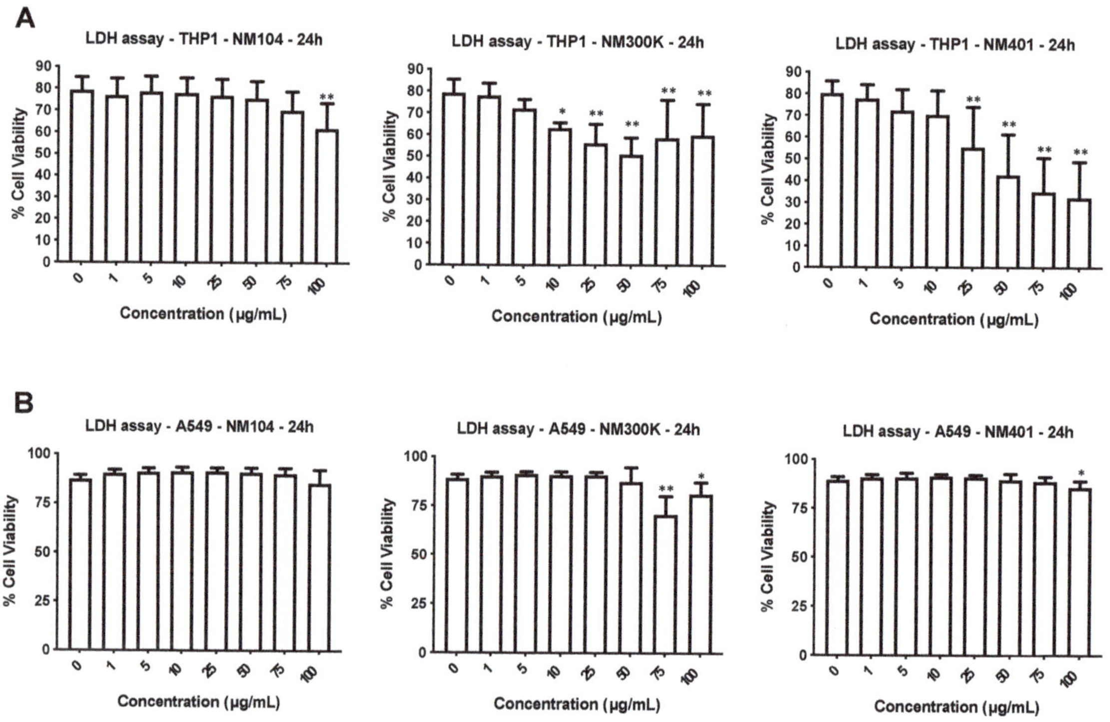

Figure 1. Cytotoxicity screening of representative nanomaterials (NMs). Human macrophage-differentiated THP-1 cells (**A**) and lung epithelium-derived A549 cells (**B**) were exposed to TiO_2 NMs (NM104), Ag NMs (NM300K), and MWCNTs (NM401) for 24 h and cell viability was evaluated by using the LDH release assay. The results shown are mean values ± S.D. of three independent experiments. * $p < 0.01$; ** $p < 0.001$.

3.3. *Cellular Uptake of Benchmark Nanomaterials*

We monitored cellular uptake by performing TEM imaging of THP-1 cells after exposure for 24 h at 25 µg/mL (a dose at which the cell viability remained >50% for all three NMs). The Ag NMs could not be visualized with certainty at this time-point, possibly due to dissolution of the NMs, as shown in previous studies [22]. The MWCNTs, on the other hand, were found to damage the microtome (Supplementary Figure S1). Therefore, results are shown for TiO_2 NMs. As seen in Figure 2A, macrophage-like THP-1 cells readily internalized large clusters of NMs in the absence of ultrastructural signs of cell death, consistent with the results of the LDH release assay.

To further explore the cellular impact of the three NMs, we monitored TNF-α production. TNF-α is a prototypic pro-inflammatory cytokine that is strongly induced by LPS. As shown in Figure 2B, while LPS triggered significant secretion of TNF-α, TiO_2 NMs had no effect, despite the considerable cellular uptake of these NMs. Furthermore, Ag NMs triggered some TNF-α production at low doses, but not at higher doses, whereas the MWCNTs triggered TNF-α production at high doses, albeit less than LPS. These results thus reveal a marginal effect of the NMs on TNF-α production in macrophage-like cells and suggest (indirectly) that these NMs are endotoxin-free, as TNF-α is a potent inducer of LPS [23].

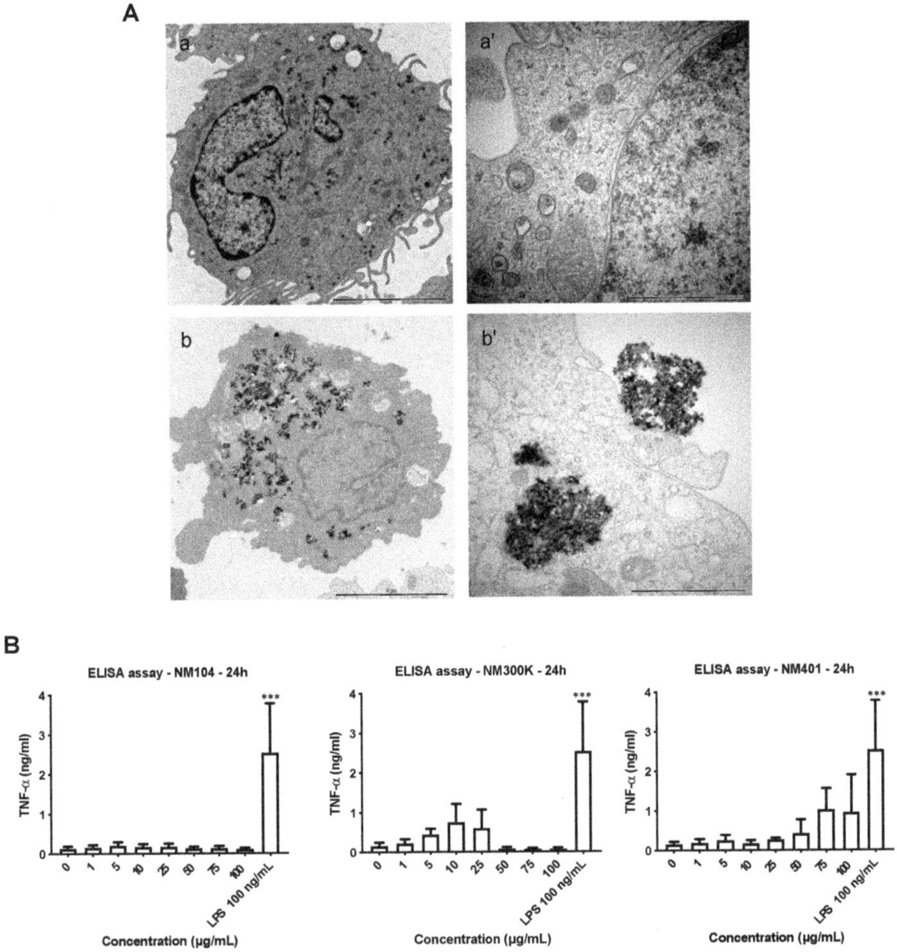

Figure 2. Cellular impact of representative NMs. (**A**) TEM images of untreated THP-1 cells (**a**,**a′**) and cells exposed to TiO_2 NMs for 24 h at 25 µg/mL (**b**,**b′**). Scale bars: 5 µm (**a**,**b**) and 1 µm (**a′**,**b′**). Refer to Figure S1 for additional findings derived from the TEM imaging. (**B**) THP-1 cells were exposed to TiO_2 NMs (NM104), Ag NMs (NM300K), and MWCNTs (NM401) for 24 h and TNF-α production was measured by ELISA. The results are mean values ± S.D. of three independent experiments. *** $p < 0.001$.

3.4. Transcriptomics Analysis of Nanomaterials

To investigate the effects of the selected NMs in more detail, we applied RNA sequencing. THP-1 cells were selected as a model. The cells were exposed for 6 h, 12 h, and 24 h to NM300K, NM104, and NM401 at 25 µg/mL in order to determine the kinetics of the transcriptomics responses. Samples were sequenced using the Illumina® HiSeq 2000 sequencing platform. RNA sequencing revealed that significant numbers of differentially expressed genes (DEGs) were affected by the NMs (NM300K: 313, NM104: 674; NM401: 124). Only DEGs with a significance level of <0.05 (FDR) and absolute fold-change ≥2 were included in the subsequent analysis. We focused the IPA analysis on immune cells and immune cell lines. The heatmap in Figure 3 shows the hierarchical cluster analysis of the top canonical pathways identified in THP-1 cells exposed to NM300K, NM104, and NM401 at various time-points. The color coding in the heatmap depicts the *p*-values for the pathways shown. The samples corresponding to the 24 h exposure to Ag (NM300K) and MWCNTs (NM401) are grouped together. To further refine the analysis, we analyzed each NM separately. The results for TiO_2 and Ag are shown in Supplementary Figures S3 and S4, respectively, while the results for MWCNTs are reported in Figure 4. The analysis shows clear time dependence insofar as the changes in gene expression are more robust (based on *p*-values) at 24 h when compared to 6 h and 12 h. We found that cell cycle related pathways were affected by all the tested NMs, and several pathways related to immune cell function were affected by MWCNTs (Figure 4) and Ag NMs (Supplementary Figure S3), but not by TiO_2 NMs (Supplementary Figure S2). Based on the activation z-scores, cell cycle pathways were deactivated, while immune related pathways were activated (data not shown).

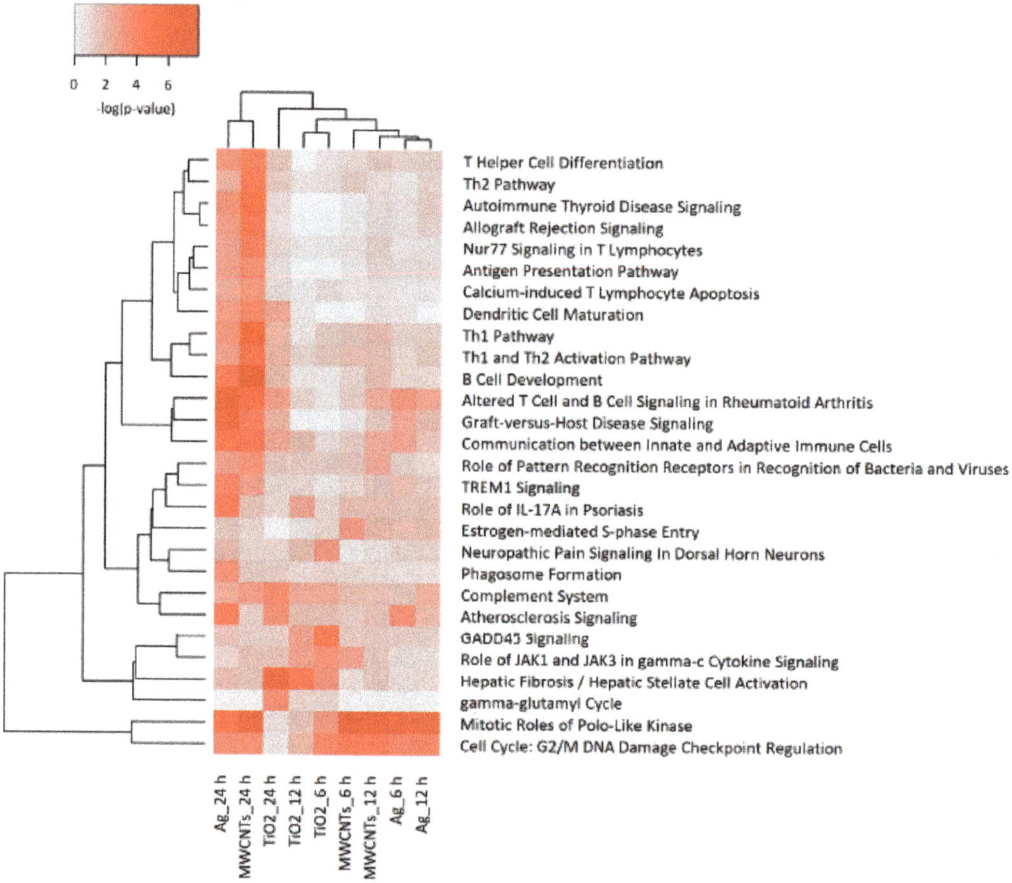

Figure 3. Pathway analysis of transcriptomics data. Macrophage-differentiated THP-1 cells were exposed to TiO_2 NMs (NM104), Ag NMs (NM300K), and MWCNTs (NM401) for 6 h, 12 h, and 24 h (25 μg/mL) and samples were subjected to RNA sequencing. The heatmap shows the canonical pathway analysis of the transcriptomics data. The significance values indicate the probability of the association of the DEGs with the respective pathway. The cutoff for the *p*-value was $p < 0.001$ for at least one of the conditions.

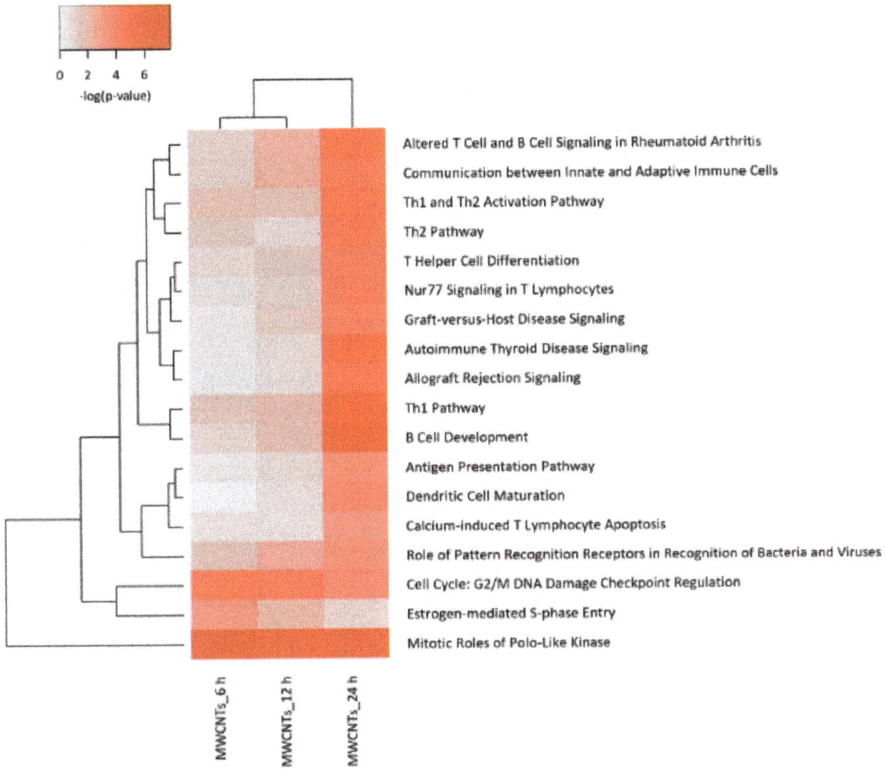

Figure 4. Canonical pathways affected by MWCNTs. The heatmap shows the results of the canonical pathway analysis of the transcriptomics data obtained from THP-1 cells exposed to MWCNTs (NM401) at 25 μg/mL at the indicated time-points. The corresponding analysis for NM401 and NM300K exposed cells is shown in Figures S2 and S3. The significance values indicate the probability of the association of DEGs with the respective pathway. The cutoff for the *p*-value was $p < 0.001$ for at least one of the conditions.

Our analysis showed that the top-most upregulated gene at every time-point in cells exposed to MWCNTs (NM401) was *CCR2*. The $\log_2$ ratio differential expression values for *CCR2* were 7.938 (6 h), 8.158 (12 h), and 13.712 (24 h). *CCR2* is a chemokine receptor encoding gene, and the corresponding receptor binds chemokine (C-C motif) ligand 2 (CCL2), also referred to as monocyte chemoattractant protein-1 (MCP-1). Figure 5A provides a graphic depiction of the network involving *CCR2* (at 24 h). It is notable that not only *CCR2*, but also *CXCR2* was significantly upregulated in cells exposed to MWCNTs. *CXCR2* is another chemokine receptor encoding gene and the corresponding protein serves as a receptor for CXCL8 (previously known as IL-8). The only downregulated gene in the network was *NLRP12*, encoding a member of the Nod-like receptor (NLR) family of proteins that have been shown to play a role in inflammasome activation [24]. However, *NLRP3* was not affected (data not shown). To validate the RNA sequencing, we checked the expression of the NLRP12 protein in THP-1 cells exposed for 24 h at 25 μg/mL, and we could confirm that the protein expression was decreased following exposure to NM401 compared to the control (Figure 5B).

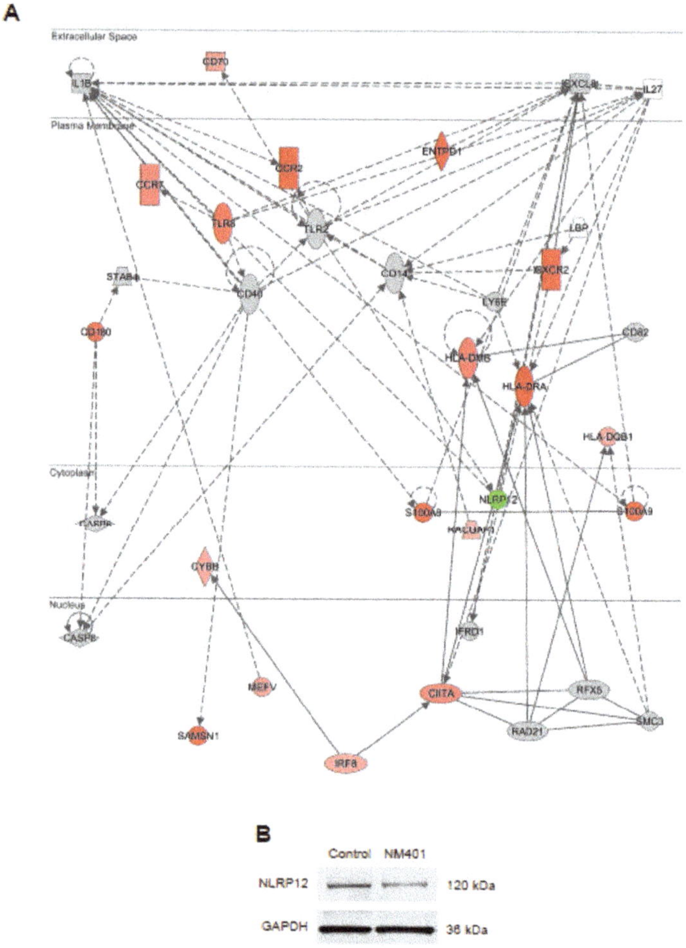

Figure 5. Impact of MWCNTs on the chemokine signaling network in macrophage-like cells. (**A**) The figure depicts the transcriptomics results for MWCNT-exposed (25 μg/mL) THP-1 cells at 24 h. The color coding shows upregulated (red) and downregulated genes (green). Data were analyzed and visualized by using the IPA software tool (Qiagen, Inc., www.qiagenbioinformatics.com/products/ingenuity-pathway-analysis). (**B**) Western blot assay for the expression of NLRP12 in THP-1 cells exposed or not to MWCNTs (25 μg/mL) for 24 h. GAPDH was included as a loading control.

3.5. *Cytokine-Chemokine Profiling of Nanomaterials*

To further corroborate the transcriptomics results and in order to add the biological context, we performed multiplex assays for the detection of cytokines (IFN-γ, IL-1β, IL-2, IL-4, IL-6, IL-8, IL-10, IL-12p70, IL-13, and TNF-α) and chemokines (Eotaxin, Eotaxin-2, Eotaxin-3, IL-8, IP-10, MCP-1, MCP-2, MCP-3, MCP-4, MDC, MIP-1α, MIP-1β, and TARC). To this end, THP-1 cells were exposed for 24 h to the different NMs (25 μg/mL). LPS (0.1 μg/mL) was included as a positive control. Three independent experiments were conducted and samples with values below the lower limit of detection were excluded from the subsequent analysis. The results confirmed the notion that the NMs did not elicit a pronounced induction of pro-inflammatory cytokines (at 25 μg/mL) (Figure S4). Hence, TNF-α and IL-8 (CXCL8) were not upregulated, while a modest induction was noted for IL-6. NM401 also triggered a modest induction of IL-1β. In contrast, several chemokines were significantly upregulated in response to NM401 (Figure S5). In particular, MCP-1 (CCL2) was upregulated, along with TARC (thymus and activation regulated chemokine, also known as CCL17) and MDC (macrophage derived chemokine, also known as CCL22). It is notable that the magnitude of these responses was similar to that of LPS. NM104 and NM300K, on the other hand, did not show such effects.

To further probe the responses of macrophage-like cells to the three NMs, we performed hierarchical cluster analysis to draw association dendrograms between cytokine and chemokine responses, respectively. LPS exposed samples (supernatants from exposed cells) were identified as separated from the other samples, both with respect to cytokine (Figure 6A) and chemokine responses (Figure 6B). However, the NM401 exposed samples clustered closer to the LPS samples in terms of chemokine responses, whereas NM104, and to some extent, NM300K, segregated with the untreated control samples (Figure 6B).

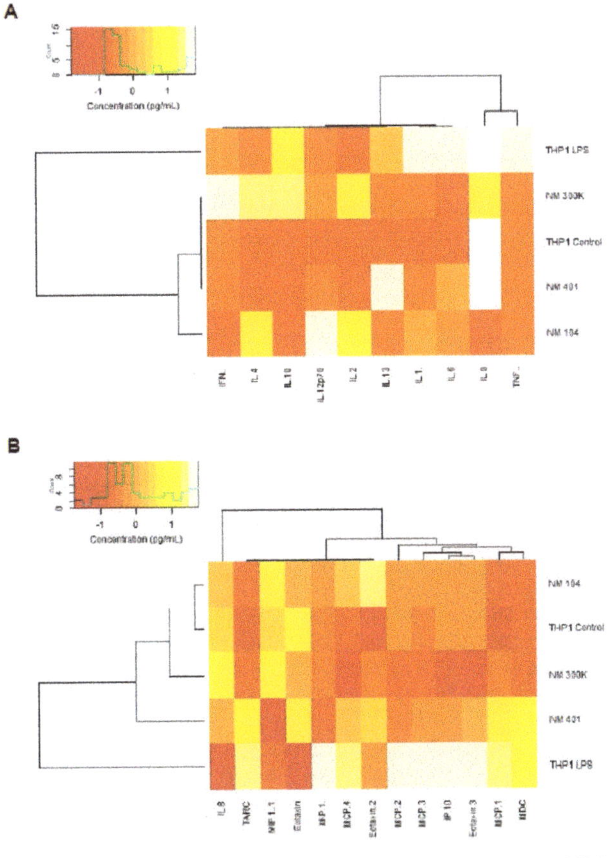

Figure 6. Profiling of cytokine and chemokine production in NM-exposed cells. Macrophage-differentiated THP-1 cells were exposed to TiO_2 NMs (NM104), Ag NMs (NM300K), and MWCNTs (NM401) for 24 h at 25 µg/mL and cytokine and chemokine production was monitored in the supernatants using multiplex assays. As a positive control, cells were exposed to 0.1 µg/mL LPS. The experiment was performed three times and results for individual biomarkers are reported in Figures S4 and S5. Hierarchical cluster analysis was performed to draw association dendrograms between cytokine (**A**) and chemokine (**B**) responses to NMs. Association clusters for exposures and biomarkers are represented by dendrograms at the **left** and at the **top** of the heatmap, respectively.

4. Discussion

Using representative NMs from the JRC nanomaterial repository, we have shown that THP-1 cells are more susceptible to NM-induced cell death than A549 cells. The differences between the two cell types could be because epithelial cells are less phagocytic when compared to macrophages. However, we did not perform a quantitative analysis of NM internalization in the present study. It is notable that A549 cells were also found to be refractory to other NMs when compared to primary human lung epithelial cells [25]. Our main finding was that several chemokines and chemokine receptors were significantly affected following a sub-lethal exposure (a dose at which the cell viability remained >50%) of THP-1 cells to MWCNTs. However, we did not observe the induction of pro-inflammatory cytokines, such as TNF-α or IL-8, at the same concentration (25 μg/mL), though MWCNT triggered TNF-α secretion was observed in THP-1 cells when tested at higher doses.

The cytotoxicity of MWCNTs towards THP-1 cells could be related to the shape of these NMs. Indeed, previous investigations have shown that long and needle-like NM401, but not short and tangled NM400 or NM402, elicited a dose-dependent loss of cell viability [12]. Furthermore, in vivo studies have demonstrated that "rod-like" MWCNTs are prone to triggering pulmonary responses with fibrosis and granuloma formation [26–28]. However, other properties or features of MWCNTs in addition to their geometric characteristics may also play a role, including the presence of metallic impurities [29–31]. We also found that Ag NMs (NM300K) triggered a loss of cell viability in THP-1 cells, while a minor effect was observed in A549 cells at the highest concentrations tested, i.e., 75 and 100 μg/mL. For the latter NMs, cellular uptake and subsequent dissolution of the particles within cells has been identified as one of the key determinants of cytotoxicity [32,33]. Hence, for different NMs, different physicochemical properties may come into play.

It is interesting to consider whether the MWCNTs might emulate some other substrate(s) to which macrophages are programmed to respond. This is presently a matter of conjecture, but we have previously reported that SWCNTs induced chemokine secretion in primary human monocyte-derived macrophages through a Toll-like receptor (TLR)-dependent signaling pathway [16], and a very recent study has provided evidence that the phosphatidylserine (PS) receptor Tim4 (T cell immunoglobulin mucin 4) contributes to the recognition of MWCNTs by murine peritoneal macrophages and plays a role in granuloma formation [34]. Thus, it appears that CNTs might "hijack" pattern recognition receptors that are otherwise deployed by macrophages to respond to microbes or dying cells.

Greco and co-workers recently employed toxicogenomics approaches to study the impact of carbon-based nanomaterials, including MWCNTs on various human cell lines [35,36]. The authors demonstrated that A549 cells are less sensitive than THP-1 cells, as evidenced by the magnitude of the molecular events [35]. In a follow-up study, the authors exposed THP-1 cells to long and rigid MWCNTs and studied genome wide transcription and gene promoter methylation in tandem [36]. Interestingly, among the 220 genes that were found to be affected both at the expression and methylation level, several chemokine encoding genes were identified. In the present study, both CCL17 and CCL22 were significantly upregulated in THP-1 cells exposed to MWCNTs. These chemokines are known to be highly expressed in the thymus and to a lesser extent by dendritic cells and macrophages in secondary lymphoid tissues [37]. Furthermore, both chemokines signal through CCR4, and both have been implicated in type 2 immune responses and were shown to play a role in asthma and in atopic dermatitis [38]. Moreover, we found that CCL2 was significantly induced by MWCNTs. CCL2 is a chemokine, which mediates monocyte chemotaxis and is involved in monocyte infiltration in inflammatory diseases such rheumatoid arthritis [39]. CCL2 acts as a ligand for CCR2, and it is notable that the gene encoding the latter receptor was the most highly upregulated gene in the present study. In a previous in vitro study, we provided evidence that the secretion of CCL3 and CCL5 by primary human monocyte-derived macrophages exposed to endotoxin-free SWCNTs occurred through a TLR2/4-MyD88-NFκB signaling pathway [16]. Furthermore, other investigators have shown that CCR5 (the receptor for CCL3, CCL4 and CCL5) plays an important role in the resolution of pulmonary inflammation in mice exposed toi SWCNTs [40]. Snyder-Talkington et al. [41] investigated in vivo responses to MWCNTs by microarray analysis and could show that several chemokine encoding genes were deregulated in the lungs of mice. Using small airway epithelial cells, the authors reported concordant results in vitro with regard to CCL2. Other investigators have shown, using the murine macrophage-like cell line J774A.1, that long (>20 μm) MWCNTs elicited CCL2 (MCP-1) secretion, even at a relatively low concentration [42]. Taken together, single- and multi-walled CNTs prominently affect chemokine signaling in immune-competent cells and especially CCL2 has been highlighted in several studies. The secretion of chemokines such as CCL2 may play a role in the granuloma formation that has been reported in the lungs following pulmonary exposure or in the pleural or abdominal cavity following intra-pleural or intra-peritoneal instillation of MWCNTs [43,44]. Moreover, Sydlik et al. [45] evaluated the biocompatibility of graphene oxide (GO) following implantation in subcutaneous and intraperitoneal tissues in mice and demonstrated a typical "foreign body" reaction (i.e., granuloma formation). The authors found that cells retrieved from these sites secreted significant amounts of monocyte chemotactic protein-1 (MCP-1) (CCL2) and macrophage inflammatory protein-1β (MIP-1β) (CCL4), providing further evidence for a role of these inflammatory chemokines in granulomatous tissue reactions. This also shows that CCL2 (MCP-1) upregulation is not specific for CNTs and is more likely part of a conserved response towards offending pathogens or xenobiotics. Indeed, we previously reported that *CCL2* was upregulated almost 90-fold in the lungs of rats exposed to CuO NMs and these findings were corroborated at the protein level [46]. Moreover, welding-related NMs (essentially, oxides of Fe, Mn and Cr) were found to induce the production of CCL2 in THP-1 cells [47]. Hence, CCL2 may be a particularly sensitive biomarker of immunological perturbations triggered by a variety of NMs.

In addition, we found that *NLRP12* was downregulated in THP-1 cells exposed to MWCNTs, and this was confirmed at the protein level. NLRP12 belongs to the NLR family of proteins involved in inflammasome activation [48]. However, unlike NLRP3, which plays an important role in IL-1β activation in response to a variety of stimuli including MWCNTs [49], NLRP12 seems to attenuate inflammation by dampening NF-κB signaling [50,51]. NLRP12 may also maintain intestinal homeostasis by modulating the gut microbiome [52]. Further studies are needed to investigate the role(s) of NLRP12 for MWCNT-triggered immune responses, and it is worth noting that NLRP12 may impinge on neutrophil function [53]. Neutrophils are a somewhat neglected cell type in nanotoxicology [54].

5. Conclusions

Using a combination of transcriptomics approaches and conventional biological assays, we have shown that sub-lethal doses of MWCNTs trigger a deregulation of chemokines and chemokine receptors in a human macrophage-differentiated cell line. These results support the emerging view that CNTs may elicit or interfere with chemokine signaling, and further our understanding of the toxicity of this class of materials [55,56]. However, it is noted that we have only studied one type of MWCNTs, and one cannot extrapolate the findings to other types of single or multi-walled CNTs. Indeed, grouping all CNTs into one material category is scientifically unjustified and may hinder innovation [57,58]. Therefore, further studies are needed to fully address the physicochemical properties that are responsible for the observed biological or toxicological effects of CNTs [10].

Supplementary Materials: The following are available online at https://www.mdpi.com/article/10.3390/nano11040883/s1, Table S1: Physicochemical characterization of the selected NMs. Figure S1: TEM imaging of cells exposed to NM401. Figure S2: Pathway analysis of transcriptomics data from cells exposed to NM104. Figure S3: Pathway analysis of transcriptomics data from cells exposed to NM300K. Figure S4: Cytokine release in cells exposed to selected NMs. Figure S5: Chemokine release in cells exposed to selected NMs.

Author Contributions: Conceptualization, coordination: B.F.; funding acquisition: B.F. and L.T.; investigation and data analysis (in vitro studies): F.T.A. and S.K.; investigation and data analysis (omics analysis): A.G., W.C. and K.R.; writing, original draft: B.F.; writing, editing: B.F. and S.K. All authors have read and agreed to the published version of the manuscript.

Funding: This research was funded by the European Commission through the FP7 project MARINA (grant agreement no. 263215) and the Horizon 2020 project BIORIMA (grant agreement no. 760928).

Data Availability Statement: The transcriptomics data were deposited at the NCBI BioProject database (PRJNA286067). Any other results are available from the authors upon reasonable request.

Acknowledgments: We thank the Joint Research Centre (JRC) for providing NMs, and Lars Haag, Electron Microscopy Core Facility, Karolinska Institutet, for assistance with TEM imaging. We also wish to thank Anil Sharma, Mayo Clinic, and visiting scientist at Karolinska Institutet, for helpful discussions, and Olesja Bondarenko, Karolinska Institutet, for assistance in collecting samples for omics analysis.

Conflicts of Interest: The authors declare no conflict of interest.

References

1. Xia, T.; Li, N.; Nel, A.E. Potential health impact of nanoparticles. *Annu. Rev. Public Health* **2009**, *30*, 137–150. [CrossRef] [PubMed]
2. Yang, W.; Wang, L.; Mettenbrink, E.M.; DeAngelis, P.L.; Wilhelm, S. Nanoparticle toxicology. *Annu. Rev. Pharmacol. Toxicol.* **2021**, *61*, 269–289. [CrossRef]
3. Paunovska, K.; Loughrey, D.; Sago, C.D.; Langer, R.; Dahlman, J.E. Using large datasets to understand nanotechnology. *Adv. Mater.* **2019**, *31*, e1902798. [CrossRef]
4. Fadeel, B.; Farcal, L.; Hardy, B.; Vázquez-Campos, S.; Hristozov, D.; Marcomini, A.; Lynch, I.; Valsami-Jones, E.; Alenius, H.; Savolainen, K. Advanced tools for the safety assessment of nanomaterials. *Nat. Nanotechnol.* **2018**, *13*, 537–543. [CrossRef]
5. Teunenbroek, T.V.; Baker, J.; Dijkzeul, A. Towards a more effective and efficient governance and regulation of nanomaterials. *Part. Fibre Toxicol.* **2017**, *14*, 54. [CrossRef]
6. Bhattacharya, K.; Kiliç, G.; Costa, P.M.; Fadeel, B. Cytotoxicity screening and cytokine profiling of nineteen nanomaterials enables hazard ranking and grouping based on inflammogenic potential. *Nanotoxicology* **2017**, *11*, 809–826. [PubMed]
7. Farcal, L.; Andón, F.T.; Di Cristo, L.; Rotoli, B.M.; Bussolati, O.; Bergamaschi, E.; Mech, A.; Hartmann, N.B.; Rasmussen, K.; Riego-Sintes, J.; et al. Comprehensive in vitro toxicity testing of a panel of representative oxide nanomaterials: First steps towards an intelligent testing strategy. *PLoS ONE* **2015**, *10*, e0127174. [CrossRef]
8. Kermanizadeh, A.; Pojana, G.; Gaiser, B.K.; Birkedal, R.; Bilanicˇová, D.; Wallin, H.; Jensen, K.A.; Sellergren, B.; Hutchison, G.R.; Marcomini, A.; et al. In vitro assessment of engineered nanomaterials using a hepatocyte cell line: Cytotoxicity, pro-inflammatory cytokines and functional markers. *Nanotoxicology* **2013**, *7*, 301–313. [CrossRef]
9. Kroll, A.; Dierker, C.; Rommel, C.; Hahn, D.; Wohlleben, W.; Schulze-Isfort, C.; Göbbert, C.; Voetz, M.; Hardinghaus, F.; Schnekenburger, J. Cytotoxicity screening of 23 engineered nanomaterials using a test matrix of ten cell lines and three different assays. *Part. Fibre Toxicol.* **2011**, *8*, 9. [CrossRef] [PubMed]
10. Kuempel, E.D.; Jaurand, M.-C.; Møller, P.; Morimoto, Y.; Kobayashi, N.; Pinkerton, K.E.; Sargent, L.M.; Vermeulen, R.C.H.; Fubini, B.; Kane, A.B. Evaluating the mechanistic evidence and key data gaps in assessing the potential carcinogenicity of carbon nanotubes and nanofibers in humans. *Crit. Rev. Toxicol.* **2017**, *47*, 1–58. [CrossRef]
11. Fraser, K.; Kodali, V.; Yanamala, N.; Birch, M.E.; Cena, L.; Casuccio, G.; Bunker, K.; Lersch, T.L.; Evans, D.E.; Stefaniak, A.; et al. Physicochemical characterization and genotoxicity of the broad class of carbon nanotubes and nanofibers used or produced in US facilities. *Part. Fibre Toxicol.* **2020**, *17*, 62. [CrossRef]
12. Di Cristo, L.; Bianchi, M.G.; Chiu, M.; Taurino, G.; Donato, F.; Garzaro, G.; Bussolati, O.; Bergamaschi, E. Comparative in vitro cytotoxicity of realistic doses of benchmark multi-walled carbon nanotubes towards macrophages and airway epithelial cells. *Nanomaterials* **2019**, *9*, 982. [CrossRef] [PubMed]
13. Gliga, A.R.; Edoff, K.; Caputo, F.; Källman, T.; Blom, H.; Karlsson, H.L.; Ghibelli, L.; Traversa, E.; Ceccatelli, S.; Fadeel, B. Cerium oxide nanoparticles inhibit differentiation of neural stem cells. *Sci. Rep.* **2017**, *7*, 9284. [CrossRef] [PubMed]
14. Gliga, A.R.; Di Bucchianico, S.; Lindvall, J.; Fadeel, B.; Karlsson, H.L. RNA sequencing reveals long-term effects of silver nanoparticles on human lung cells. *Sci. Rep.* **2018**, *8*, 6668. [CrossRef] [PubMed]
15. Rasmussen, K.; Rauscher, H.; Mech, A.; Sintes, J.R.; Gilliland, D.; González, M.; Kearns, P.; Moss, K.; Visser, M.; Groenewold, M.; et al. Physico-chemical properties of manufactured nanomaterials-characterisation and relevant methods. An outlook based on the OECD testing programme. *Regul. Toxicol. Pharmacol.* **2018**, *92*, 8–28. [CrossRef] [PubMed]
16. Mukherjee, S.P.; Bondarenko, O.; Kohonen, P.; Andón, F.T.; Brzicová, T.; Gessner, I.; Mathur, S.; Bottini, M.; Calligari, P.; Stella, L.; et al. Macrophage sensing of single-walled carbon nanotubes via Toll like receptors. *Sci. Rep.* **2018**, *8*, 1115. [CrossRef]
17. Libalová, H.; Costa, P.M.; Olsson, M.; Farcal, L.; Ortelli, S.; Blosi, M.; Topinka, J.; Costa, A.L.; Fadeel, B. Toxicity of surface-modified copper oxide nanoparticles in a mouse macrophage cell line: Interplay of particles, surface coating and particle dissolution. *Chemosphere* **2018**, *196*, 482–493. [CrossRef]

18. Klöditz, K.; Fadeel, B. Three cell deaths and a funeral: Macrophage clearance of cells undergoing distinct modes of cell death. *Cell Death Discov.* **2019**, *5*, 65. [CrossRef] [PubMed]
19. Mukherjee, S.P.; Gupta, G.; Klöditz, K.; Wang, J.; Rodrigues, A.F.; Kostarelos, K.; Fadeel, B. Next-generation sequencing reveals differential responses to acute *versus* long-term exposures to graphene oxide in human lung cells. *Small* **2020**, *16*, e1907686. [CrossRef]
20. Krämer, A.; Green, J.; Pollard, J.; Tugendreich, S. Causal analysis approaches in Ingenuity Pathway Analysis. *Bioinformatics* **2014**, *30*, 523–530. [CrossRef]
21. Gallud, A.; Klöditz, K.; Ytterberg, J.; Östberg, N.; Katayama, S.; Skoog, T.; Gogvadze, V.; Chen, Y.-Z.; Xue, D.; Moya, S.; et al. Cationic gold nanoparticles elicit mitochondrial dysfunction: A multi-omics study. *Sci. Rep.* **2019**, *9*, 4366. [CrossRef]
22. Gliga, A.; De Loma, J.; Di Bucchianico, S.; Skoglund, S.; Keshavan, S.; Odnevall Wallinder, I.; Karlsson, H.L.; Fadeel, B. Silver nanoparticles modulate lipopolysaccharide-triggered Toll like receptor signaling in immune-competent human cell lines. *Nanoscale Adv.* **2020**, *2*, 648–658. [CrossRef]
23. Mukherjee, S.P.; Lozano, N.; Kucki, M.; Del Rio-Castillo, A.E.; Newman, L.; Vázquez, E.; Kostarelos, K.; Wick, P.; Fadeel, B. Detection of endotoxin contamination of graphene based materials using the TNF-α expression test and guidelines for endotoxin-free graphene oxide production. *PLoS ONE* **2016**, *11*, e0166816. [CrossRef]
24. Broz, P.; Dixit, V.M. Inflammasomes: Mechanism of assembly, regulation and signalling. *Nat. Rev. Immunol.* **2016**, *16*, 407–420. [CrossRef]
25. Wilkinson, K.E.; Palmberg, L.; Witasp, E.; Kupczyk, M.; Feliu, N.; Gerde, P.; Seisenbaeva, G.A.; Fadeel, B.; Dahlén, S.E.; Kessler, V.G. Solution-engineered palladium nanoparticles: Model for health effect studies of automotive particulate pollution. *ACS Nano* **2011**, *5*, 5312–5324. [CrossRef]
26. Rydman, E.M.; Ilves, M.; Koivisto, A.J.; Kinaret, P.A.; Fortino, V.; Savinko, T.S.; Lehto, M.T.; Pulkkinen, V.; Vippola, M.; Hämeri, K.J.; et al. Inhalation of rod-like carbon nanotubes causes unconventional allergic airway inflammation. *Part. Fibre Toxicol.* **2014**, *11*, 48. [CrossRef] [PubMed]
27. Rydman, E.M.; Ilves, M.; Vanhala, E.; Vippola, M.; Lehto, M.; Kinaret, P.A.; Pylkkänen, L.; Happo, M.; Hirvonen, M.R.; Greco, D.; et al. A single aspiration of rod-like carbon nanotubes induces asbestos-like pulmonary inflammation mediated in part by the IL-1 receptor. *Toxicol. Sci.* **2015**, *147*, 140–155. [CrossRef] [PubMed]
28. Duke, K.S.; Thompson, E.A.; Ihrie, M.D.; Taylor-Just, A.J.; Ash, E.A.; Shipkowski, K.A.; Hall, J.R.; Tokarz, D.A.; Cesta, M.F.; Hubbs, A.F.; et al. Role of p53 in the chronic pulmonary immune response to tangled or rod-like multi-walled carbon nanotubes. *Nanotoxicology* **2018**, *12*, 975–991. [CrossRef] [PubMed]
29. Aldieri, E.; Fenoglio, I.; Cesano, F.; Gazzano, E.; Gulino, G.; Scarano, D.; Attanasio, A.; Mazzucco, G.; Ghigo, D.; Fubini, B. The role of iron impurities in the toxic effects exerted by short multi-walled carbon nanotubes (MWCNT) in murine alveolar macrophages. *J. Toxicol. Environ. Health A* **2013**, *76*, 1056–1071. [CrossRef]
30. Vitkina, T.I.; Yankova, V.I.; Gvozdenko, T.A.; Kuznetsov, V.L.; Krasnikov, D.V.; Nazarenko, A.V.; Chaika, V.V.; Smagin, S.V.; Tsatsakis, A.M.; Engin, A.B.; et al. The impact of multi-walled carbon nanotubes with different amount of metallic impurities on immunometabolic parameters in healthy volunteers. *Food Chem. Toxicol.* **2016**, *87*, 138–147. [CrossRef]
31. Lee, D.K.; Jeon, S.; Jeong, J.; Yu, I.J.; Song, K.S.; Kang, A.; Yun, W.S.; Kim, J.S.; Cho, W.S. Potential role of soluble metal impurities in the acute lung inflammogenicity of multi-walled carbon nanotubes. *Nanomaterials* **2020**, *10*, 379. [CrossRef] [PubMed]
32. Veronesi, G.; Aude-Garcia, C.; Kieffer, I.; Gallon, T.; Delangle, P.; Herlin-Boime, N.; Rabilloud, T.; Carrière, M. Exposure-dependent Ag+ release from silver nanoparticles and its complexation in AgS2 sites in primary murine macrophages. *Nanoscale* **2015**, *7*, 7323–7330. [CrossRef] [PubMed]
33. Veronesi, G.; Deniaud, A.; Gallon, T.; Jouneau, P.H.; Villanova, J.; Delangle, P.; Carrière, M.; Kieffer, I.; Charbonnier, P.; Mintz, E.; et al. Visualization, quantification and coordination of Ag+ ions released from silver nanoparticles in hepatocytes. *Nanoscale* **2016**, *8*, 17012–17021. [CrossRef]
34. Omori, S.; Tsugita, M.; Hoshikawa, Y.; Morita, M.; Ito, F.; Yamaguchi, S.I.; Xie, Q.; Noyori, O.; Yamaguchi, T.; Takada, A.; et al. Tim4 recognizes carbon nanotubes and mediates phagocytosis leading to granuloma formation. *Cell Rep.* **2021**, *34*, 108734. [CrossRef]
35. Scala, G.; Kinaret, P.; Marwah, V.; Sund, J.; Fortino, V.; Greco, D. Multi-omics analysis of ten carbon nanomaterials effects highlights cell type specific patterns of molecular regulation and adaptation. *NanoImpact* **2018**, *11*, 99–108. [CrossRef]
36. Saarimäli, L.A.; Kinaret, P.A.; Scala, G.; del Giudice, G.; Federico, A.; Serra, A.; Greco, D. Toxicogenomics analysis of dynamic dose-response in macrophages highlights molecular alterations relevant for multi-walled carbon nanotube-induced lung fibrosis. *NanoImpact* **2020**, *20*, 100274. [CrossRef]
37. Griffith, J.W.; Sokol, C.L.; Luster, A.D. Chemokines and chemokine receptors: Positioning cells for host defense and immunity. *Annu. Rev. Immunol.* **2014**, *32*, 659–702. [CrossRef]
38. Lloyd, C.M.; Snelgrove, R.J. Type 2 immunity: Expanding our view. *Sci. Immunol.* **2018**, *3*, eaat1604. [CrossRef] [PubMed]
39. Miyabe, Y.; Lian, J.; Miyabe, C.; Luster, A.D. Chemokines in rheumatic diseases: Pathogenic role and therapeutic implications. *Nat. Rev. Rheumatol.* **2019**, *15*, 731–746. [CrossRef]
40. Park, E.J.; Roh, J.; Kim, S.N.; Kim, Y.; Han, S.B.; Hong, J.T. CCR5 plays an important role in resolving an inflammatory response to single-walled carbon nanotubes. *J. Appl. Toxicol.* **2013**, *33*, 845–853. [CrossRef] [PubMed]

41. Snyder-Talkington, B.N.; Dymacek, J.; Porter, D.W.; Wolfarth, M.G.; Mercer, R.R.; Pacurari, M.; Denvir, J.; Castranova, V.; Qian, Y.; Guo, N.L. System-based identification of toxicity pathways associated with multi-walled carbon nanotube-induced pathological responses. *Toxicol. Appl. Pharmacol.* **2013**, *272*, 476–489. [CrossRef] [PubMed]
42. Boyles, M.S.; Young, L.; Brown, D.M.; MacCalman, L.; Cowie, H.; Moisala, A.; Stone, V.; Smail, F.; Smith, P.J.W.; Proudfoot, L.; et al. Multi-walled carbon nanotube induced frustrated phagocytosis, cytotoxicity and pro-inflammatory conditions in macrophages are length dependent and greater than that of asbestos. *Toxicol. In Vitro* **2015**, *29*, 1513–1528. [CrossRef] [PubMed]
43. Morimoto, Y.; Horie, M.; Kobayashi, N.; Shinohara, N.; Shimada, M. Inhalation toxicity assessment of carbon-based nanoparticles. *Acc. Chem. Res.* **2013**, *46*, 770–781. [CrossRef] [PubMed]
44. Donaldson, K.; Poland, C.A.; Murphy, F.A.; MacFarlane, M.; Chernova, T.; Schinwald, A. Pulmonary toxicity of carbon nanotubes and asbestos-similarities and differences. *Adv. Drug Deliv. Rev.* **2013**, *65*, 2078–2086. [CrossRef] [PubMed]
45. Sydlik, S.A.; Jhunjhunwala, S.; Webber, M.J.; Anderson, D.G.; Langer, R. In vivo compatibility of graphene oxide with differing oxidation states. *ACS Nano* **2015**, *9*, 3866–3874. [CrossRef]
46. Costa, P.M.; Gosens, I.; Williams, A.; Farcal, L.; Pantano, D.; Brown, D.M.; Stone, V.; Cassee, F.R.; Halappanavar, S.; Fadeel, B. Transcriptional profiling reveals gene expression changes associated with inflammation and cell proliferation following short-term inhalation exposure to copper oxide nanoparticles. *J. Appl. Toxicol.* **2018**, *38*, 385–397. [CrossRef] [PubMed]
47. Andujar, P.; Simon-Deckers, A.; Galateau-Sallé, F.; Fayard, B.; Beaune, G.; Clin, B.; Billon-Galland, M.-A.; Durupthy, O.; Pairon, J.-C.; Doucet, J.; et al. Role of metal oxide nanoparticles in histopathological changes observed in the lung of welders. *Part. Fibre Toxicol.* **2014**, *11*, 23. [CrossRef] [PubMed]
48. Tuncer, S.; Fiorillo, M.T.; Sorrentino, R. The multifaceted nature of NLRP12. *J. Leukoc. Biol.* **2014**, *96*, 991–1000. [CrossRef]
49. Palomäki, J.; Välimäki, E.; Sund, J.; Vippola, M.; Clausen, P.A.; Jensen, K.A.; Savolainen, K.; Matikainen, S.; Alenius, H. Long, needle-like carbon nanotubes and asbestos activate the NLRP3 inflammasome through a similar mechanism. *ACS Nano* **2011**, *5*, 6861–6870. [CrossRef] [PubMed]
50. Zaki, M.H.; Vogel, P.; Malireddi, R.K.; Body-Malapel, M.; Anand, P.K.; Bertin, J.; Green, D.R.; Lamkanfi, M.; Kanneganti, T.D. The NOD-like receptor NLRP12 attenuates colon inflammation and tumorigenesis. *Cancer Cell* **2011**, *20*, 649–660. [CrossRef]
51. Allen, I.C.; Wilson, J.; Schneider, M.; Lich, J.; Roberts, R.; Arthur, J.; Woodford, R.; Davis, B.; Uronis, J.; Herfarth, H.; et al. NLRP12 suppresses colon inflammation and tumorigenesis through the negative regulation of noncanonical NF-κB signaling. *Immunity* **2012**, *36*, 742–754. [CrossRef]
52. Chen, L.; Wilson, J.E.; Koenigsknecht, M.J.; Chou, W.-C.; Montgomery, S.A.; Truax, A.D.; Brickey, W.J.; Packey, C.D.; Maharshak, N.; Matsushima, G.K.; et al. NLRP12 attenuates colon inflammation by maintaining colonic microbial diversity and promoting protective commensal bacterial growth. *Nat. Immunol.* **2017**, *18*, 541–551. [CrossRef]
53. Ulland, T.K.; Jain, N.; Hornick, E.E.; Elliott, E.I.; Clay, G.M.; Sadler, J.J.; Mills, K.A.M.; Janowski, A.M.; Volk, A.P.D.; Wang, K.; et al. Nlrp12 mutation causes C57BL/6J strain-specific defect in neutrophil recruitment. *Nat. Commun.* **2016**, *7*, 13180. [CrossRef] [PubMed]
54. Keshavan, S.; Calligari, P.; Stella, L.; Fusco, L.; Delogu, L.G.; Fadeel, B. Nano-bio interactions: A neutrophil-centric view. *Cell Death Dis.* **2019**, *10*, 569. [CrossRef]
55. Bhattacharya, K.; Andón, F.T.; El-Sayed, R.; Fadeel, B. Mechanisms of carbon nanotube-induced toxicity: Focus on pulmonary inflammation. *Adv. Drug Deliv. Rev.* **2013**, *65*, 2087–2097. [CrossRef] [PubMed]
56. Liu, Y.; Zhao, Y.; Sun, B.; Chen, C. Understanding the toxicity of carbon nanotubes. *Acc. Chem. Res.* **2013**, *46*, 702–713. [CrossRef] [PubMed]
57. Fadeel, B.; Kostarelos, K. Grouping all carbon nanotubes into a single substance category is scientifically unjustified. *Nat. Nanotechnol.* **2020**, *15*, 164. [CrossRef]
58. Heller, D.A.; Jena, P.V.; Pasquali, M.; Kostarelos, K.; Delogu, L.G.; Meidl, R.E.; Rotkin, S.V.; Scheinberg, D.A.; Schwartz, R.E.; Terrones, M.; et al. Banning carbon nanotubes would be scientifically unjustified and damaging to innovation. *Nat. Nanotechnol.* **2020**, *15*, 164–166. [CrossRef]

nanomaterials

MDPI

Article

Serum Lowers Bioactivity and Uptake of Synthetic Amorphous Silica by Alveolar Macrophages in a Particle Specific Manner

Martin Wiemann [1,*], Antje Vennemann [1], Cornel Venzago [2], Gottlieb-Georg Lindner [3], Tobias B. Schuster [2] and Nils Krueger [2]

[1] IBE R&D Institute for Lung Health gGmbH, Mendelstr. 11, 48149 Münster, Germany; vennemann@ibe-ms.de
[2] Evonik Operations GmbH, Rodenbacher Chaussee 4, 63457 Hanau-Wolfgang, Germany; cornel.venzago@evonik.com (C.V.); tobias.schuster@evonik.com (T.B.S.); nils.krueger@evonik.com (N.K.)
[3] Evonik Operations GmbH, Brühler Straße 2, 50389 Wesseling, Germany; gottlieb-georg.lindner@evonik.com
* Correspondence: martin.wiemann@ibe-ms.de; Tel.: +49-251-9802340

Abstract: Various cell types are compromised by synthetic amorphous silica (SAS) if they are exposed to SAS under protein-free conditions in vitro. Addition of serum protein can mitigate most SAS effects, but it is not clear whether this is solely caused by protein corona formation and/or altered particle uptake. Because sensitive and reliable mass spectrometric measurements of SiO_2 NP are cumbersome, quantitative uptake studies of SAS at the cellular level are largely missing. In this study, we combined the comparison of SAS effects on alveolar macrophages in the presence and absence of foetal calf serum with mass spectrometric measurement of ^{28}Si in alkaline cell lysates. Effects on the release of lactate dehydrogenase, glucuronidase, TNFα and H_2O_2 of precipitated (SIPERNAT® 50, SIPERNAT® 160) and fumed SAS (AEROSIL® OX50, AEROSIL® 380 F) were lowered close to control level by foetal calf serum (FCS) added to the medium. Using a quantitative high resolution ICP-MS measurement combined with electron microscopy, we found that FCS reduced the uptake of particle mass by 9.9% (SIPERNAT® 50) up to 83.8% (AEROSIL® OX50). Additionally, larger particle agglomerates were less frequent in cells in the presence of FCS. Plotting values for lactate dehydrogenase (LDH), glucuronidase (GLU) or tumour necrosis factor alpha (TNFα) against the mean cellular dose showed the reduction of bioactivity with a particle sedimentation bias. As a whole, the mitigating effects of FCS on precipitated and fumed SAS on alveolar macrophages are caused by a reduction of bioactivity and by a lowered internalization, and both effects occur in a particle specific manner. The method to quantify nanosized SiO_2 in cells is a valuable tool for future in vitro studies.

Keywords: nanomaterials; synthetic amorphous silica; in vitro testing; NR8383 alveolar macrophage; ICP-MS analysis of cell bound SiO_2

Citation: Wiemann, M.; Vennemann, A.; Venzago, C.; Lindner, G.-G.; Schuster, T.B.; Krueger, N. Serum Lowers Bioactivity and Uptake of Synthetic Amorphous Silica by Alveolar Macrophages in a Particle Specific Manner. *Nanomaterials* **2021**, *11*, 628. https://doi.org/10.3390/nano11030628

Academic Editor: Eleonore Fröhlich

Received: 24 January 2021
Accepted: 26 February 2021
Published: 3 March 2021

Publisher's Note: MDPI stays neutral with regard to jurisdictional claims in published maps and institutional affiliations.

1. Introduction

Synthetic amorphous silica (SAS) form a major group of industrially relevant nanomaterials (NMs) [1–3]. They are produced either from aqueous solutions of sodium silicate to form colloidal silica, silica gels, and precipitated silica, or may be synthesized from the gaseous phase of $SiCl_4$ to form fumed (pyrogenic) silica [3,4]. Due to the production process, pyrogenic and precipitated silica form indivisible aggregates, which have no physical boundaries among their primary structures. These aggregates have external dimensions that are highly variable in nature with some particles being in the nano-size range [3,5]. Since most SAS materials come as dry powders, a non-intentional uptake into the body may occur via inhalation [6,7]. Animal studies have shown that SAS can induce transient inflammatory responses in the rat lung [6–10] whereas fibrogenic or genotoxic effects, as induced by crystalline silica, such as quartz or cristobalite, were not induced even at high lung burden [11,12].

To describe and predict the bioactivity of the multitude of SAS, in vitro assays using different cell types and incubation conditions have been published [13–17]. Recently, the effects of SAS from all major production processes were tested using rat alveolar macrophages (NR8383) in vitro [18]. A major finding was that SAS, irrespective of the production method, elicit highly uniform responses, e.g., with respect to the release of lactate dehydrogenase (LDH), glucuronidase (GLU), tumour necrosis factor alpha (TNFα) or induction of H_2O_2 release [18]. In these experiments, cells were exposed to SAS under protein-free standard conditions, i.e., in the absence of serum proteins. This is a well-established testing procedure reflecting the circumstance that particles entering into lung alveoli are primarily protein-free entities. Furthermore, the protein-free in vitro conditions allow to study particle effects linked, e.g., to surface properties of nanoparticles [19]. However, for most SAS, the half maximal effective concentration (EC50) for several endpoints is comparatively low under protein-free conditions (e.g., 10–20 µg/mL for the release of LDH) [18], a finding which does not correspond to the in vivo effects of SAS especially when effects of amorphous and crystalline silica are compared [12]. On the other hand, the bioactivity of SAS in vitro is strongly reduced when particles (i) are administered in the presence of serum [20], (ii) are protein-treated prior to exposure [21–24] or (iii) are dispersed by extensive ultrasonic energy in the presence of low concentrations of albumin [25]. All aforementioned protein-treatments inevitably lead to the formation of a protein corona [26,27]. However, they also influence particle dispersion, gravitational settling and uptake by cells. Studies with fluorescent silica probes showed a decreased gravitational settling in the presence of protein, whereas larger precipitates of SAS settled onto the cells in the absence of protein [21,22,28]. The direct contact with the cell membrane and/or the uptake of particles is a prerequisite at least for poorly soluble particles to elicit cellular effects. Therefore, a lower rate of gravitational settling can reduce the effects of nanoparticles under submersed in vitro conditions [29]. Interestingly, the addition of protein has no uniform effect on the uptake of SAS particles and this appears to be especially relevant for macrophages. In RAW264.7 macrophages, addition of FCS enabled the uptake of SAS but mitigated cytotoxic effects [21]. In contrast, albumin-coating of NM-200, a precipitated SAS and of the pyrogenic NM-203 led to more cytotoxicity in THP-1 cells, but lowered the cytotoxicity in RAW264.7 cells [25]. Another unexpected result was provided by Binnemars–Postma and co-workers, who showed that human M1 macrophages ingested more silica nanoparticles in the absence of serum, whereas the presence of serum increased the uptake of SAS by M2 macrophage [30]. Although not yet fully elucidated, these discrepancies may be due to the presence of surface receptors involved in particle uptake, such as the scavenger receptor expressed in RAW264.7 cells [31]. Together, these results show that the effects of FCS on bioactivity and uptake of SAS are cell-type specific and need to be explored more thoroughly, especially when different types of macrophages are compared.

In the present paper, we aim to close this gap for NR8383 alveolar macrophages from rat lung using fumed and precipitated SAS with small and large specific surface areas, which were chosen to represent the large number of different SAS on the market. The well-established NR8383 cell line is widely used to analyse the bioactivity of particles in the lung: in the so-called macrophage model, NR8383 cells are exposed to settling particles under submersed conditions. The particles' bioactivity in the lung is then predicted from a set of assays carried out with the cell culture supernatant [19,32–36]. However, because SAS particles are small, their gravitational settling followed by cellular uptake may be incomplete counteracting a reliable dosimetry. Although elaborated models may predict the fraction of gravitationally settled of SAS in a time-dependent manner [37], there is still a need for quantitative measurements of SAS in cells. The quantification of SAS in cells requires a sensitive and valid analytical method. Since the mass spectrometric measurement of silicon suffers from N_2 interference, an instrument with a high mass resolution is needed. Moreover, the conventional solubilisation of silica particles in organic matter with hydrofluoric acid (HF) is subject to critical handling guidelines and requires specialized labs and personnel [38]. Recently, Bossert et al. (2019) proposed a HF-free hot alkaline lysis followed by acid treatment to dissolve silica particles; silicon was then detected by ICP-OES or by a colorimetric method with a limit of detection (LOD) being in the range of 40–100 mg/L [39]. Of note, cells exposed in vitro to approximately 10 µg SAS per mL likely underscore this LOD by at least one order of magnitude, unless the cell number is scaled up to very high amounts. To meet more conventional dimensions of cell culture testing, i.e., testing of several million cells per well, here we present a sufficiently sensitive method for SAS quantification, combining alkaline dissolution, acid neutralization and high resolution ICP-MS. By this, the amount of cellular SAS was measured and compared with the subcellular distribution of SAS in NR8383 cells in the absence and presence of foetal calf serum (FCS). This way the effect of FCS, known to reduce the bioactivity of SAS on macrophages in vitro, could be analysed for the first time on the basis of quantitative uptake data.

2. Materials and Methods

2.1. Materials

The materials were provided by Evonik Operations GmbH (Hanau-Wolfgang, Germany) as dry powders and had been extensively characterized in a previous publication [18]. The main data are summarized in Table 1.

Table 1. Material properties of the synthetic amorphous silica (SAS) used in the study.

Material	Size of Primary Structures (nm) [(1)]	Aggregate Size (nm) [(1)]	BET (m^2/g) [(2)]	Zeta Potential (mV) [(3)]	Solubility (mg/L) [(4)]	pH [(5)]	SEARs No. [(6)]
AEROSIL® 380F	8.0 ± 2.7	101.9	390	−36	226.0	4.2	14.5
AEROSIL® OX50	41.4 ± 18.3	233.7	45	−40	117.9	4.6	1.8
SIPERNAT® 50	3.1. ± 0.7	59.8	460	−21	113.9	6.3	16.3
SIPERNAT® 160	12.2. ± 2.7	58.3	180	−53	112.1	6.1	11.1

[(1)] As measured by transmission electron microscopy. [(2)] Specific surface area measured by N_2 adsorption. [(3)] Zeta potential and point of zero charge. [(4)] Measured according to enhanced OECD 105 Test Guideline on solubility. [(5)] Measured in 5% solution; [(6)] a measure for the number of silanol groups on the surface of silica according. For details, see [18].

2.2. Preparation of Particle Suspensions

The main goal of the study was to compare effects of SAS in the absence and presence of foetal calf serum, after particles had been dispersed according to a previously established protocol [18]. In brief, particles were suspended in sterile H_2O (Aqua ad injectabilia, Braun Melsungen, Germany) at a concentration of 2 mg/mL. Suspensions were vortexed, stirred with a magnetic bar for 90 min and passed through a sterile polyamide gauze with a nominal pore width of 5 µm (Bückmann, Mönchengladbach, Germany) (see [4] for filtration characteristics). 5 mL of each filtrate was then transferred to a 20 mL glass vial and subjected to an ultrasonic dispersion energy 270 J/mL [4]. Dispersed masses amounted to 70–100% the original masses, as determined by gravimetric analysis. The stock aqueous stock suspensions of SIPERNAT® 160, SIPERNAT® 50, AEROSIL® OX50 and AEROSIL® 380 F were adjusted to 360 µg/mL, and stored at 4 °C for up to 4 weeks. Immediately before experiments, aqueous stock suspensions were mixed with an equal volume double concentrated KRPG buffer (see below) or F-12K media to obtain a physiologic medium composition.

2.3. Cultivation of NR8383 Macrophages and Cell Culture Assays

NR8383 cells (ATCC, Manassas, VA, USA; ATCC® Number: CRL-2192TM) were maintained in F-12K cell culture medium (Sigma-Aldrich, Taufkirchen, Germany) supplemented with 15% foetal calf serum (FCS), 1% penicillin/streptomycin and 1% L-glutamine (all from PAN Biotech, Aidenbach, Gremany) under cell culture conditions (37 °C and 5% CO_2) [32]. For the assay, 3×10^5 cells were seeded per well of a 96-well plate, and covered with 200 µL F-12K cell culture medium plus 5% (v/v) FCS to foster cell adherence. The next day, the medium was replaced by serum-free or FCS (10%)-containing F-12K medium containing increasing concentrations of each material (11.25, 22.5, 45 or 90 µg/mL). After 16 h, supernatant was retrieved to determine LDH, GLU and TNFα. To measure the release of H_2O_2, materials were equivalently diluted in KRPG buffer (129 mM NaCl, 4.86 mM KCl, 1.22 mM $CaCl_2$, 15.8 mM NaH_2PO_4, 5–10 mM glucose; pH 7.3–7.4).

Assays were carried out as described [32]. In brief, H_2O_2 was quantified with the Amplex Red® assay by photometrically measuring formed resorufin at 570 nm (reference value: 620 nm) with a plate reader (Tecan Infinite F200Pro, Tecan GmbH, Crailsheim, Germany); positive controls were run with 360 µg/mL zymosan (Sigma-Aldrich, Taufkirchen, Germany). Measurements were corrected for background absorbance of cell free-particle controls and converted into concentrations of H_2O_2 as described. LDH activity was measured with the Roche Cytotoxicity Kit (Sigma-Aldrich, Taufkirchen, Germany) according to the manufacturer's protocol. GLU activity was detected with p-nitrophenyl-D-glucuronide dissolved in 0.2 M sodium acetate buffer (pH 5) containing 0.1% Triton X-100. Both the LDH- and GLU-based values were corrected for cell-free absorption and normalised to the positive control (0.1% Triton X-100 in F-12K) which was set to 100%. Tumour necrosis factor α (TNF α) was determined with a specific enzyme-linked immosorbent assay (ELISA) for rat TNFα (Quantikine ELISA Kit) according to the manufacturer's protocol (Bio-Techne GmbH, Wiesbaden-Nordenstadt, Germany). The TNFα-forming capacity of NR8383 cells was tested with 0.5 µg/mL lipopolysaccharide (LPS, Sigma-Aldrich, Taufkirchen, Germany). Notably, aliquots for measuring LDH, GLU and TNFα were taken from the same well.

2.4. *Particle Size Determination under Cell Culture Conditions with Particle Tracking Analysis*

The hydrodynamic diameter was determined by optical tracking analyses using a NanoSight LM10 instrument equipped with a violet laser (405 nm), an Andor CCD camera, and particle tracking software NTA3.0 (all from: Malvern Instruments GmbH, Herrenberg, Germany). Starting with the aqueous particle stock suspension, dilutions were prepared in KRPG and F-12K medium in the absence and presence of 10% FCS. Concentration was uniformly set to 90 µg/mL. Suspensions were incubated under cell culture conditions (37 °C, 5% CO_2, 100% humidity) for 90 min (KRPG) and 16 h (F-12K), respectively. Suspensions were further diluted to obtain measurable concentrations, approximately in the range of 5×10^8 particle/mL.

2.5. *Electron Microscopy of NR8383 Macrophages*

NR8383 cells were seeded onto small discs (diameter 6 mm) of Melinex film (Plano, Wetzlar, Germany) placed in the wells of a 96-well plate, subjected to particle treatment for 16 h as described in paragraph 2.4. Then, media were withdrawn and cells were immediately covered with 2.5% glutardialdehyde in 0.1 M sodium phosphate buffer (SPB, pH 7.3) for 60 min. Cells were washed three times with SPB, post-fixed in 1% OsO_4, dehydrated in ethanol to the 70% step, and stained en bloc with uranium acetate (1%). Cells were dehydrated via ethanol/propylene oxide, and embedded in Epon 812 (Sigma Aldrich, Taufkirchen, Germany). Ultrathin sections (50–60 nm) were viewed with a Tecnai G2 electron microscope operated at 100 or 120 kV; images were taken with a Quemesa digital camera (Olympus Soft Imaging Solutions, Münster, Germany).

2.6. *Quantification of Cell-Associated SiO_2 NP by High Resolution ICP-MS*

To quantitate the amount of cell-associated SiO_2 NP, 2.8×10^6 NR8383 cells were seeded into each well of a 6-well plate and incubated in 6 mL F-12K medium containing 11.25 µg/mL of each SiO_2 samples, both in the absence and presence of 10% FCS. After 16 h, the culture medium was completely withdrawn and replaced by 1 mL phosphate buffered saline (PBS). Cells were detached from the plates by vigorous pipetting and transferred into a 15 mL test tube (Falcon) pre-loaded with 6 mL fresh F-12K medium. Cells were spun down (200× *g*, 10 min), washed with 2 mL KRPG buffer, pelleted again (200× *g*, 10 min), and finally re-suspended in 130–230 µL KRPG buffer. A defined volume (90%) of this final suspension was dehydrated at 60 °C for 12 h for analysis.

To measure the SiO_2 content, each sample was dissolved with 50 µL of 20% NaOH and heated to 120 °C for 2 h. Lysates were diluted with 5 mL ultrapure H_2O. In further dilution steps, 4% (v/v) of a HNO_3 solution was added. Measurements of Si were carried out with a double focusing magnetic sector field ICP-MS instrument in the medium resolution mode (Element 2™, Thermo Fisher Scientific, Meerbusch, Germany) equipped with a quartz spray chamber and a quartz injection device (sample loop: 500 µL, ESI-Fastvalve). ^{115}In was used as an internal standard. To calibrate the ICP-MS signal for ^{28}Si, a Si standard stock solution of 100 mg/L (Labkings, Hilversum, The Netherlands) was diluted with 4% (v/v) of a HNO_3-solution and an equivalent amount of NaOH as mentioned above to obtain a calibration range of 0.5–100 µg/L. Final SiO_2 concentrations were obtained by multiplying measured Si concentrations with the stoichiometric factor of 2.1393.

2.7. Statistical Evaluation

For in vitro testing, i.e., effects on LDH, GLU, H_2O_2, and TNFα, three independent repetitions were carried out; data were expressed as mean ± standard deviation (SD). To find significant differences, values from each concentration step were compared to the respective vehicle-treated control using 2-way analysis of variance (ANOVA) with Dunnett's multiple comparisons test. Calculations were carried out with GraphPad Prism software. A value of $p \leq 0.05$ was considered significant. Calculation of hydrodynamic diameters were carried out with NTA 3.0 software.

3. Results

3.1. Particle Characterization

Two precipitated and two fumed SAS were selected for this study, whose major physical-chemical properties are shown in Table 1. A smaller and a larger particle type was selected for each group, also reflected by the BET values which, overall, span more than one order of magnitude. Acidity of the SAS powders was low but more pronounced for both AEROSIL®s. The SEARs No., which is a measure for the number of silanol groups at the particles' surface, was similar for three SAS but lower for AEROSIL® OX50. Solubility was very similar (112.1 to 117.9 mg/L) but slightly higher for AEROSIL® 380 F.

The addition of FCS to a SAS dispersion is likely to change the particles' surface charge and agglomeration behaviour which is highly relevant for in vitro testing. Therefore, the hydrodynamic diameter (HD) of all four SAS was measured with particle tracking analysis (PTA) in H_2O, and in the absence and presence of 10% foetal calf serum (FCS) in KRPG and F-12K medium, to mimic testing conditions (Table S1). In the case of SIPERNAT® 160 and SIPERNAT® 50, the HD (mode values) obtained in KRPG and F-12K were only slightly increased (<15%) compared to H_2O; HD values also hardly increased upon of 10% FCS. AEROSIL® 380 F particles were too small to be measured in H_2O but measurable agglomerates were found in F-12K medium especially in the presence of FCS. The size of AEROSIL® OX50 agglomerates increased in KRPG only. Overall, the effects of FCS on the hydrodynamic diameter of the particle fraction measurable by PTA were low. Nevertheless, the addition of FCS led to the formation of agglomerates visible by light microscopy at the bottom of the culture vessels (Figure 1). This effect was pronounced for AEROSIL® 380 F (Figure 1a,b), but low for AEROSIL® OX50 (Figure 1e,f), SIPERNAT® 160 (Figure 1i,j) and SIPERNAT® 50 (Figure 1m,n).

3.2. Quantification of Particle Uptake by NR8383 Cells

To measure the cell-associated SAS fraction which comprises internalized plus surface-bound particulate matter, we administered the lowest concentration of SAS particles (11.25 µg/mL) to a defined number of cells for 16 h (2.8×10^6 per well). As expected, this treatment led to a low amount of dead cells in the absence (4.2–10.6%) and nearly no dead cells in the presence of serum (1.5–2.5%, see Table S2). Table 2 shows the cell-associated SiO_2

masses measured by ICP-MS: Control cells contained low, though measurable amounts of ^{28}Si. All SAS-treated cells showed a cell-associated SiO_2 mass above background level, which could not be lowered, e.g., by avoiding SiO_2 containing cell culture material (data not shown). In the presence of 10% FCS, values for the precipitated SAS SIPERNAT® 50 and SIPERNAT® 160 were higher than those for the fumed SAS AEROSIL® OX50 and AEROSIL® 380 F and this difference was not obvious under FCS-free conditions (Table 2). The cell-associated amount of SiO_2 was reduced in the presence of 10% FCS-free conditions. The effect was pronounced for AEROSIL® 380 F (−69.5%), AEROSIL® OX50 (−83.8%), and SIPERNAT® 160 (−62.3%), but comparatively small for SIPERNAT® 50 (−9.9%).

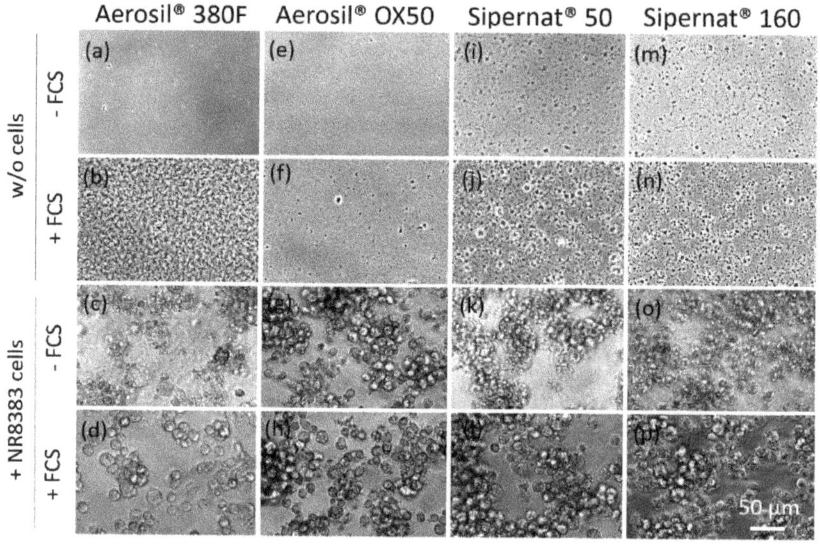

Figure 1. Sedimentation and uptake of precipitates by NR8383 cells which were formed in the presence of AEROSIL® 380 F (**a–d**), AEROSIL® OX50 (**e–h**), SIPERNAT® 50 (**i–l**) and SIPERNAT® 160 (**m–p**). Micrographs were taken 16 h after administration of particles (180 µg/mL) in the absence (w/o cells) and presence of cells (+NR8383). Foetal calf serum (FCS) led to the formation of agglomerates. In the absence of serum, many cells appeared deteriorated.

Table 2. Quantification of SiO_2 uptake in the absence and presence of foetal calf serum (FCS).

	10% FCS		FCS-Free		
Material	**Cell-Associated SiO_2 (µg)** (1)	% Total (2)	**Cell-Associated SiO_2 (µg)** (1)	% Total (2)	**Ratio FCS-Free/10% FCS** (3)
AEROSIL® 380 F	4.4/4.4	6.6/6.6	13.3/15.6	19.9/23.4	3.28
AEROSIL® OX50	5.7/5.8	8.4/8.6	33.3/37.8	49.5/56.2	6.18
SIPERNAT® 50	25.5/26.7	42.3/44.3	27.8/30.1	46.1/49.9	1.11
SIPERNAT® 160	13.3/14.4	21.1/22.8	34.4/38.9	54.5/61.6	2.65
Control (4)	1.2/1.6	-/-	1.2/1.3	-/-	-

(1) Amounts of SiO_2 in the cell pellet after 16 h, as measured by ICP-MS; values measured in duplicates are separated by a slash. (2) Cell-associated SiO_2 in percent of the total added mass (67.5 µg SAS per 6 mL medium; weigh in of each SAS was individually corrected for its water content measured as loss on ignition [18]. (3) Ratios were calculated from mean values of columns 2 and 4. (4) ^{28}Si values from control cells were assumed to represent SiO_2 and were converted equivalently.

3.3. *In Vitro Toxicity Determination of SAS and Electron Microscopic Study*

In vitro toxicity of SAS was measured in the absence and presence of FCS with the well-established alveolar macrophage assay. The activity of lactate dehydrogenase (LDH) and glucuronidase (GLU), as well as the concentration of tumour necrosis factor α (TNFα), were determined in the cell culture supernatant. Corundum and quartz DQ12 particles were included as negative and positive particle controls, respectively. Numerical results are shown in Table S3. The subcellular distribution of particles was investigated by transmission electron microscopy (TEM) of cells treated with the lowermost particle concentration of the study (11.25 µg/mL) and matched the particle concentration used above for the quantification experiments.

3.3.1. AEROSIL® 380 F and AEROSIL® OX50

Both AEROSIL®s showed a high biologic activity under FCS-free conditions (Figure 2a,b), indicated by the dose-dependent release of LDH, GLU and TNFα. As for most SAS particles the release of H_2O_2 was low and became significant at the highest doses only. In the presence of 10% FCS, all aforementioned responses were abolished (H_2O_2) or drastically lowered, as indicated by the flattened curves for the release of LDH, GLU and TNFα. The degree of reduction and the shift in the low observed adverse effect concentration (LOAEC) are provided in Table 3.

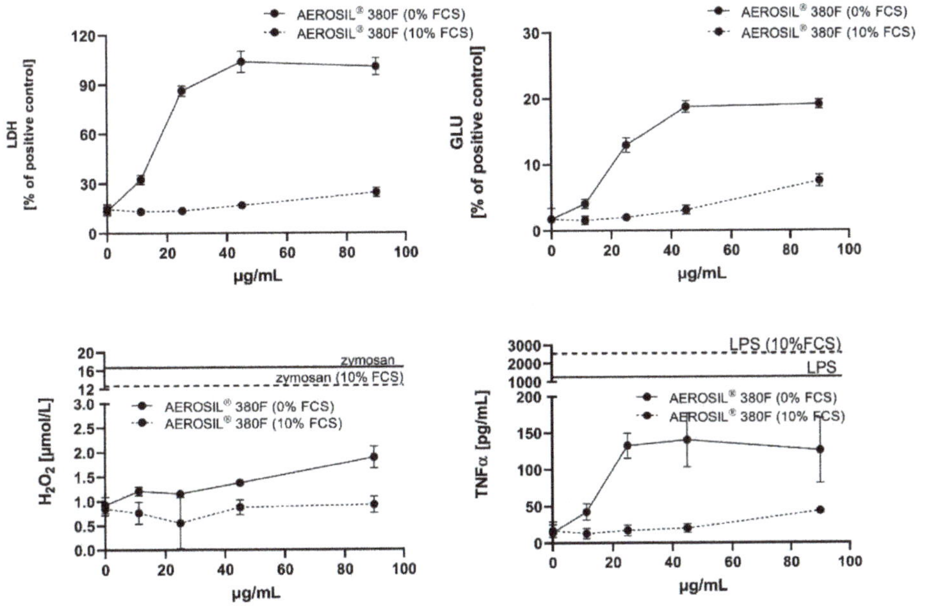

(a)

Figure 2. *Cont.*

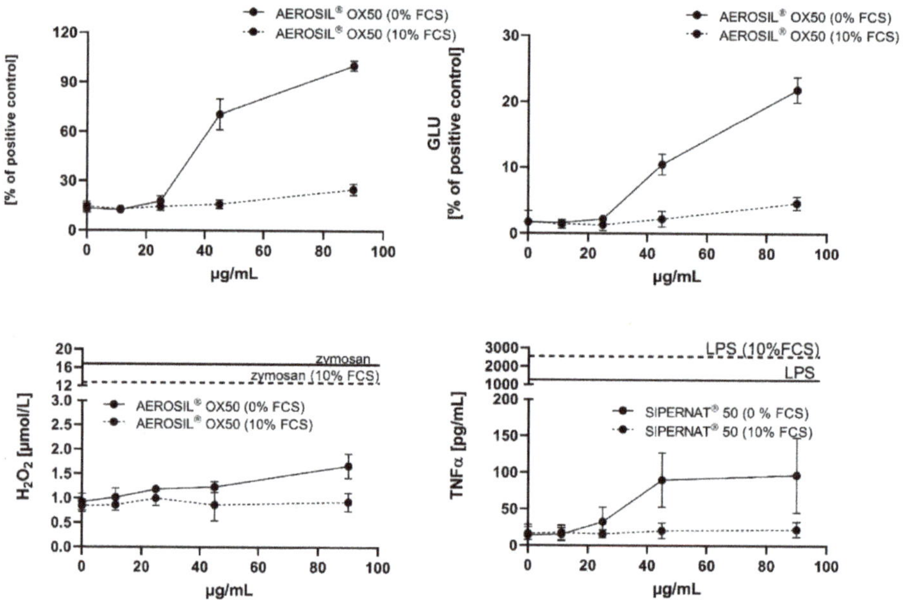

(**b**)

Figure 2. In vitro response of NR8383 alveolar macrophages to AEROSIL® 380 F and to AEROSIL® OX50 in the absence or in the presence of 10% FCS (dashed lines). Lactate dehydrogenase activity (LDH), glucuronidase activity (GLU), H_2O_2 concentration, and tumour necrosis factor alpha (TNFα) were measured in the supernatant from NR8383 cells exposed to AEROSIL® 380 F (**a**) or AEROSIL® OX50 (**b**). Effects of zymosan and lipopolysaccharide (LPS) on the formation of H_2O_2 and TNFα, respectively, are indicated by vertical lines.

The TEM investigation of NR8383 cells laden with AEROSIL® 380 F in the absence of FCS cells is shown in Figure 3a–d. Although minor portions of the material were regularly found at the outer cell membrane (Figure 3b), larger assemblies occurred within phagosomes (Figure 3a,c). Small particle deposits were found in lysosomes (Figure 3d) and autophagosomes, together with condensed cellular material (Figure 3d). Of note, small and often branched aggregates/agglomerates of AEROSIL® 380 F particles occurred in the cytoplasm; neither mitochondria nor the cell nucleus were found to contain particles. In the *presence of FCS*, particles (aggregates/agglomerates) of AEROSIL® 380 F were not found at the outer cell membrane or within the cytoplasm. Additionally, heavily laden phagosomes were not found. Instead, cells contained large phagosomes filled with fine granular material of low-to-medium electron density (Figure 4a). Particles were mainly found in lysosomes (Figure 4b).

AEROSIL® OX50 was found as single particles or small groups thereof within endosomes, most likely presenting lysosomes, and phagosomes (Figure 5a–c). Although the presence of FCS did not lead to a major change of this pattern, smaller aggregates appeared to be more frequent (Figure 6a–c). Typical uptake-figures (Figure 6b) showed single particles close to a membrane invagination, suggesting that particles enter into cells via small endosomes. The material was also found in autophagosomes.

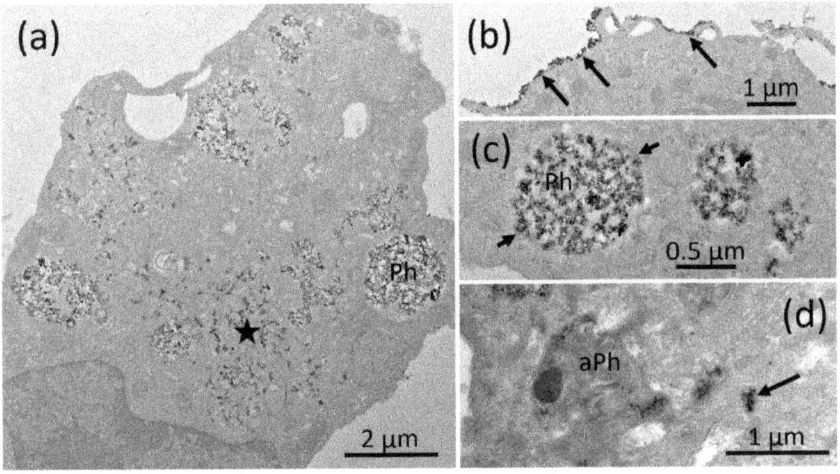

Figure 3. Electron microscopy of NR8383 cells laden with AEROSIL® 380 F (11.25 μg/mL) in the absence of FCS for 16 h. (**a**) Overview of a cell containing particle filled phagosomes (Ph) and branched particle assemblies in distinct regions of the cytoplasm (asterisk). The cytoplasm of this cell appears condensed. (**b**) Particles adhering to a section of the outer cell membrane (arrows). (**c**) Particle filled phagosomes; arrows point to the enclosing membrane. (**d**) An autophagosome (aPh) filled with condensed matter together with several electron dense lysosomes (arrow); both compartments contain small amounts of the typical, small electron dense AEROSIL® 380 F particles.

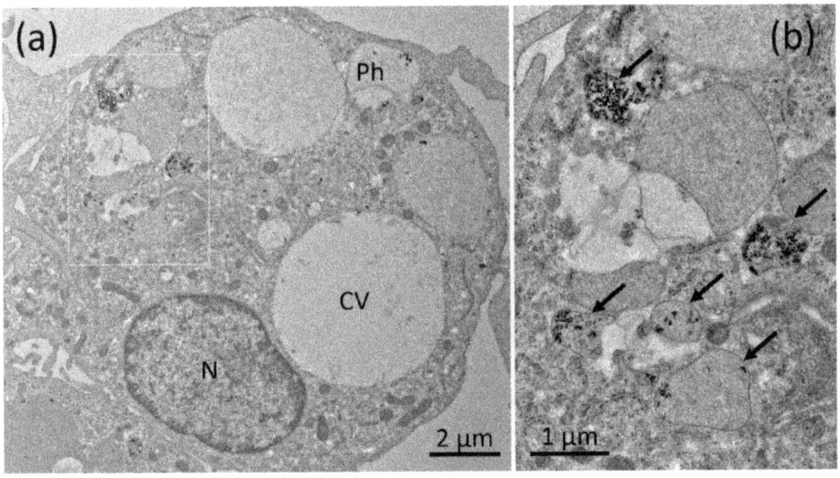

Figure 4. Electron microscopy of NR8383 cells laden with AEROSIL® 380 F (11.25 μg/mL) in the presence of FCS for 16 h. (**a**) Aspect from a cell with typical phagosomes (Ph) mainly filled with fine granular material, particle laden lysosomes and a clear vacuole (CV). (**b**) Boxed area from (**a**) showing several particle-laden lysosomes (arrows).

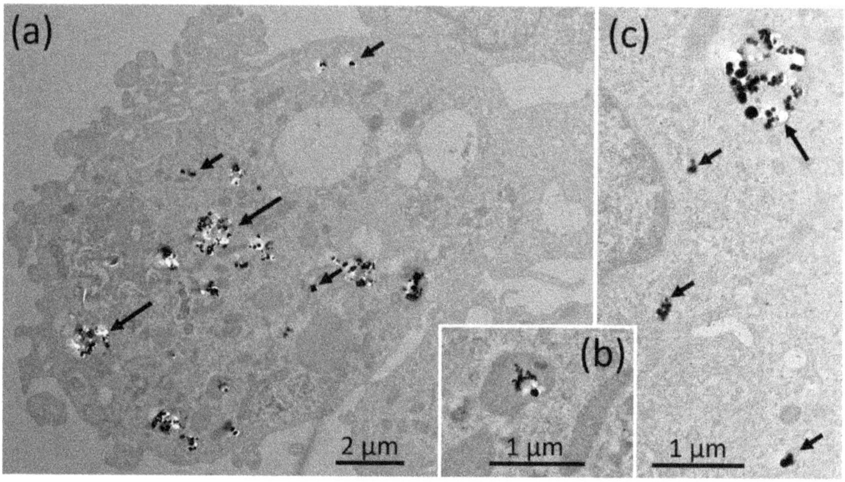

Figure 5. Electron microscopy of NR8383 cells laden with AEROSIL® OX50 F in the absence of FCS for 16 h. Electron lucent areas close to particles are interpreted as cutting artefacts. (**a**) Overview of a cells with particle-containing phagosomes (large arrows) and smaller endosomes (small arrows). (**b**) shows a typical particle-laden; (**c**) shows a higher magnification of a phagosome (large arrow) and three small endosomes (small arrows) and arrows point to membrane continuities.

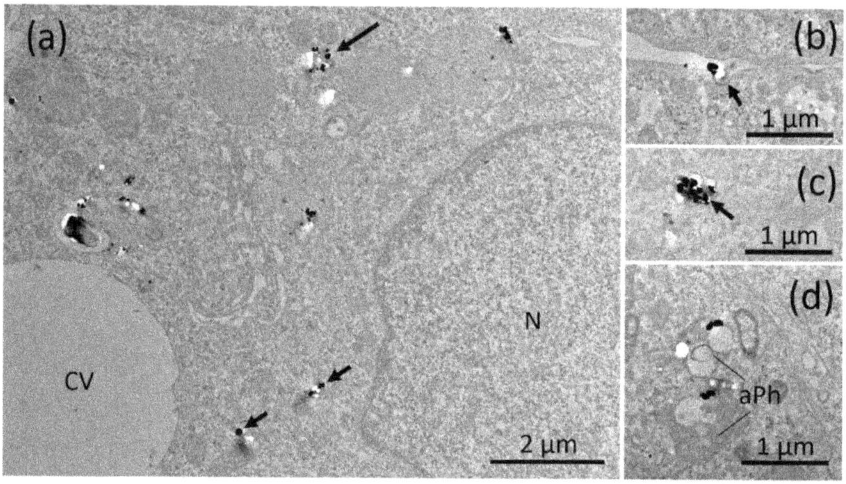

Figure 6. Electron microscopy of NR8383 cells laden with AEROSIL® OX50 F in the presence of FCS for 16 h. Electron lucent areas close to particles are interpreted as cutting artefacts. (**a**) Overview of a cell with particle-containing phagosomes (large arrows) and smaller endosomes (small arrows). (**b**) A membrane invagination (arrow) underneath a particle attached to the cell membrane, interpreted as an early uptake figure. (**c**) A small particle-filled endosome; (**d**) shows two particle-containing autophagosomes (aPh).

3.3.2. SIPERNAT® 50 and SIPERNAT® 160

The biological activity of SIPERNAT® 50 and SIPERNAT® 160 was very similar to that of the AEROSIL®s (Figure 7a,b), though the dose-dependent release of LDH, GLU and TNFα was more pronounced for SIPERNAT® 160. Again, 10% FCS abolished the H_2O_2 response and strongly reduced the cytotoxic effect (LDH, GLU) and also TNFα formation.

There was a strong reduction of bioactivity in the presence of FCS. The shift in LOAEC upon FCS treatment are provided in Table 3.

The electron microscopic examination revealed no major differences with respect to the endosomal compartments crowed by SIPERNAT® 50 or SIPERNAT® 160 particles. Even the fine structure of agglomerates within phagosomes appeared indistinguishable (Figures S1 and S2). With respect to SIPERNAT® 160, endosomes with larger particle assemblies appeared less frequent (Figures S3 and S4).

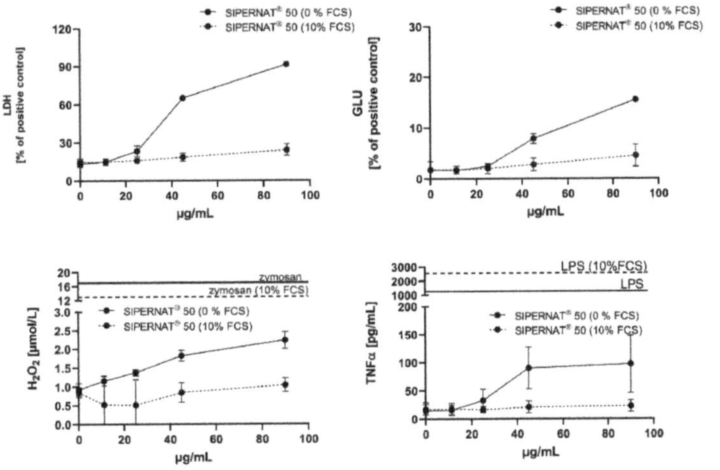

(a)

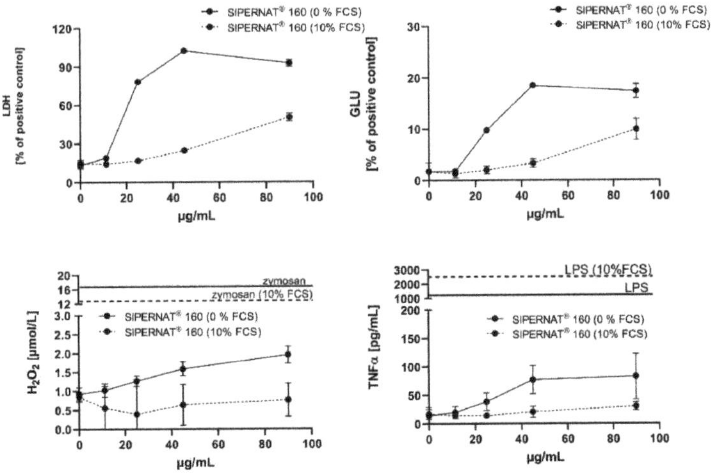

(b)

Figure 7. In vitro response of NR8383 alveolar macrophages to SIPERNAT® 50 and SIPERNAT® 160 in the absence or in the presence of FCS (dashed lines). Lactate dehydrogenase activity (LDH), glucuronidase activity (GLU), H_2O_2 concentration and tumour necrosis factor alpha (TNFα) were measured in the supernatant from NR8383 cells exposed to SIPERNAT® 50 (**a**) or SIPERNAT® 160 (**b**). Effects of zymosan and lipopolysaccharide (LPS) on the formation of H_2O_2 and TNFα, respectively, are indicated by vertical lines.

Table 3. Apparent reduction of the bioactivity of SAS nanoparticles upon addition of FCS.

				Low Observed Adverse Effect Concentration (LOAEC) Shift (µg/mL) [(2)]			
Material	**LDH** [(1)]	**GLU** [(1)]	**TNFα** [(1)]	**LDH**	**GLU**	**H_2O_2**	**TNFα**
AEROSIL® 380F	−92.6%	−81.2%	−87.4%	11.25⟶90	11.25⟶90	90⟶≥90	45⟶≥90
AEROSIL® OX50	−68.9%	−65.9%	−81.2%	45⟶90	45⟶90	90⟶≥90	45⟶≥90
SIPERNAT® 50	−72.3%	−64.1%	−81.9%	22.5⟶90	45⟶90	45⟶≥90	45⟶≥90
SIPERNAT® 160	−79.6%	−71.6%	−79.6%	11.25⟶45	22.5⟶90	90⟶≥90	45⟶≥90

[(1)] Measured at 90 µg/mL by linear interpolation; [(2)] LOAEC with and without FCS as derived from Table S3. LDH: Lactate dehydrogenase, GLU: glucuronidase, TNFα: tumor necrosis factor α.

3.4. Evaluation of Data Using the Cell-Associated SiO_2 Mass as a Dose Metric

Finally, we plotted the release of LDH, GLU and TNFα (Table S1) against the cell-associated particle mass. Except for AEROSIL® 380 F, which partly adhered to the cell surface in the absence of FCS (Figure 3), the cell-associated particle mass in fact reflects fully internalized particles. Because a meaningful determination of SiO_2 uptake relative to administered SAS concentration had to rely on non-compromised cells (i.e., at low cytotoxicity), we background corrected the "% total" values from Table 3 and extrapolated them to the maximum theoretical cell burden at a given concentration step (i.e., 7.5, 15, 30 and 60 pg/cell; see Supplementary Information for calculation).

These uptake-corrected abscissa values were then plotted against the released enzyme activities the absence and presence of FCS (Figure 8). The FCS-mediated reduction in particle uptake is reflected by a shortening of the curves and the lowered slopes seen for the releases of LDH, GLU and TNFα indicate the FCS-mediated reduction of biological activity. The slope reductions (LDH, GLU and TNFα curves) appeared largely uniform for each singly SAS but differed in the order SIPERNAT® 50 > SIPERNAT® 160 = AEROSIL® 380 F. AEROSIL® OX50 was not evaluable due to a strong shortening of the respective curve. Resulting EC50 values were calculated for the FCS-free administration of SAS (Table S4) and will be discussed below. Overall, the curves shown in Figure 8 reveal that the reduced bioactivity of SAS in the presence of FCS is material dependent and due, at least in parts, to cellular processes secondary to particle uptake.

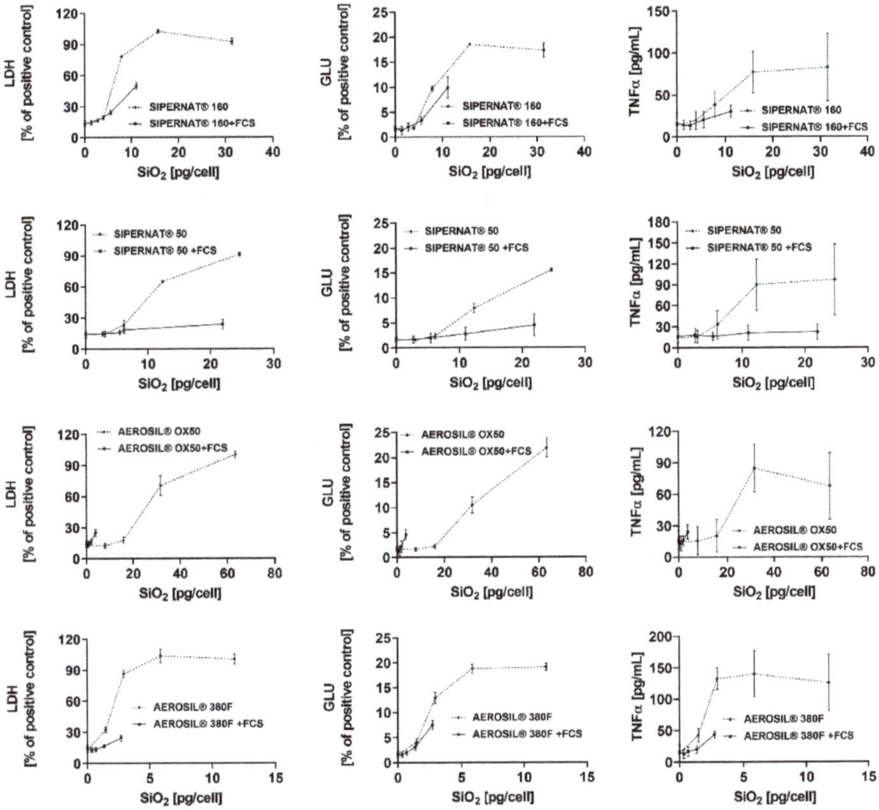

Figure 8. In vitro response of NR8383 alveolar macrophages to the cell-associated masses of SIPERNAT® 160, SIPERNAT® 50, AEROSIL® OX50 and AEROSIL® 380 F in the absence and presence of FCS. Values (from Table S1) for lactate dehydrogenase activity (LDH), glucuronidase activity (GLU), H_2O_2 concentration, and tumour necrosis factor alpha (TNFα) from were plotted against the cell-associated masses of SAS which were measured for a low SAS concentration and then extrapolated to higher values.

4. Discussion

In this investigation, we analysed the effect of FCS on the apparent bioactivity of fumed and precipitated SAS using an established alveolar macrophage model. For the first time, the uptake of SAS by alveolar macrophages was quantified with a high resolution ICP-MS technique. This enabled us to attribute the effect of FCS to both an influence on particle adhesion and subsequent uptake by cells, and an influence on the bioactivity of the cell-associated, i.e., ingested SAS material.

The reduction of particle uptake in the presence of FCS was largest for both AEROSIL®s (69.5 to 83.5%): TEM analyses strongly suggest that the lower content of the AEROSIL®s in cells in the presence of FCS was mainly due to less particles captured within large phagosomes, whereas lysosomes or autophagosomes contained similar loads of particles under both conditions and, therefore, appear to be of minor relevance for the mitigating effect of FCS on the SAS effects. This appears to be different from the changing numbers of autophagosomes and lysosomes observed in alveolar macrophages treated with crystalline silica [40]. The failure to form larger particle-filled phagosomes may by explained, at least in part, by an absence of binding of AEROSIL® 380 F to the cell surface in the presence of FCS. The lack of large particle-filled and afterwards disrupted phagosomes may have also prevented AEROSIL® 380 F particles from entering into the cytoplasm under protein-free conditions, a mode of particle uptake strongly suggested by the patchy distribution pattern of SiO_2 nanoparticles (Figure 3a). The reduced uptake of AEROSIL® 380 F in the presence of FCS is seemingly in contrast to the strongly increased aggregate/agglomerate size (up to several hundred micrometers, see Table S1) and to the large number of precipitates visible with phase contrast optics (Figure 1a,b). We assume, however, that these particulates mainly consist of precipitated proteins which were cleared from the culture bottom most likely via ingestion by the NR8383 cells. Evidence for this assumption comes from numerous large vacuoles filled with low-contrast material possibly representing protein but only few silica particles (Figure 4a). Overall, the presence of FCS led to an enlargement of the AEROSIL® 380 F particles' HD, a reduced uptake into phagosomes, followed by an altered subcellular localization and reduced the biological activity.

The influence of FCS on the uptake of both precipitated SAS was not uniform. While FCS reduced the uptake of SIPERNAT® 160, most likely again by reducing the formation of particle-filled phagosomes, it had nearly no influence on the uptake of SIPERNAT® 50. The lack of ultrastructural changes seen for SIPERNAT® 50 upon FCS treatment was in line with the quantitative ICP-MS measurement. Therefore, the pronounced reduction of biologic activity seen for SIPERNAT® 50 was more directly attributable to a change of biological particle properties. Of note, SIPERNAT® 50 exhibited the smallest primary structures, the largest specific surface area, and also the highest number of reactive silanol groups as reflected by SEAR's number (see Table 1). Reactive silanol groups of SAS are believed to contribute to the bioactivity of crystalline silica [41,42]. A protein corona, which will inevitably form around SAS in the presence of FCS [26,27], may keep biological structures at a distance from reactive structures at the SAS surface and this protective effect, as illustrated by the reduced slopes of LDH, GLU and TNFα release (Figure 8), may be larger for highly reactive SAS.

Interestingly, the reduction of biological activity by FCS found for ingested AEROSIL® OX50 appeared to be solely due to the reduction in particle uptake (Figure 8). Unlike all other SAS nanomaterials, the slope of the shortened curve reflecting the effect of the ingested AEROSIL® OX50 was not reduced, suggesting that FCS had a minor effect on the biologic activity of ingested AEROSIL® OX50. Although a protein corona formation around this material is highly likely, its effect may be relatively small, possibly because AEROSIL® OX50 had the smallest specific surface and the smallest SEAR's number. Of note, the addition of protein to nanoparticles does not change or attenuate their biologic activity in general, as shown, e.g., for CeO_2 [43], TiO_2 or Fe_2O_3 [24]. Therefore, the specific surface reactivity of a given material needs to be taken into account if the effect of protein coating has to be predicted.

It may also be speculated that the primary particle size and/or the specific surface (BET value) correlates to the protective effect of FCS, because the highest reduction in bioactivity (80–90%) was found for AEROSIL® 380 F (see Table 3). However, despite large differences in size and/or BET surface, the mitigating effects of FCS on all other SAS were highly similar (70–80%), arguing against a simple correlation of primary particles size and FCS-mediated reduction of bioactivity. On the other hand, there may be a size and/or surface-dependent influence of FCS on the uptake of SAS, which was more reduced for AEROSIL® 380 F and also for the SIPERNAT® 160 both of which exhibit the largest specific surface of the fumed and precipitated SAS, respectively (see Table 2: Ratio FCS-free/10% FCS). However, this effect may be indirectly caused via an influence of FCS on particle settling.

In a previous test of the four SAS with the macrophage model, we found that the EC50 values for the release of LDH span a comparatively narrow range (from 13.2 µg/mL (AEROSIL® 380 F) to 31.7 µg/mL (SIPERNAT® 50). As shown here, this range becomes larger when the EC50 values are expressed as pg per cell (2.03 pg/cell (AEROSIL® 380 F) to 28 pg/cell (AEROSIL® OX50); see compilation in Table S4). The disparity of the EC50 values based on the cellular dose is likely to be more relevant because it is measured directly and is not deduced from particle agglomeration and settling. However, the knowledge of cell-associated particle burden helps not only to compare different experimental conditions. It is also urgently needed to better compare in vitro and in vivo data with the aim to refine in vitro tests by using adequate cellular doses. At present, in vivo experiments have mostly been evaluated for organ burden of nanoparticles. Values at the single cell level are rare, although some progress has been made, e.g., for silver laden phagocytes in lymph nodes, whose silver content has been estimated to reach up to 140 pg per cell [44].

The question of which type of protein coating in vitro adequately mimics the situation of particles in the lung is still unresolved. While it is beyond dispute that nanoparticles in body fluids such as blood or extracellular fluid carry a protein corona [13,43,45], protein corona formation in the lung parenchyma is more complex. At least in theory, a respirable (SAS) particle will first contact and adsorb biomolecules of the lung surfactant (phospholipids, various surfactant proteins) before it enters into the lung lining fluid with its multitude of different proteins [46–48]. During inhalation exposure, the dose rate is typically low and the binding of surfactant and protein components to inhaled particles may be complete and more or less well-structured. In contrast, the administration of a particle-containing fluid into the lung, i.e., a high dose rate, may locally disturb the lung's surfactant layer and lead to unconventionally coated or even uncoated particles. In the case of colloidal SAS, this leads to a more intense inflammatory reaction of the rat lung during the first days after particle administration compared to inhalation exposure [36]. It is also noteworthy that in the case of an acute lung inflammation upon SAS, the protein concentration of the lung lining fluid will rise [33], which may limit the bioactivity of SAS as observed in vitro.

Based on these considerations and on the findings of this study, the way of in vitro testing being most predictive for the in vivo outcome remains a matter of discussion. Depending on the starting conditions, alveolar macrophages in vivo may engulf uncoated as well as protein-coated particles. However, we suggest that the well-established alveolar macrophage assay with NR8383 cells, which was originally developed and validated as a protein-free approach [32] and, as such, has been successfully incorporated into a tiered grouping strategy for nanomaterials [49], may be expanded for effects of proteins on the in vitro bioactivity of nanomaterials. As shown here for SAS, protein-free and protein-supplemented exposure of cells may differ substantially and the effects of both treatments should be understood as corner points possibly spanning the full range of responses of alveolar macrophages in situ. In any case, the additional inclusion of protein-containing assays needs to be supported by a quantification of nanomaterials' uptake to avoid unwarranted conclusions. To this end, the method introduced here is applied as a reliable tool to quantify SAS nanomaterials at the cell culture level.

Supplementary Materials: The following are available online at https://www.mdpi.com/2079-4991/11/3/628/s1, Figure S1. Electron microscopy of NR8383 cells laden with SIPERNAT® 50 in the absence of FCS for 16 h. Figure S2. Electron microscopy of NR8383 cells laden with SIPERNAT® 50 in the presence of FCS for 16 h. Figure S3. Electron microscopy of NR8383 cells laden with SIPERNAT® 160 in the absence of FCS for 16 h. Figure S4. Electron microscopy of NR8383 cells laden with SIPERNAT® 160 in the presence of FCS for 16 h. Table S1. Hydrodynamic diameter of SAS in H2O and cell culture media. Table S2. Trypan Blue Exclusion Test and cell numbers of SAS-treated cells used for mass spectrometric. Table S3. Numerical values from in vitro tests with the Alveolar Macrophage Model. Table S4. EC50 values for cell-associated SAS causing the release of LDH, GLU and TNFα. Table S5. EC50 values calculated for extrapolated intracellular SAS concentrations.

Author Contributions: M.W., T.B.S., G.-G.L. and N.K. designed the study, A.V. and M.W. conceived and performed the cell experiments and wrote the manuscript. C.V. performed the quantification of SAS. All authors contributed to the final manuscript. All authors have read and agreed to the published version of the manuscript.

Funding: The study was sponsored by Evonik Industries GmbH. M.W. and A.V. received funding from the German Federal Ministry of Education and Research (BMBF), grant number 03XP0213A.

Institutional Review Board Statement: Not applicable.

Informed Consent Statement: Not applicable.

Data Availability Statement: The data presented in this study are available in the article or in the Supplementary Material.

Acknowledgments: The cell culture work of Oliver Gräb is gratefully acknowledged.

Conflicts of Interest: M.W. and A.V. declare no conflict of interest. G.-G.L., T.B.S., C.V., and N.K. are employees of Evonik Industries GmbH, a company which produces and sells amorphous silica products.

References

1. Stark, W.J.; Stoessel, P.R.; Wohlleben, W.; Hafner, A. Industrial Applications of Nanoparticles. *Chem. Soc. Rev.* **2015**, *44*, 5793–5805. [CrossRef]
2. Winkler, H.C.; Suter, M.; Naegeli, H. Critical Review of the Safety Assessment of Nano-Structured Silica Additives in Food. *J. Nanobiotechnol.* **2016**, *14*, 1–9. [CrossRef] [PubMed]
3. Dekkers, S.; Krystek, P.; Peters, R.J.B.; Lankveld, D.P.K.; Bokkers, B.G.H.; van Hoeven-Arentzen, P.H.; Bouwmeester, H.; Oomen, A.G. Presence and Risks of Nanosilica in Food Products. *Nanotoxicology* **2011**, *5*, 393–405. [CrossRef] [PubMed]
4. Retamal Marín, R.; Babick, F.; Lindner, G.-G.; Wiemann, M.; Stintz, M. Effects of Sample Preparation on Particle Size Distributions of Different Types of Silica in Suspensions. *Nanomaterials* **2018**, *8*, 454. [CrossRef] [PubMed]
5. *Bio-Nanotechnology: A Revolution in Food, Biomedical, and Health Sciences*; Bagchi, D. (Ed.) Functional Food Science and Technology series; Wiley-Blackwell: Chichester, UK; Ames, IA, USA, 2013; ISBN 978-0-470-67037-8.
6. Lorenz, C.; Von Goetz, N.; Scheringer, M.; Wormuth, M.; Hungerbühler, K. Potential Exposure of German Consumers to Engineered Nanoparticles in Cosmetics and Personal Care Products. *Nanotoxicology* **2011**, *5*, 12–29. [CrossRef] [PubMed]
7. Napierska, D.; Thomassen, L.C.; Lison, D.; Martens, J.A.; Hoet, P.H. The Nanosilica Hazard: Another Variable Entity. *Part. Fibre Toxicol.* **2010**, *7*, 39. [CrossRef] [PubMed]
8. Brinker, C.J.; Scherer, G.W. *Sol.-Gel Science: The Physics and Chemistry of Sol.-Gel Processing*; Academic Press: Boston, MA, USA, 1990; ISBN 978-0-12-134970-7.
9. Taeger, D.; McCunney, R.; Bailer, U.; Barthel, K.; Küpper, U.; Brüning, T.; Morfeld, P.; Merget, R. Cross-Sectional Study on Nonmalignant Respiratory Morbidity Due to Exposure to Synthetic Amorphous Silica. *J. Occup. Environ. Med.* **2016**, *58*, 376–384. [CrossRef]
10. Arts, J.H.E.; Muijser, H.; Duistermaat, E.; Junker, K.; Kuper, C.F. Five-Day Inhalation Toxicity Study of Three Types of Synthetic Amorphous Silicas in Wistar Rats and Post-Exposure Evaluations for up to 3 Months. *Food Chem. Toxicol.* **2007**, *45*, 1856–1867. [CrossRef] [PubMed]
11. Murugadoss, S.; Lison, D.; Godderis, L.; Van Den Brule, S.; Mast, J.; Brassinne, F.; Sebaihi, N.; Hoet, P.H. Toxicology of Silica Nanoparticles: An Update. *Arch. Toxicol.* **2017**, *91*, 2967–3010. [CrossRef] [PubMed]
12. Johnston, C.J.; Driscoll, K.E.; Finkelstein, J.N.; Baggs, R.; O'Reilly, M.A.; Carter, J.; Gelein, R.; Oberdörster, G. Pulmonary Chemokine and Mutagenic Responses in Rats after Subchronic Inhalation of Amorphous and Crystalline Silica. *Toxicol. Sci.* **2000**, *56*, 405–413. [CrossRef]
13. Nel, A.E.; Mädler, L.; Velegol, D.; Xia, T.; Hoek, E.M.V.; Somasundaran, P.; Klaessig, F.; Castranova, V.; Thompson, M. Understanding Biophysicochemical Interactions at the Nano-Bio Interface. *Nat. Mater.* **2009**, *8*, 543–557. [CrossRef]
14. Rushton, E.K.; Jiang, J.; Leonard, S.S.; Eberly, S.; Castranova, V.; Biswas, P.; Elder, A.; Han, X.; Gelein, R.; Finkelstein, J.; et al. Concept of Assessing Nanoparticle Hazards Considering Nanoparticle Dosemetric and Chemical/Biological Response Metrics. *J. Toxicol. Environ. Health Part. A* **2010**, *73*, 445–461. [CrossRef] [PubMed]
15. Cho, W.-S.; Duffin, R.; Bradley, M.; Megson, I.L.; MacNee, W.; Lee, J.K.; Jeong, J.; Donaldson, K. Predictive Value of in Vitro Assays Depends on the Mechanism of Toxicity of Metal Oxide Nanoparticles. *Part. Fibre Toxicol.* **2013**, *10*, 55. [CrossRef] [PubMed]
16. Han, X.; Corson, N.; Wade-Mercer, P.; Gelein, R.; Jiang, J.; Sahu, M.; Biswas, P.; Finkelstein, J.N.; Elder, A.; Oberdörster, G. Assessing the Relevance of in Vitro Studies in Nanotoxicology by Examining Correlations between in Vitro and in Vivo Data. *Toxicology* **2012**, *297*, 1–9. [CrossRef] [PubMed]
17. Driscoll, K.E.; Higgins, J.M.; Leytart, M.J.; Crosby, L.L. Differential Effects of Mineral Dusts on the in Vitro Activation of Alveolar Macrophage Eicosanoid and Cytokine Release. *Toxicol. Vitro* **1990**, *4*, 284–288. [CrossRef]
18. Wiemann, M.; Vennemann, A.; Stintz, M.; Retamal Marín, R.R.; Babick, F.; Lindner, G.-G.; Schuster, T.B.; Brinkmann, U.; Krueger, N. Effects of Ultrasonic Dispersion Energy on the Preparation of Amorphous SiO_2 Nanomaterials for In Vitro Toxicity Testing. *Nanomaterials* **2018**, *9*, 11. [CrossRef] [PubMed]
19. Vennemann, A.; Alessandrini, F.; Wiemann, M. Differential Effects of Surface-Functionalized Zirconium Oxide Nanoparticles on Alveolar Macrophages, Rat Lung, and a Mouse Allergy Model. *Nanomaterials* **2017**, *7*, 280. [CrossRef]
20. Bianchi, M.G.; Chiu, M.; Taurino, G.; Ruotolo, R.; Marmiroli, N.; Bergamaschi, E.; Cubadda, F.; Bussolati, O. Pyrogenic and Precipitated Amorphous Silica Nanoparticles Differentially Affect Cell Responses to LPS in Human Macrophages. *Nanomaterials* **2020**, *10*, 1395. [CrossRef] [PubMed]

21. Leibe, R.; Hsiao, I.-L.; Fritsch-Decker, S.; Kielmeier, U.; Wagbo, A.M.; Voss, B.; Schmidt, A.; Hessman, S.D.; Duschl, A.; Oostingh, G.J.; et al. The Protein Corona Suppresses the Cytotoxic and Pro-Inflammatory Response in Lung Epithelial Cells and Macrophages upon Exposure to Nanosilica. *Arch. Toxicol.* **2019**, *93*, 871–885. [CrossRef] [PubMed]
22. Peuschel, H.; Ruckelshausen, T.; Cavelius, C.; Kraegeloh, A. Quantification of Internalized Silica Nanoparticles via STED Microscopy. *BioMed Res. Int.* **2015**, *2015*, 1–16. [CrossRef]
23. Al-Rawi, M.; Diabaté, S.; Weiss, C. Uptake and Intracellular Localization of Submicron and Nano-Sized SiO2 Particles in HeLa Cells. *Arch. Toxicol.* **2011**, *85*, 813–826. [CrossRef]
24. Panas, A.; Marquardt, C.; Nalcaci, O.; Bockhorn, H.; Baumann, W.; Paur, H.-R.; Mülhopt, S.; Diabaté, S.; Weiss, C. Screening of Different Metal Oxide Nanoparticles Reveals Selective Toxicity and Inflammatory Potential of Silica Nanoparticles in Lung Epithelial Cells and Macrophages. *Nanotoxicology* **2013**, *7*, 259–273. [CrossRef] [PubMed]
25. Marucco, A.; Aldieri, E.; Leinardi, R.; Bergamaschi, E.; Riganti, C.; Fenoglio, I. Applicability and Limitations in the Characterization of Poly-Dispersed Engineered Nanomaterials in Cell Media by Dynamic Light Scattering (DLS). *Materials* **2019**, *12*, 3833. [CrossRef] [PubMed]
26. Monopoli, M.P.; Aberg, C.; Salvati, A.; Dawson, K.A. Biomolecular Coronas Provide the Biological Identity of Nanosized Materials. *Nat. Nanotechnol.* **2012**, *7*, 779–786. [CrossRef] [PubMed]
27. Docter, D.; Westmeier, D.; Markiewicz, M.; Stolte, S.; Knauer, S.K.; Stauber, R.H. The Nanoparticle Biomolecule Corona: Lessons Learned—Challenge Accepted? *Chem. Soc. Rev.* **2015**, *44*, 6094–6121. [CrossRef] [PubMed]
28. Halamoda-Kenzaoui, B.; Ceridono, M.; Colpo, P.; Valsesia, A.; Urbán, P.; Ojea-Jiménez, I.; Gioria, S.; Gilliland, D.; Rossi, F.; Kinsner-Ovaskainen, A. Dispersion Behaviour of Silica Nanoparticles in Biological Media and Its Influence on Cellular Uptake. *PLoS ONE* **2015**, *10*, e0141593. [CrossRef] [PubMed]
29. Hinderliter, P.M.; Minard, K.R.; Orr, G.; Chrisler, W.B.; Thrall, B.D.; Pounds, J.G.; Teeguarden, J.G. ISDD: A Computational Model of Particle Sedimentation, Diffusion and Target Cell Dosimetry for in Vitro Toxicity Studies. *Part. Fibre Toxicol.* **2010**, *7*, 36. [CrossRef] [PubMed]
30. Binnemars-Postma, K.A.; ten Hoopen, H.W.; Storm, G.; Prakash, J. Differential Uptake of Nanoparticles by Human M1 and M2 Polarized Macrophages: Protein Corona as a Critical Determinant. *Nanomedicine* **2016**, *11*, 2889–2902. [CrossRef]
31. Orr, G.A.; Chrisler, W.B.; Cassens, K.J.; Tan, R.; Tarasevich, B.J.; Markillie, L.M.; Zangar, R.C.; Thrall, B.D. Cellular Recognition and Trafficking of Amorphous Silica Nanoparticles by Macrophage Scavenger Receptor A. *Nanotoxicology* **2011**, *5*, 296–311. [CrossRef] [PubMed]
32. Wiemann, M.; Vennemann, A.; Sauer, U.G.; Wiench, K.; Ma-Hock, L.; Landsiedel, R. An in Vitro Alveolar Macrophage Assay for Predicting the Short-Term Inhalation Toxicity of Nanomaterials. *J. Nanobiotechnol* **2016**, *14*, 16. [CrossRef] [PubMed]
33. Großgarten, M.; Holzlechner, M.; Vennemann, A.; Balbekova, A.; Wieland, K.; Sperling, M.; Lendl, B.; Marchetti-Deschmann, M.; Karst, U.; Wiemann, M. Phosphonate Coating of SiO2 Nanoparticles Abrogates Inflammatory Effects and Local Changes of the Lipid Composition in the Rat Lung: A Complementary Bioimaging Study. *Part. Fibre Toxicol.* **2018**, *15*, 31. [CrossRef] [PubMed]
34. Van Landuyt, K.L.; Cokic, S.M.; Asbach, C.; Hoet, P.; Godderis, L.; Reichl, F.X.; Van Meerbeek, B.; Vennemann, A.; Wiemann, M. Interaction of Rat Alveolar Macrophages with Dental Composite Dust. *Part. Fibre Toxicol.* **2016**, *13*, 62. [CrossRef] [PubMed]
35. Wiemann, M.; Vennemann, A.; Wohlleben, W. Lung Toxicity Analysis of Nano-Sized Kaolin and Bentonite: Missing Indications for a Common Grouping. *Nanomaterials* **2020**, *10*, 204. [CrossRef] [PubMed]
36. Wiemann, M.; Sauer, U.G.; Vennemann, A.; Bäcker, S.; Keller, J.-G.; Ma-Hock, L.; Wohlleben, W.; Landsiedel, R. In Vitro and In Vivo Short-Term Pulmonary Toxicity of Differently Sized Colloidal Amorphous SiO_2. *Nanomaterials* **2018**, *8*. [CrossRef] [PubMed]
37. Thomas, D.G.; Smith, J.N.; Thrall, B.D.; Baer, D.R.; Jolley, H.; Munusamy, P.; Kodali, V.; Demokritou, P.; Cohen, J.; Teeguarden, J.G. ISD3: A Particokinetic Model for Predicting the Combined Effects of Particle Sedimentation, Diffusion and Dissolution on Cellular Dosimetry for in Vitro Systems. *Part. Fibre Toxicol.* **2018**, *15*, 6. [CrossRef]
38. Aureli, F.; Ciprotti, M.; D'Amato, M.; do Nascimento da Silva, E.; Nisi, S.; Passeri, D.; Sorbo, A.; Raggi, A.; Rossi, M.; Cubadda, F. Determination of Total Silicon and SiO2 Particles Using an ICP-MS Based Analytical Platform for Toxicokinetic Studies of Synthetic Amorphous Silica. *Nanomaterials* **2020**, *10*, 888. [CrossRef] [PubMed]
39. Bossert, D.; Urban, D.A.; Maceroni, M.; Ackermann-Hirschi, L.; Haeni, L.; Yajan, P.; Spuch-Calvar, M.; Rothen-Rutishauser, B.; Rodriguez-Lorenzo, L.; Petri-Fink, A.; et al. A Hydrofluoric Acid-Free Method to Dissolve and Quantify Silica Nanoparticles in Aqueous and Solid Matrices. *Sci. Rep.* **2019**, *9*, 7938. [CrossRef] [PubMed]
40. Tan, S.; Chen, S. Macrophage Autophagy and Silicosis: Current Perspective and Latest Insights. *IJMS* **2021**, *22*, 453. [CrossRef] [PubMed]
41. Turci, F.; Pavan, C.; Leinardi, R.; Tomatis, M.; Pastero, L.; Garry, D.; Anguissola, S.; Lison, D.; Fubini, B. Revisiting the Paradigm of Silica Pathogenicity with Synthetic Quartz Crystals: The Role of Crystallinity and Surface Disorder. *Part. Fibre Toxicol.* **2015**, *13*, 1–12. [CrossRef] [PubMed]
42. Fubini, B.; Zanetti, G.; Altilia, S.; Tiozzo, R.; Lison, D.; Saffiotti, U. Relationship between Surface Properties and Cellular Responses to Crystalline Silica: Studies with Heat-Treated Cristobalite. *Chem. Res. Toxicol.* **1999**, *12*, 737–745. [CrossRef]
43. Yokel, R.A.; Hancock, M.L.; Cherian, B.; Brooks, A.J.; Ensor, M.L.; Vekaria, H.J.; Sullivan, P.G.; Grulke, E.A. Simulated Biological Fluid Exposure Changes Nanoceria's Surface Properties but Not Its Biological Response. *Eur. J. Pharm. Biopharm.* **2019**, *144*, 252–265. [CrossRef] [PubMed]

44. Wiemann, M.; Vennemann, A.; Blaske, F.; Sperling, M.; Karst, U. Silver Nanoparticles in the Lung: Toxic Effects and Focal Accumulation of Silver in Remote Organs. *Nanomaterials* **2017**, *7*, 441. [CrossRef] [PubMed]
45. Mathé, C.; Devineau, S.; Aude, J.-C.; Lagniel, G.; Chédin, S.; Legros, V.; Mathon, M.-H.; Renault, J.-P.; Pin, S.; Boulard, Y.; et al. Structural Determinants for Protein Adsorption/Non-Adsorption to Silica Surface. *PLoS ONE* **2013**, *8*, e81346. [CrossRef]
46. Wattiez, R.; Hermans, C.; Bernard, A.; Lesur, O.; Falmagne, P. Human Bronchoalveolar Lavage Fluid: Two-Dimensional Gel Electrophoresis, Amino Acid Microsequencing and Identification of Major Proteins. *Electrophoresis* **1999**, *20*, 1634–1645. [CrossRef]
47. Noël-Georis, I.; Bernard, A.; Falmagne, P.; Wattiez, R. Database of Bronchoalveolar Lavage Fluid Proteins. *J. Chromatogr. B* **2002**, *771*, 221–236. [CrossRef]
48. Geiser, M.; Kreyling, W.G. Deposition and Biokinetics of Inhaled Nanoparticles. *Part. Fibre Toxicol.* **2010**, *7*, 2. [CrossRef] [PubMed]
49. Wohlleben, W.; Hellack, B.; Nickel, C.; Herrchen, M.; Hund-Rinke, K.; Kettler, K.; Riebeling, C.; Haase, A.; Funk, B.; Kühnel, D.; et al. The NanoGRAVUR Framework to Group (Nano)Materials for Their Occupational, Consumer, Environmental Risks Based on a Harmonized Set of Material Properties, Applied to 34 Case Studies. *Nanoscale* **2019**, *11*, 17637–17654. [CrossRef]

nanomaterials

MDPI

Article

Scavenger Receptor A1 Mediates the Uptake of Carboxylated and Pristine Multi-Walled Carbon Nanotubes Coated with Bovine Serum Albumin

Mai T. Huynh [1], Carole Mikoryak [2], Paul Pantano [1] and Rockford Draper [1,2,*]

[1] Department of Chemistry and Biochemistry, The University of Texas at Dallas, 800 West Campbell Road, Richardson, TX 75080-3021, USA; Mai.t.Huynh@utdallas.edu (M.T.H.); pantano@utdallas.edu (P.P.)
[2] Department of Biological Sciences, The University of Texas at Dallas, 800 West Campbell Road, Richardson, TX 75080-3021, USA; mikoryak@utdallas.edu
* Correspondence: draper@utdallas.edu; Tel.: +1-972-883-2512

Abstract: Previously, we noted that carboxylated multi-walled carbon nanotubes (cMWNTs) coated with Pluronic® F-108 (PF108) bound to and were accumulated by macrophages, but that pristine multi-walled carbon nanotubes (pMWNTs) coated with PF108 were not (Wang et al., *Nanotoxicology* **2018**, *12*, 677). Subsequent studies with Chinese hamster ovary (CHO) cells that overexpressed scavenger receptor A1 (SR-A1) and with macrophages derived from mice knocked out for SR-A1 provided evidence that SR-A1 was a receptor of PF108-cMWNTs (Wang et al., *Nanomaterials* (Basel) **2020**, *10*, 2417). Herein, we replaced the PF108 coat with bovine serum albumin (BSA) to investigate how a BSA corona affected the interaction of multi-walled carbon nanotubes (MWNTs) with cells. Both BSA-coated cMWNTs and pMWNTs bound to and were accumulated by RAW 264.7 macrophages, although the cells bound two times more BSA-coated cMWNT than pMWNTs. RAW 264.7 cells that were deleted for SR-A1 using CRISPR-Cas9 technology had markedly reduced binding and accumulation of both BSA-coated cMWNTs and pMWNTs, suggesting that SR-A1 was responsible for the uptake of both MWNT types. Moreover, CHO cells that ectopically expressed SR-A1 accumulated both MWNT types, whereas wild-type CHO cells did not. One model to explain these results is that SR-A1 can interact with two structural features of BSA-coated cMWNTs, one inherent to the oxidized nanotubes (such as COOH and other oxidized groups) and the other provided by the BSA corona; whereas SR-A1 only interacts with the BSA corona of BSA-pMWNTs.

Keywords: carbon nanotube; macrophages; scavenger receptor; phagocytosis; protein corona; bovine serum albumin

Citation: Huynh, M.T.; Mikoryak, C.; Pantano, P.; Draper, R. Scavenger Receptor A1 Mediates the Uptake of Carboxylated and Pristine Multi-Walled Carbon Nanotubes Coated with Bovine Serum Albumin. *Nanomaterials* **2021**, *11*, 539. https://doi.org/10.3390/nano11020539

Academic Editor: Olesja Bondarenko

Received: 30 January 2021
Accepted: 15 February 2021
Published: 20 February 2021

1. Introduction

The interaction of engineered nanoparticles (ENPs) with cells is influenced by a corona of macromolecules that deposit on the ENP surface from the surrounding biological fluid. What macromolecules (often proteins) adhere to the ENP depends on the properties of the macromolecules and on the ENP surface structure, charge, hydrophobicity, and geometry [1–4]. Corona components may provide dominant features controlling the interaction of ENPs with specific cell surface binding sites, often followed by ENP internalization and a subsequent response by the cells. Understanding what corona components are present on an ENP and how they interface with cells is thus important to provide rational approaches for promoting positive responses, such as targeted drug delivery, or mitigating negative responses, such as toxicity. However, understanding ENP coronas is challenging because the potential corona components in complex biological environments are diverse and the properties of ENP surfaces vary widely. Single-walled carbon nanotubes (SWNTs) and multi-walled carbon nanotubes (MWNTs) are ENPs whose production is increasing due to a wide variety of commercial applications [5–8]. Nevertheless, there is ample evidence that carbon nanotubes can be toxic to organisms and the environment, but how their coronas contribute to toxicity is not well understood [9–11].

We previously noted that carboxylated MWNTs (cMWNTs) coated with Pluronic® F-108 (PF108) preferentially bind to and are accumulated by cells, whereas PF108-coated pristine MWNTs (pMWNTs) do not bind and are poorly accumulated [12]. This suggested that surface receptors on macrophages selectively bind cMWNTs but not pMWNTs. Class A scavenger receptors (SR-As) are membrane glycoproteins that bind polyanionic compounds and modified proteins [13–15], and several observations in the literature implicate SR-As as potential carbon nanotube receptors. For example, there is evidence that SWNTs coated with bovine serum albumin (BSA) are targeted to SR-As [16]. There are also numerous reports where antagonists of class A-type 1 scavenger receptors (SR-A1s) affect cell responses to MWNTs: The accumulation of cMWNTs by RAW 264.7 macrophages correlated with the extent of carboxylation and was inhibited by the SR-A1 antagonist dextran sulfate [17]; the rate of apoptosis induced by MWNTs could be reduced by treating the cells with poly I, another SR-A antagonist [18]; and the accumulation of FITC-BSA-coated MWNTs by THP-1 macrophages was inhibited by the SR-A antagonist fucoidan [19]. In addition, Hirano et al. found that MWNTs suspended in the surfactant Pluronic® F-68 bind to MARCO (SR-A6) receptors on Chinese hamster ovary (CHO) cells overexpressing MARCO [20]. We also observed that dextran sulfate reduced the binding of PF108-coated cMWNTs by macrophages [12].

Recently, we reported that alveolar macrophages derived from SR-A1 knockout mice did not bind or accumulate PF108-cMWNTs whereas they were accumulated by CHO cells that ectopically expressed SR-A1 [21]—strong evidence that SR-A1 is a receptor for PF108-coated cMWNTs. An interesting feature of PF108-coated cMWNTs is that they bind strongly to cells in the absence of serum or any exogenous protein, suggesting that a protein corona is not required for cMWNT binding to SR-A1 [12]. Thus, some inherent structural feature of oxidized MWNTs, perhaps carboxyl groups, carbonyl groups, or hydroxyl groups, appear sufficient for interaction with SR-A1.

Herein, we replaced the PF108 coat with BSA and studied the interaction of cMWNTs and pMWNTs bearing a BSA corona with CHO cells that ectopically express SR-A1 and with RAW 264.7 cells that were deleted for SR-A1 using CRISPR-Cas9 technology. CHO cells expressing SR-A1, but not wild-type (WT) CHO cells, accumulated both BSA-coated cMWNTs and pMWNTs, but the amount of cMWNTs accumulated was 2–3 times more than pMWNTs. WT RAW 264.7 cells also accumulated approximately 2 times more BSA-coated cMWNTs than pMWNTs. Moreover, in binding studies with RAW 264.7 cells at 4 °C in the absence of serum, more BSA-cMWNTs than BSA-pMWNTs were bound. These data suggest that there are more binding sites on the RAW 264.7 cell surface for BSA-cMWNTs than BSA-pMWNTs. To assess what effect the absence of SR-A1 would have, the binding and accumulation of BSA-coated cMWNTs and pMWNTs to SR-A1 knockout RAW 264.7 cells at 4 °C in medium without serum and at 37 °C was measured. The amount of bound or accumulated BSA-MWNTs in the knockout SR-A1 cells was significantly decreased for both BSA-pMWNTs and BSA-cMWNTs compared to the WT RAW 264.7 cells. These observations suggest that pMWNTs coated with a BSA protein corona gain the capacity to bind SR-A1. Overall, BSA-cMWNTs have enhanced binding to SR-A1 above that observed with BSA-pMWNTs, emphasizing the differences between how BSA-coated cMWNTs and pMWNTs interact with receptors. Models to account for the differences are presented.

2. Materials and Methods

2.1. Nanomaterials

The pMWNT (product 1236-YJS, lot 2015-041709) and cMWNT (product 1256-YJF, lot 2015-070510) powders were purchased from Nanostructured & Amorphous Materials, Inc. (Houston, TX). pMWNTs and cMWNTs were synthesized using a Fe/Co/Ni-catalyzed chemical vapor deposition process. Caution should be taken, and a fine particulate respirator and other appropriate personal protective equipment should be worn when handling dry MWNT powders. Both MWNT products were reported by the manufacturer to be >95% in purity and to contain MWNTs with outer diameters of 10–20 nm, inner diameters of 5–10 nm, and lengths of 0.5–2 µm. The cMWNT powder was oxidized using sulfuric acid and potassium permanganate and comprised 1.9–2.1% by weight carboxylic acid groups. Elemental analyses of MWNTs were performed using a previously described combustion analysis technique [22]. The combined carbon, hydrogen, nitrogen, sulfur, and oxygen elemental analyses of the pMWNTs and cMWNTs were 99.52% and 98.18%, respectively, indicative of MWNT powders that are essentially metal-free. An extensive physical and chemical characterization of the pMWNTs and cMWNTs powders appears elsewhere [23]. The major similarities of the pMWNTs and cMWNTs were their outer diameters (18 ± 3 nm and 19 ± 5 nm, respectively) and inner diameters (5.6 ± 1.3 and 5.7 ± 1.7 nm, respectively), as determined using transmission electron microscopy. The key difference was the presence of a carbonyl vibrational stretching mode associated with carboxyl groups in the infrared spectra of cMWNTs that was not observed in the pMWNT spectra.

2.2. Chemicals and Solutions

Dulbecco's modified Eagle medium (DMEM) and Ham's F-12K complete medium were purchased from Gibco (Grand Island, NY, USA), fetal bovine serum (FBS) from Atlanta Biologicals (Flowery Branch, GA, USA), Geneticin® selective antibiotic G418 sulfate from Calbiochem (San Diego, CA, USA), and Accumax™ from Innovative Cell Technologies (San Diego, CA, USA). SR-AI/MSR Alexa Fluor® 488-conjugated antibody and rat IgG2B Alexa Fluor® 488-conjugated Isotype Control were purchased from R&D Systems (Minneapolis, MN, USA). Bovine serum albumin (BSA), dextran sulfate (product # D6001), chondroitin sulfate (product # C9819), penicillin (10,000 U/mL), streptomycin (10 mg/mL), and all other chemicals were purchased from Millipore Sigma (Burlington, MA, USA). All chemicals were used as received. Deionized water (18.3 MΩ·cm) was obtained using a Milli-Q® Integral water purification system (Billerica, MA, USA). Phosphate buffered saline (PBS; 0.8 mM phosphate, 150 mM NaCl, pH 7.4) was sterilized by autoclaving at 121 °C for 45 min. Stock solutions of 100 mg/mL BSA were prepared by dissolving 10 g of BSA in 100 mL of deionized water and adjusting the pH to 7.4. Working solutions of 0.10 mg/mL BSA were prepared by diluting stock BSA solutions with aqueous 10 mM HEPES (pH 7.4) and filtering the solutions through a 0.22-µm pore membrane; stock and working solutions of BSA were stored at 4 °C in the dark.

2.3. Cell lines and Cell Culture

Abelson murine leukemia virus transformed RAW 264.7 macrophages were purchased from the American Type Culture Collection (ATCC® TIB-71™; Manassas, VA, USA). A scavenger receptor A1 (SR-A1) knockout RAW 264.7 cell pool was purchased from Synthego Corporation (Silicon Valley, CA, USA). The cell pool was generated using CRISPR-Cas9 technologies with the guide RNA sequence CAGCAUCCUCUCGUUCAUGA. Synthego validated, via genome sequencing, that 70% of the SR-A1 knockout pool of RAW 264.7 cells had insertion(s) or deletion(s) between base pairs 41 and 42 of the SR-A1 gene. Because the site of alteration is at the beginning of the gene, expression of SR-A1.1, which is a splice variant of SR-A1, would also be affected. A dilution scheme was used to clone cells that did not express SR-A1 receptors on their surface. Serial dilutions of the SR-A1 knockout RAW 264.7 cell pool were plated in 96-well plates and incubated for 7 days. Cells that had arisen from a single colony were grown for several passages before selecting clones that lacked surface SR-A1 expression using immunofluorescence microscopy and flow cytometry. All RAW 264.7 cells and SR-A1 knockout RAW 264.7 cells were grown in DMEM supplemented with 1.5 mg/mL sodium bicarbonate, 10 mM HEPES (pH 7.4), and 10% (*v/v*) FBS.

Chinese hamster ovary (CHO) cells stably transfected with mouse SR-A1 cDNA (CHO[mSR-AI] cells) were generously provided by Professor Monty Krieger (Massachusetts Institute of Technology) [24]. The control WT CHO cell line for CHO[mSR-AI] cells were CHO-K1 cells (ATCC® CCL-61™). All CHO cells were grown in Ham's F-12K medium supplemented with 2.0 mg/mL sodium bicarbonate, 10 mM HEPES (pH 7.4), 10% (*v/v*) FBS, 100 units/mL penicillin, and 100 µg/mL streptomycin; the mSR-AI cells were additionally maintained under 0.25 mg/mL G418. The standard incubation conditions for all cell lines were 37 °C in a 5% CO_2 and 95% air environment.

2.4. *Preparation of BSA-MWNT Suspensions*

The sonication and centrifugation protocol described in our previous works [12,25] was used with slight modifications to prepare purified BSA-coated MWNT suspensions, as summarized in Scheme 1. MWNTs were coated with BSA to match the albumin in the FBS used in growth media. A total of 10.0 mg of pMWNT or cMWNT powder was weighed into a pre-cleaned 20-mL glass vial and baked at 200 °C for 2 h to inactivate potential endotoxin contaminants [26]. Next, 10 mL of a 0.10 mg/mL BSA working solution was added to the vial and the mixture was sonicated. Specifically, a single vial was secured in a hanging rack and sonicated for 240 min using an ultrasonic bath sonicator (Elmasonic P30H; Elma Ultrasonic, Singen, Germany) that was operated at 120 W and 37 kHz in a 4 °C cold room. During sonication, the temperature of the bath water was maintained below 18 °C by using a refrigerated water bath circulator (Isotemp 1006S). After sonication, the solution was divided by transferring 1-mL aliquots into ten 1.5-mL centrifuge tubes. One of the 1-mL aliquots of each non-centrifuged BSA-pMWNT or BSA-cMWNT suspension was set aside as the standard suspension, and each standard solution was serially diluted with a 0.10 mg/mL-BSA working solution. The absorbance at 500 nm of the dilutions determined using a BioTek SynergyMx plate reader (Winooski, VT, USA) was used to construct pMWNT or cMWNT calibration curves. The remaining nine aliquots were centrifuged at 20,000 RCF for 5 min at 4 °C using an Eppendorf 5417R centrifuge to remove MWNT bundles and other impurities, as demonstrated in our previous work [27]. The top 900 µL from each supernatant was collected without disturbing the pellet and combined in a sterile vial to afford ~9 mL of a purified BSA-pMWNT or BSA-cMWNT suspension. The concentration of MWNTs in each purified suspension was determined using the measured absorbance at 500 nm and the calibration curves described above. Purified BSA-MWNT suspensions were stored at 4 °C in the dark.

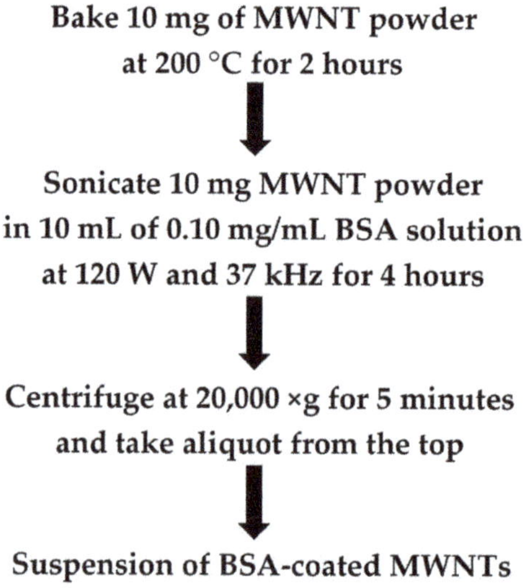
Bake 10 mg of MWNT powder
at 200 °C for 2 hours
Sonicate 10 mg MWNT powder
in 10 mL of 0.10 mg/mL BSA solution
at 120 W and 37 kHz for 4 hours
Centrifuge at 20,000 ×g for 5 minutes
and take aliquot from the top
Suspension of BSA-coated MWNTs

Scheme 1. Preparation of purified BSA-coated MWNT suspensions by sonication and centrifugation.

2.5. Characterization of MWNT Suspensions

The particle size distributions, in terms of hydrodynamic diameter, of BSA-MWNT suspensions were determined by dynamic light scattering (DLS). In brief, aliquots of purified pMWNT or cMWNT suspensions were diluted 1:10 in a 0.10 mg/mL BSA working solution and analyzed using a 633-nm laser and a backscatter measurement angle of 173° (Zetasizer Nano-ZS 3600, Malvern Instruments, Worcestershire, UK). The instrument was calibrated with Polybead® standards (Polysciences, Warrington, PA, USA) and ten consecutive 30-s runs were taken per measurement at 25 °C. The hydrodynamic diameter was calculated using a viscosity and refractive index of 0.8872 cP and 1.330, respectively, for deionized water, and an absorption and refractive index of 0.010 and 1.891, respectively, for MWNTs. Zeta potential values were also determined for purified BSA-coated MWNT suspensions that were diluted 1:10 with deionized water, medium with serum, or serum-free medium. In addition, DLS and zeta potential analyses were performed periodically on purified MWNT suspensions stored at 4 °C to detect any changes. Typically, MWNT suspensions were stable in storage for months, indicated by the lack of aggregates detected by DLS and constant zeta potential results.

2.6. Crystal Violet Cell Proliferation Assay

For the assays with RAW 264.7 cells, purified BSA-MWNT suspensions were first diluted with a freshly prepared 0.10 mg/mL-BSA working solution to a concentration twice the desired MWNT concentration to be tested. The diluted MWNT suspensions were then mixed 1:1 in equal volumes with 2X-concentrated medium that contained 3.0 mg/mL sodium bicarbonate, 20 mM HEPES (pH 7.4), 20% (*v/v*) FBS, 200 units/mL penicillin, and 0.2 mg/mL streptomycin. The result is a test medium with the same concentration of 10 mM HEPES and 10% FBS as the control medium. A total of ~3.5×10^4 RAW 264.7 cells/well were seeded in 48-well plates and incubated at 37 °C overnight before the medium was replaced with freshly prepared control medium or test medium containing MWNTs and incubated for 24 h. At the end of the incubation, cells were washed 3 times with fresh medium, 2 times with PBS, air-dried, and fixed with 4% (*w/v*) paraformaldehyde in PBS. Cell proliferation was determined using a standardized crystal violet assay, as described in our previous work where it was demonstrated that MWNTs do not interfere with the assay [28].

2.7. Quantitation of MWNTs Extracted from Cell Lysates by SDS-PAGE

The SDS-PAGE method with optical detection [29], previously validated by a large-area Raman scan technique [12], was used for quantifying MWNTs extracted from RAW 264.7 cells or CHO cells. In brief, aliquots of known amounts of pMWNT or cMWNT standard suspensions, lysates of control cells, and lysates of cells treated with MWNTs were mixed with 5% 2-mercaptoethanol, 10% glycerol, 62.5 mM Tris-HCl, pH 6.2, and 2X-concentrated SDS sample loading buffer to a final concentration of 2% SDS, and boiled for 3 min. Samples at various dilutions and volumes were subsequently loaded into the wells of an SDS-polyacrylamide gel composed of a 4% stacking gel on top of a 10% resolving gel. An electric current was applied at a constant 100 V for 2 h. MWNTs in standard suspensions and in the lysates bind SDS in the sample loading buffer to become negatively charged and migrate toward the anode upon electrophoresis. The large aspect ratio of MWNTs prevents them from sieving through the pores of a 4% polyacrylamide gel mesh; thus, the MWNTs accumulate at the bottom of the sample loading well during electrophoresis and form a sharp dark band. Following electrophoresis, optical images of the gels were obtained using a flatbed scanner (HP Scanjet G3110, Hewlett Packard Enterprise, Fort Collin, CO, USA), and the pixel intensity of each dark band was quantified using ImageJ software (NIH ImageJ system, Bethesda, MD, USA). The known amount of MWNTs in the standards and their corresponding pixel intensities form a linear calibration curve that was used to determine the unknown amount of MWNTs in cell lysates, based on the pixel intensities of lysate bands loaded in the same gel as the standards.

2.8. Accumulation of MWNTs by Cells at 37 °C

The following procedure was used to detect the accumulation of pMWNTs and cMWNTs by RAW 264.7 or CHO cells at 37 °C for 24 h. MWNT suspensions were first diluted in a freshly prepared 0.10 mg/mL BSA working solution to twice the desired final MWNT concentrations specified in the experiment. The diluted MWNT suspension samples were then mixed 1:1 with the appropriate 2X-concentrated medium. A total of ~3.5×10^5 cells/well were seeded in 6-well plates and incubated in medium at 37 °C overnight to allow the cells to adhere to the plates. The medium was removed the next day and 2 mL of the appropriate freshly prepared control medium that contained no MWNTs or test medium that contained an MWNT suspension at a specified concentration was added to each well. Cells were incubated in a control or test medium at 37 °C for 24 h, as described in each experiment. At the end of the incubation, the control and test media were removed by aspiration and the cells were washed 3 times with fresh medium followed by 2 washes with PBS. Cells were then lifted off the well using 0.5 mL Accumax^{TM}, transferred to a centrifuge tube, and the well was rinsed with 1.5 mL PBS that was subsequently added to the tube to make a final cell suspension of 2 mL/well/tube. Three aliquots of cell suspension, 100 μL each, were used to determine cell counts in each sample using a Beckman Coulter particle counter (Miami, FL, USA) and the cells in the remaining 1.7-mL cell suspension were collected by centrifugation at 1000× *g* for 5 min at 4 °C. The cells in the pellet were lysed in 200 μL of cell lysis buffer that contained 0.25 M Tris-HCl (pH 6.8), 8% (*w/v*) SDS, and 20% (*v/v*) 2-mercaptoethanol. To ensure complete lysis of the cells, the lysate samples were heated in a boiling water bath for 2 h and then stored at 4 °C. The amounts of MWNTs in the cell lysate samples were determined using the SDS-PAGE method, as described previously herein.

2.9. Surface Binding of MWNTs to Cells at 4 °C

To detect and compare the association of pMWNTs and cMWNTs to the surface of RAW 264.7 cells in the absence of endocytic or phagocytic activity, ~5.0×10^5 RAW 264.7 cells/well were first seeded in 6-well plates and incubated in the appropriate medium at 37 °C overnight. Then, the cells were incubated in the appropriate serum-free medium for 2 h at 37 °C to deplete the serum in the cells. In order to incubate cells at a low temperature outside of the 37 °C incubator, the medium was replaced with the respective serum-free medium that additionally did not contain sodium bicarbonate. The 6-well plates were then placed on a shallow ice-water bath and incubated in a 4 °C cold room for 30 min. The appropriate 2X-concentrated, serum- and sodium bicarbonate-free medium was pre-chilled to 4 °C before mixing 1:1 with a MWNT suspension, such that the final test medium contained MWNTs at the desired concentration specified in the experiment. After chilling down to 4 °C, the cells were incubated for 1 h at 4 °C with the appropriate pre-chilled serum- and sodium bicarbonate-free medium that did not contain MWNTs (control), or test serum- and sodium bicarbonate-free medium that contained a MWNT suspension at the specified final MWNT concentration. Because phagocytosis and endocytosis are blocked at low temperature, MWNTs in the test medium were free to interact with cell surface components without subsequently entering the vacuolar compartment of the cells. After incubation, the cells were washed, harvested, and the subsequent procedures for cell counting and lysate preparation were followed, as described in the previous sections. The amounts of cell-surface bound MWNTs in the cell lysate samples were determined using the SDS-PAGE method, as described previously herein.

2.10. Dissociation of Bound BSA-cMWNTs and BSA-pMWNTs from RAW 264.7 Cells at 4 °C

MWNTs suspended in a 0.10 mg/mL BSA working solution were mixed with an equal volume of 2X-concentrated, serum- and sodium bicarbonate-free medium to give a final MWNT concentration of 100 μg/mL. Equivalent number of RAW 264.7 cells were seeded in 6-well plates and incubated at 37 °C under standard cell culture conditions for 24 h prior to the experiment. Next, the cells were pre-incubated with serum-free medium (in the absence of MWNTs) for 2 h at 37 °C to deplete the serum in the cells. The cells were then pre-chilled to 4 °C and incubated at 4 °C for 1 h in serum- and sodium bicarbonate-free medium that contained either BSA-pMWNTs or BSA-cMWNTs. Finally, the cells were then incubated with serum- and sodium bicarbonate-free medium for an additional 20, 40, 60, 90, or 120 min, and then washed 3 times with serum- and sodium bicarbonate-free medium, then 2 times with PBS. After incubation, surface-bound MWNTs were extracted and quantified by the SDS-PAGE method, as described previously herein.

2.11. Additive Binding Test for BSA-cMWNTs and BSA-pMWNTs to RAW 264.7 Cells

To determine whether BSA-cMWNTs and BSA-pMWNTs use independent surface binding sites, ~5.0×10^5 RAW 264.7 cells/well were first seeded in 6-well plates and incubated in medium at 37 °C overnight. Cells were then incubated in a serum-free medium for 2 h at 37 °C to deplete the serum in the cells. Next, this medium was replaced with a serum-free medium that did not contain sodium bicarbonate. The 6-well plates were placed on a shallow ice-water bath and incubated in a 4 °C cold room for 30 min. A 2X-concentrated, serum- and sodium bicarbonate-free medium was pre-chilled to 4 °C before mixing 1:1 with a MWNT suspension such that the final test serum- and sodium bicarbonate-free medium contained 100 µg/mL MWNTs. After chilling to 4 °C, the cells were incubated with either BSA-cMWNTs or BSA-pMWNTs separately at 4 °C for 90 min or simultaneously with both ligands at 4 °C for 90 min. In a slightly different experimental design, the ligands were added sequentially, first BSA-cMWNTs for 45 min at 4 °C followed by washing the cells and the addition of BSA-pMWNTs, for 45 min at 4 °C for a total incubation time of 90 minutes. The order of the ligand addition was then reversed with another set of cells. The amounts of cell-surface bound MWNTs in the cell lysate samples were determined using the SDS-PAGE method, as described previously herein.

2.12. Surface Binding of MWNTs to RAW 264.7 Cells in the Presence of Dextran Sulfate, an SR-A1 Antagonist

To determine the effects of dextran sulfate on the association of pMWNTs and cMWNTs to the surfaces of RAW 264.7 cells, ~5.0×10^5 RAW 264.7 cells/well were seeded in 6-well plates and incubated in medium at 37 °C overnight. Then, RAW 264.7 cells were incubated in serum-free medium for 2 h at 37 °C to deplete the serum in the cells. To incubate cells at low temperature outside of the 37 °C incubator, the serum-free medium was replaced with serum-free medium that did not contain sodium bicarbonate. The 6-well plates were then placed on a shallow ice-water bath and incubated in a 4 °C cold room for 30 min. A 2X-concentrated, serum- and sodium bicarbonate-free medium was pre-chilled to 4 °C before mixing 1:1 with a MWNT suspension followed by the addition of dextran sulfate (or chondroitin sulfate, a control that is not an SR-A1 antagonist) at various concentrations such that the final test serum- and sodium bicarbonate-free medium contained 100 µg/mL MWNTs. After chilling down to 4 °C, the cells were incubated for 1 h at 4 °C with test serum- and sodium bicarbonate-free medium that contained 100 µg/mL MWNTs, washed 3 times with serum- and sodium bicarbonate-free medium, and then washed 2 times with PBS. In all cases, the amounts of cell-surface bound MWNTs in the cell lysate samples were determined using the SDS-PAGE method, as described previously herein.

2.13. Immunofluorescence Microscopy of WT and SR-A1 Knockout RAW 264.7 Cells

A total of ~2×10^4 RAW 264.7 cells were seeded on coverslips in 4-well plates and incubated in medium at 37 °C for 48 h to allow the cells to adhere to the plates. RAW 264.7 cells were incubated in serum-free medium for 1 h at 37 °C to deplete the serum in the cells. The cells were washed three times with media and 2 times with PBS. Then the cells were fixed with 4% paraformaldehyde at room temperature for 20 min followed by washing with PBS. The cells were incubated in blocking buffer containing 4% fish gelatin in PBS at room temperature for 1 hour to block non-specific protein-protein interactions. The cells were incubated with mouse SR-AI/MSR Alexa Fluor® 488-conjugated antibody or a rat IgG2B Alexa Fluor® 488-conjugated monoclonal antibody as the isotype control at room temperature for 1 h in the dark; control cells were not treated with any antibody. After rinsing, cell nuclei were stained with Hoechst 33342 dye for 10 min at room temperature. Then the cells were washed two times with PBS to remove excess dye. The coverslips were mounted on the glass slide using Fluoromount-G™. Images were taken with a Nikon Eclipse TE-2000 fluorescence microscope using a 60× oil-immersion objective with a NA of 1.4; the images for Hoechst 33342 (Ex. 350 nm; Em. 435–485 nm) and Alexa Fluor®488 (Ex. 488 nm; Em. 520–550 nm) were overlaid using ImageJ software.

2.14. Flow Cytometry for Surface Receptor(s) on WT and SR-A1 Knockout RAW 264.7 Cells

A total of ~2 × 10^6 RAW 264.7 cells were seeded in 10-mm plates and incubated in medium at 37 °C for 48 h to allow the cells to adhere to the plates. The cells were rinsed and harvested with warm FACS staining buffer (1% BSA in PBS) in 15 mL centrifuge tube followed by centrifugation (1000× g) for 5 min. The cells were suspended in 1 mL of FACS staining buffer, then three 100 µL-aliquots of the cell suspension were used to determine cell counts in each aliquot using a Beckman Coulter particle counter. A total of ~1 × 10^6 cells in 100 µL FACS staining buffer were aliquoted into 2 mL tubes. The cells were incubated in blocking buffer containing 5 µg IgG for 15 min at 4 °C to block non-specific protein interactions. The cells were stained with 5 µg mouse SR-AI/MSR Alexa Fluor® 488-conjugated antibody (R&D Systems cat. No. FAB1797G) or a rat IgG2B Alexa Fluor® 488-conjugated monoclonal antibody (R&D Systems cat. No. IC013G) as the isotype control for 30 min at 4 °C in the dark. Unbound antibody was removed by washing and re-suspending the cells in 1.5 mL FACS staining buffer thrice. The cells were re-suspended in 500 µL of FACS staining buffer for the final flow cytometric analysis. Flow cytometry analysis and data processing were performed using BD Accuri™ C6 Plus flow cytometer and CSampler™ Plus software (Becton and Dickinson Company, Franklin Lakes, NJ, USA) to determine the mean fluorescent index of each sample using a 518–548 nm emission filter.

3. Results

3.1. Characterization of BSA-MWNT Suspensions

The sonication and centrifugation protocol used to prepare purified BSA-coated MWNT suspensions is shown in Scheme 1. The initial baking step is to inactivate lipopolysaccharide derived from bacteria, should any be present. DLS and zeta potential analyses were used as part of a quality control routine for the preparation of all MWNT suspensions, as previously described [25,27]. Table 1 shows few differences in the particle size distributions of BSA-pMWNT and BSA-cMWNT suspensions, and that the zeta potentials for the BSA-cMWNTs in deionized water were slightly more negative than those for the BSA-pMWNTs. Zeta potentials were also determined for BSA-pMWNTs and BSA-cMWNTs in cell culture medium with and without 10% serum. In both matrices, the values were less negative for both MWNT samples in medium than in water as expected due to the increase in salt and/or serum proteins; the BSA-cMWNTs still had a slightly more negative zeta potential than the BSA-pMWNTs as expected due to the presence of ionized carboxyl groups on the cMWNTs.

3.2. BSA-pMWNTs and BSA-cMWNTs Are Not Significantly Toxic to RAW 264.7 Cells

The cell proliferation of RAW 264.7 cells incubated with BSA-pMWNTs or cMWNTs was measured after 24-h exposure to different concentrations of MWNTs up to 200 µg/mL using a previously standardized crystal violet assay [28]. The control in each case was cells exposed to BSA alone. Figure 1 shows no significant decline in cell proliferation for RAW 264.7 cells with either BSA-pMWNTs or cMWNTs at the highest concentrations tested (200 µg/mL); however, exposures longer than 24 h could reveal toxicity. Except where noted, a MWNT concentration of 100 µg/mL was chosen for the majority of experiments involving a constant MWNT concentration.

Table 1. Dynamic light scattering (DLS) particle size and zeta potential analyses of BSA-MWNT suspensions.

MWNT Suspension	DLS [1]		Zeta Potential [2] (mV)		
	HDD (nm)	PDI	Water	Medium + FBS	Medium − FBS
BSA-pMWNTs	83.23	0.20	−31.2	−5.7	−5.6
BSA-cMWNTs	84.18	0.19	−32.5	−6.6	−6.1

[1] Aliquots of purified pristine multi-walled carbon nanotubes (pMWNT) or carboxylated multi-walled carbon nanotubes (cMWNT) suspensions were diluted 1:10 in 0.10 mg/mL BSA working solutions. HDD is the hydrodynamic diameter, and PDI is the polydispersity index. [2] Aliquots of purified pMWNT or cMWNT suspensions were diluted 1:10 in deionized water, medium with fetal bovine serum (FBS), or FBS-free medium.

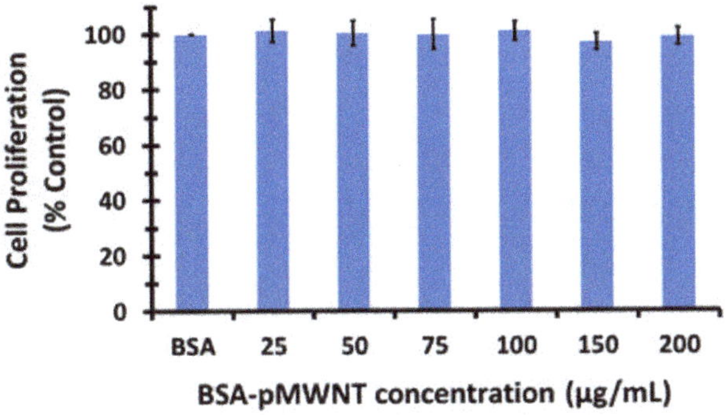

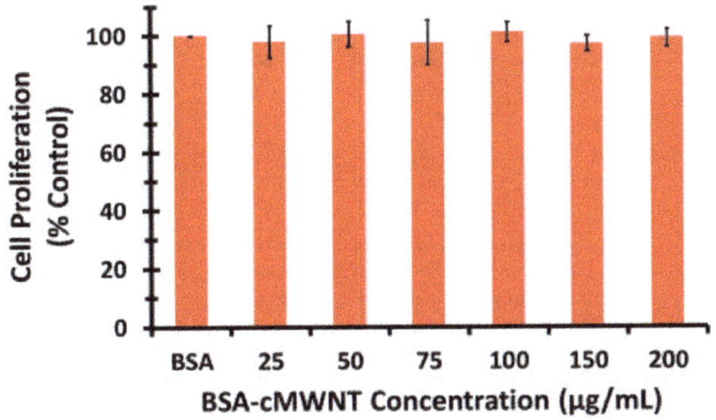

Figure 1. Cell proliferation of RAW 264.7 cells cultured with BSA-MWNTs. MWNTs suspended in a 0.10 mg/mL BSA working solution were mixed with an equal volume of 2X-concentrated medium to produce MWNT concentrations shown on the x-axes of the graphs. An equivalent number of cells were seeded in 48-well plates and incubated at 37 °C under standard cell culture conditions for 24 h prior to the experiment. Cell proliferation after incubation with control and test media for 24 h at 37 °C was determined by the crystal violet assay as described in the Methods, where the proliferation of control cells exposed to BSA in the absence of MWNTs was set to 100%. (**Top**) RAW 264.7 macrophage cell proliferation post 24-h incubation with various concentrations of BSA-pMWNTs. (**Bottom**) RAW 264.7 macrophage cell proliferation post 24-h incubation with various concentrations of BSA-cMWNTs. Both data sets are the mean of quadruple samples in three independent experiments ± the standard deviation (SD).

3.3. Evidence for BSA-MWNT Receptors on RAW 264.7 Cells

The accumulation of MWNTs by RAW 264.7 cells at 37 °C as a function of the applied BSA-MWNT concentrations between 0 and 200 µg/mL at 37 °C for 24 h was determined for BSA-pMWNTs and cMWNTs (Figure 2 top). For both, the uptake was linear to ~100 µg/mL and then began to decline as the concentration approached 200 µg/mL, consistent with a saturable receptor-mediated uptake process. To determine whether the receptors could be saturated when bound MWNTs were not internalized and in the absence of serum that otherwise could complicate the interpretation of the results, MWNT binding to cells was performed at 4 °C in medium without serum. RAW 264.7 cells were incubated with different concentrations of BSA-MWNTs (0–200 µg/mL) at 4 °C for 1 h in serum- and sodium bicarbonate-free medium. As shown in Figure 2 bottom, these experiments directly demonstrated that the binding of both MWNT types to the cell surface was a saturable function of the applied MWNT concentration, supporting the idea that there are receptors that bind BSA-coated MWNTs. Note also that more BSA-cMWNTs were bound than BSA-pMWNTs, suggesting that there are differences in the receptor interactions between the two MWNT types.

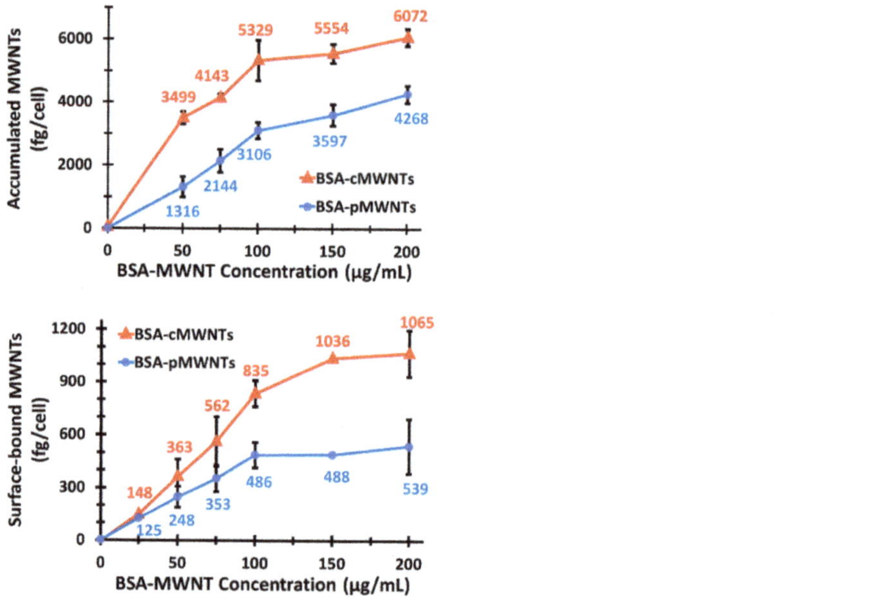

Figure 2. Accumulation at 37 °C and surface binding at 4 °C of BSA-MWNTs by RAW 264.7 cells as a function of the applied BSA-MWNT concentration. MWNTs suspended in a 0.10 mg/mL BSA working solution were mixed with an equal volume of 2X-concentrated medium to produce MWNT concentrations shown in the x-axes of the graphs. Exposure to a 0.10 mg/mL BSA working solution alone (in the absence of MWNTs) was the control. (**Top**) RAW 264.7 cells in 6-well plates were incubated at 37 °C for 24 h in complete medium with serum that contained either BSA alone, BSA-pMWNTs (blue line), or BSA-cMWNTs (red line). After incubation, MWNTs were extracted from cells and quantified by the SDS-PAGE method. (**Bottom**) Cells in 6-well plates were pre-incubated with serum-free medium (in the absence of BSA-MWNTs) for 2 h at 37 °C to deplete the serum in the cells. The cells were then pre-chilled to 4 °C and incubated at 4 °C for 1 h in serum- and sodium bicarbonate-free medium that contained either a 0.10 mg/mL BSA working solution without MWNTs, with BSA-pMWNTs (blue line), or with BSA-cMWNTs (red line). After incubation, surface-bound MWNTs were extracted and quantified by the SDS–PAGE method. For both data sets the numbers above the data points are the mean femtograms of MWNTs/cell; each data point is the mean of ≥3 independent experiments ± SD.

To further characterize the ligand/receptor properties of bound BSA-coated MWNTs, the dissociation of bound BSA-cMWNTs and BSA-pMWNTs from cells was measured in the absence of serum at 4 °C. Briefly, RAW 264.7 cells were incubated with BSA-coated MWNTs to allow binding at 4 °C, washed, and further incubated in medium without serum to allow dissociation, followed by quantitating the amount of cell-bound MWNTs as a function of dissociation time. BSA-pMWNTs dissociated very slowly from cells, with more than 80% of the material still bound after 120 min (Figure 3, inset). This slow dissociation is not surprising considering that BSA is likely a major determinant of receptor interaction, and there are multiple copies of BSA on each nanotube that may simultaneously interact with multiple receptors, decreasing the probability of dissociation. BSA-cMWNTs' dissociation was biphasic, with about 50% of the bound material dissociating within the first hour, followed by a slowly dissociating component, suggesting that BSA-cMWNTs may contain two binding sites for cells that have different dissociation rates from the two receptor sites. Further, the slowly dissociating component seen with BSA-cMWNTs might share features with the slowly dissociating material observed with BSA-pMWNTs. Regardless of mechanistic details, these data emphasize that the receptor interaction characteristics of BSA-cMWNTs and BSA-pMWNTs are not identical.

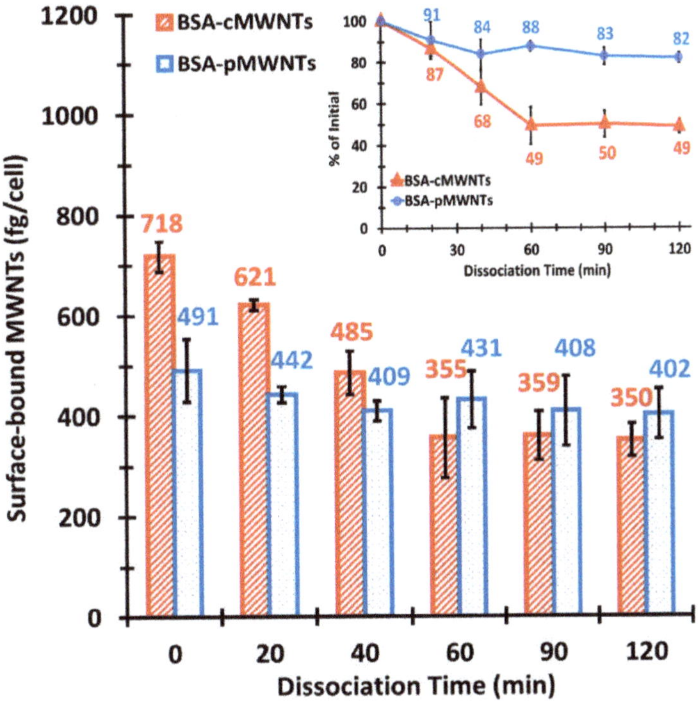

Figure 3. Dissociation of bound BSA-cMWNTs and BSA-pMWNTs from RAW 264.7 cells at 4 °C. A total of 100 μg/mL of BSA-cMWNTs or BSA-pMWNTs in serum- and sodium bicarbonate-free medium were incubated with RAW 264.7 cells at 4 °C for 1 h to achieve binding, then washed and incubated in serum- and sodium bicarbonate-free medium for the indicated times, as described in Methods. Surface-bound MWNTs were extracted and quantified by the SDS-PAGE method. The numbers above the bars are the mean femtograms of MWNTs/cell. **Inset:** The data are plotted as the percentage of the initial surface-bound MWNTs at t = 0 min. Data are the mean of ≥3 independent experiments ± SD.

One explanation for the apparent differences between BSA-cMWNTs and BSA-pMWNTs in the number of cell surface binding sites and the differing dissociation kinetics is that there are two independent receptors on these cells—one for BSA-coated cMWNTs and another for BSA-coated pMWNTs. If so, then their binding should be additive at saturation; that is, if BSA-cMWNTs and BSA-pMWNTs are both added simultaneously, the total cell-associated MWNTs should be the sum of the amount for each when added alone. As shown in Figure 4, when cells were incubated with both BSA-cMWNTs and BSA-pMWNTs, the amount bound by cells was greater than for BSA-pMWNTs alone, but did not exceed that of BSA-cMWNTs alone, which is not fully additive. In a slightly different experimental design to test additive binding, the cells were exposed to the ligands sequentially—an experimental design that avoids the possible interaction of cMWNTs and pMWNTs when they are together in medium during binding. Cells were first exposed for 45 min to BSA-cMWNTs alone, followed by washing and exposure for 45 min to BSA-pMWNTs. The order of the two sequential ligand additions was then reversed, with results seen in the last two bars of Figure 4. When BSA-cMWNTs were added first, followed by BSA-pMWNTs, there was no additional binding compared to BSA-cMWNTs alone, suggesting that there were no further open sites for BSA-pMWNTs. When BSA-pMWNTs were added first, followed by BSA-cMWNTs, there was additional binding compared to pMWNTs alone, but binding did not exceed that of BSA-cMWNTs alone. Altogether, these data do not fit a simple model of additive binding with two independent receptors each interacting autonomously with the two ligands. Rather, they suggest a semi-additive situation where BSA-cMWNTs can occupy all the sites that BSA-pMWNTs may interact with, but that there are sites for BSA-cMWNTs to which BSA-pMWNTs do not bind.

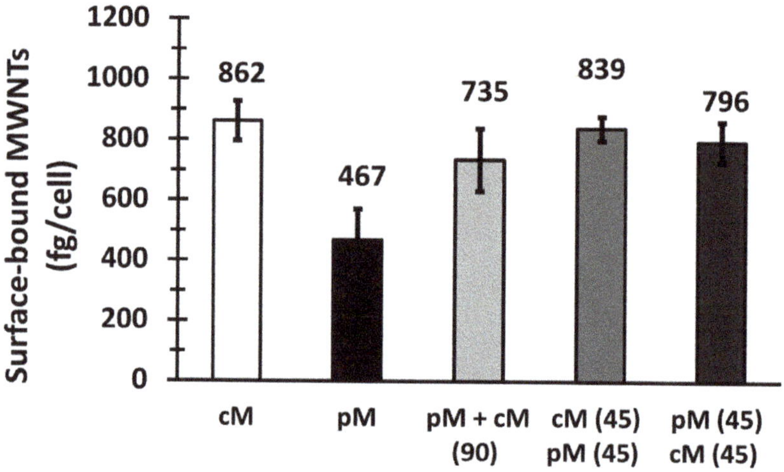

Figure 4. Test for additive binding of BSA-cMWNTs and BSA-pMWNTs to cells. Equivalent numbers of RAW 264.7 cells were seeded in 6-well plates and incubated at 37 °C under standard cell culture conditions for 24 h prior to the experiment in preparation for the additive binding studies as described in Methods. Cells were exposed to serum- and sodium bicarbonate-free media containing either 100 µg/mL BSA-pMWNTs or BSA-cMWNTs (labelled pM and cM in the graph) followed by incubation at 4 °C for 90 min to establish the amount of each bound when separate. Additive binding was tested by exposing the cells simultaneously to both BSA-cMWNTs and BSA-pMWNTs for 90 min. In a slightly different experimental design, the cells incubated with either BSA-cMWNTs or BSA-pMWNTs at 4 °C for 45 min, washed, and incubated with BSA-pMWNTs or BSA-cMWNTs, respectively, at 4 °C for 45 min for a total incubation time of 90 minutes. Surface-bound MWNTs were extracted and quantified using the SDS-PAGE method. The numbers above the bars are the mean femtograms of MWNTs/cell, and each data point is the mean of $\geq$3 independent experiments $\pm$ SD.

3.4. An SR-A Antagonist Reduces Binding of BSA-MWNTs to RAW 264.7 Cells

SR-As are involved in the binding of anionic ligands and certain modified proteins, such as oxidized LDL and maleylated albumin [30–33]. Moreover, the interaction of BSA with several nanoparticles causes conformation changes in BSA that expose cryptic SR-A1 binding sites [34–36]. In addition, there is indirect evidence that SRs bind carbon nanotubes [20]. Work from our lab also provided evidence that PF108-cMWNTs, but not PF108-pMWNTs, interact with SR-A1 [12,21]. Thus, SR-A1 is a potential receptor for BSA-MWNTs. This was initially explored by determining whether dextran sulfate, a known antagonist of SR-As, interferes with the binding of BSA-coated MWNTs. Chondroitin sulfate, an anionic polysaccharide that is not a SR-A1 inhibitor, was used as the control. RAW 264.7 cells were exposed to 100 µg/mL of BSA-MWNTs in serum- and sodium bicarbonate-free medium at 4 °C in the presence or absence of dextran sulfate or chondroitin sulfate, as indicated in Figure 5. The amount of BSA-cMWNTs bound to the cells declined as a function of dextran sulfate concentration and leveled off to about 50% compared to cells not exposed to the antagonist, whereas the amount of BSA-pMWNTs bound appeared to monotonically decline to a final level of ~25% of the control at the highest dextran sulfate concentration. These data again emphasize the differences in the receptor binding properties of the two BSA-MWNT types and further suggest that binding of both MWNTs types to receptors are sensitive to an SR-A1 antagonist; however, interpreting the data is not straightforward because the inhibition was partial, especially for BSA-cMWNTs. Therefore, studies were performed with cells that over- or under-express SR-A1 to clarify whether SR-A1 might interact with BSA-cMWNTs or BSA-pMWNTs, or both.

3.5. Evidence That SR-A1 Mediates the Uptake of Both BSA-cMWNTs and BSA-pMWNTs in CHO Cells Overexpressing SR-A1

CHO cells stably transfected with mouse SR-A1 cDNA (CHO[mSR-AI] cells) [24] were studied to determine whether the expression of SR-A1 in a cell line that does not normally express the receptor results in the accumulation of BSA-coated MWNTs by the cells. CHO[mSR-AI] cells overexpressing SR-A1 were incubated at 37 °C for 24 h with 100 µg/mL of BSA-pMWNTs or cMWNT dispersions. Similarly treated wild-type CHO-K1 cells were the control. The results showed that the SR-A1 overexpressing CHO-K1 cells accumulated BSA-pMWNTs and BSA-cMWNTs two and three times more, respectively, compared to the control cells (Figure 6). This evidence supports the idea that SR-A1 is a receptor for both BSA-cMWNTs and BSA-pMWNTs, and also recapitulates the observation in Figure 2 that BSA-cMWNTs were accumulated to a greater extent than BSA-pMWNTs.

3.6. SR-A1 Knockout RAW 264.7 Cells Bind and Accumulate Far Less BSA-MWNTs Than WT Cells

Another approach to understanding the role that SR-A1 has in the uptake and binding of BSA-MWNTs is to knock out the SR-A1 gene using CRISPR-Cas9 technology. A RAW 264.7 cell knockout pool was obtained that contained a high proportion of cells with a mutation in the SR-A1 gene at a site near the beginning of the DNA sequence. This ensured that both SR-A1 as well as SR-A1.1 protein expression would be affected. A dilution cloning strategy was used to obtain 10 cell clones that did not express SR-A1 receptors on their surface as validated by immunofluorescence microscopy and flow cytometry. Both techniques showed that WT RAW 264.7 cells had high expression of SR-A1 receptors, whereas two knockout clones selected for study (termed C4 and B11) had negligible surface receptors (Figure 7).

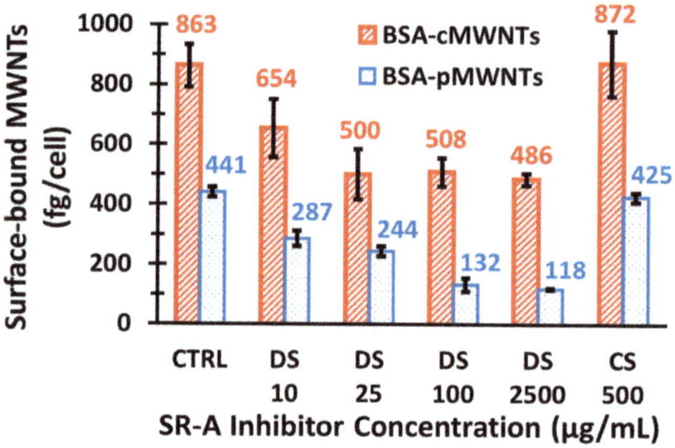

Figure 5. Effect of dextran sulfate on BSA-MWNT binding to RAW 264.7 cells at 4 °C. MWNTs suspended in a 0.10 mg/mL BSA working solution were mixed with an equal volume of 2X-concentrated, serum- and sodium bicarbonate-free medium to give a MWNT concentration of 100 µg/mL followed by the addition of chondroitin sulfate (CS) or the SR-A1 antagonist dextran sulfate (DS) at various concentrations as described in the Methods. The serum- and sodium bicarbonate-free medium control contained the same 100 µg/mL BSA-MWNTs, but without CS or DS. After initial plating and attachment to the substrate, cells were pre-incubated with serum-free medium (in the absence of MWNTs) for 2 h at 37 °C to deplete the serum in the cells. The cells were then pre-chilled to 4 °C and incubated at 4 °C for 1 h in serum- and sodium bicarbonate-free test medium that contained either a 0.10 mg/mL BSA working solution without MWNTs, with BSA-pMWNTs ± DS or CS (blue bars and line), or with BSA-cMWNTs ± DS or CS (red bars and line). Surface-bound MWNTs were extracted and quantified using the SDS-PAGE method. The numbers above the bars are the mean femtograms of MWNTs/cell. Data are the mean of ≥3 independent experiments ± SD.

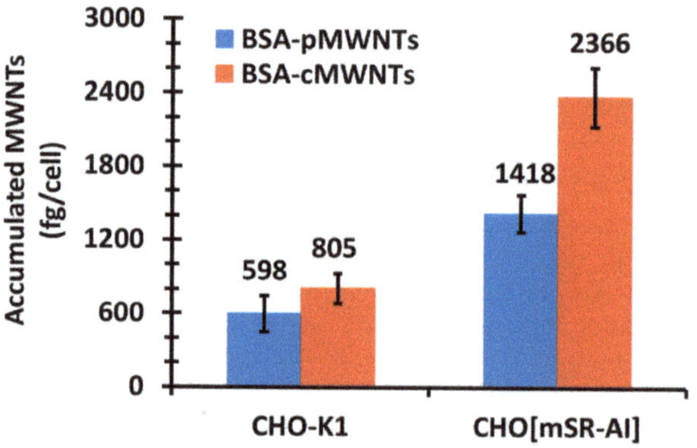

Figure 6. Accumulation of BSA-MWNTs by wild-type Chinese hamster ovary (WT CHO)-K1 control cells and Chinese hamster ovary (CHO) cells that overexpress SR-A1 receptors (CHO[mSR-AI] cells) at 37 °C. Equivalent numbers of each cell line were seeded in 6-well plates and incubated at 37 °C under standard cell culture conditions for 24 h prior to the experiment. The cells were then incubated at 37 °C for 24 h in medium that contained BSA-pMWNTs (blue bars) or BSA-cMWNTs (red bars) each at 100 µg/mL. After incubation, MWNTs were extracted from the cells and quantified by the SDS-PAGE method. The numbers above the data points are the mean femtograms of MWNTs/cell, and each data point is the mean of ≥3 experiments ± SD.

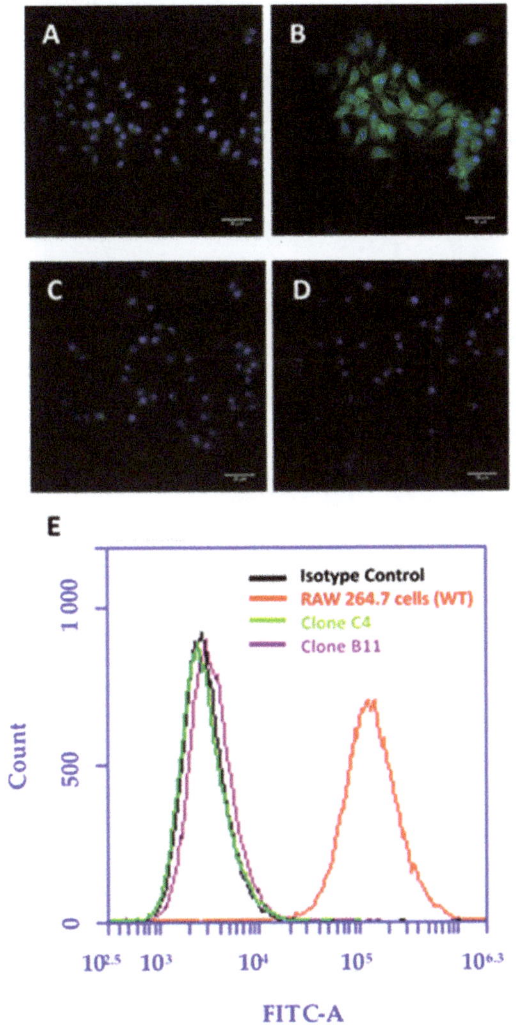

Figure 7. Immunofluorescence microscopy and flow cytometric analysis of WT and SR-A1 knockout RAW 264.7 cells. Immunofluorescence images of **(A)** control WT RAW 264.7 cells without mouse anti-SR-AI/MSR Alexa Fluor® 488-conjugated antibody, **(B)** WT RAW 264.7 cells incubated with mouse anti SR-AI/MSR Alexa Fluor® 488-conjugated antibody, and **(C,D)** two different clones (C4 and B11) of SR-A1 knockout RAW 264.7 cells incubated with anti-mouse SR-AI/MSR Alexa Fluor® 488-conjugated antibody. Hoechst 33342 staining is shown in blue and Alexa Fluor® 488 staining is shown in green. All images are normalized to the same intensity scale, and the scale bars represent 20 μm. **(E)** Flow cytometry analyses where the black line represents WT RAW 264.7 cells incubated with the rat IgG2B Alexa Fluor® 488-conjugated monoclonal antibody as the isotype control, the red line represents WT RAW 264.7 cells incubated with mouse anti-SR-AI/MSR Alexa Fluor® 488-conjugated antibody, and the green and purple lines represent two different clones (C4 and B11, respectively) of SR-A1 knockout RAW 264.7 cells incubated with mouse anti-SR-AI/MSR Alexa Fluor® 488-conjugated antibody. The x-axis denotes fluorescence detected in the 518–548 nm spectral region, and the y-axis denotes the number of events for each analysis.

To assess the recognition of BSA-pMWNTs and BSA-cMWNTs by SR-A1 receptors, the accumulation of 100 µg/mL BSA-coated pMWNTs or cMWNTs was measured using knockout clones C4 and B11 with the corresponding WT RAW 264.7 cells for comparison. The cells were incubated at 37 °C for 24 h with 100 µg/mL BSA-MWNTs and the accumulated MWNTs were measured using SDS-PAGE. As shown in Figure 8, the amount of accumulated MWNTs in the knockout SR-A1 cell lines was significantly decreased for both BSA-pMWNTs and BSA-cMWNTs compared to the WT RAW 264.7 cells.

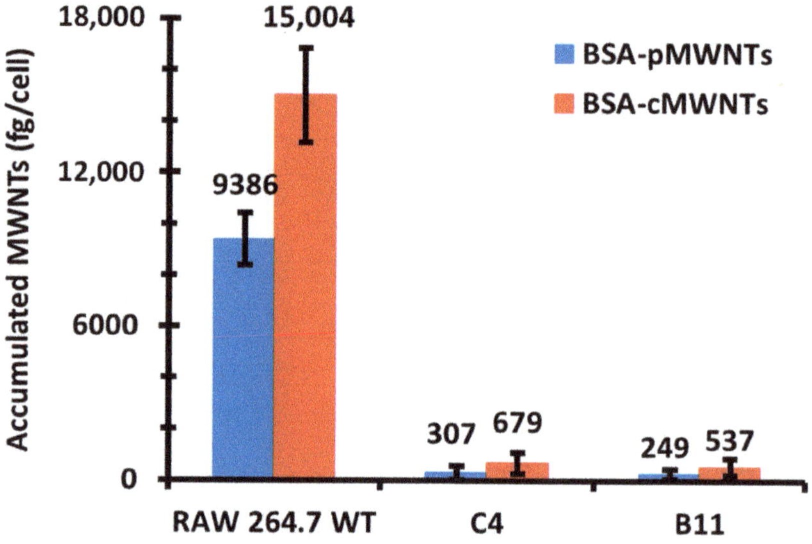

Figure 8. Accumulation of BSA-MWNTs by WT and SR-A1 knockout RAW 264.7 cells at 37 °C. MWNTs suspended in a 0.10 mg/mL BSA working solution were mixed with an equal volume of 2X-concentrated medium to produce MWNT concentrations of 100 µg/mL. Equivalent numbers of WT and SR-A1 knockout RAW 264.7 cells were seeded in 6-well plates and incubated at 37 °C under standard cell culture conditions for 24 h prior to the experiment. The cells were then incubated at 37 °C for 24 h in medium that contained BSA-pMWNTs (blue bars) or BSA-cMWNTs (red bars). After incubation, MWNTs were extracted from cells and quantified by the SDS-PAGE method. The numbers above the data points are the mean femtograms of MWNTs/cell. Data are the mean of $\geq$3 experiments $\pm$ SD.

The binding of 100 µg/mL BSA-coated cMWNTs and pMWNTs by RAW 264.7 cells was also studied using the same knockout SR-A1 clones (C4 and B11) and corresponding WT RAW 264.7 cells at 4 °C in the absence of serum, conditions under which MWNT binding by macrophages can be directly measured where the influence of protein coronas and cell uptake are controlled. The results indicated that there is a significant decrease in binding of BSA-pMWNTs and BSA-cMWNTs by SR-A1 knockout RAW 264.7 cells compared to WT RAW 264.7 cells (Figure 9). Interestingly, 20% of the surface-bound BSA-cMWNTs were still present on the SR-A1 knockout cells, suggesting that a low binding capacity for BSA-cMWNTs still remained. Taken together, the observation that CHO cells expressing SR-A1 do bind BSA-MWNTs and the finding that RAW 264.7 cells lacking SR-A1 have greatly reduced binding, suggest that SR-A1 has a dominant role in the binding and accumulation of both BSA-MWNTs types.

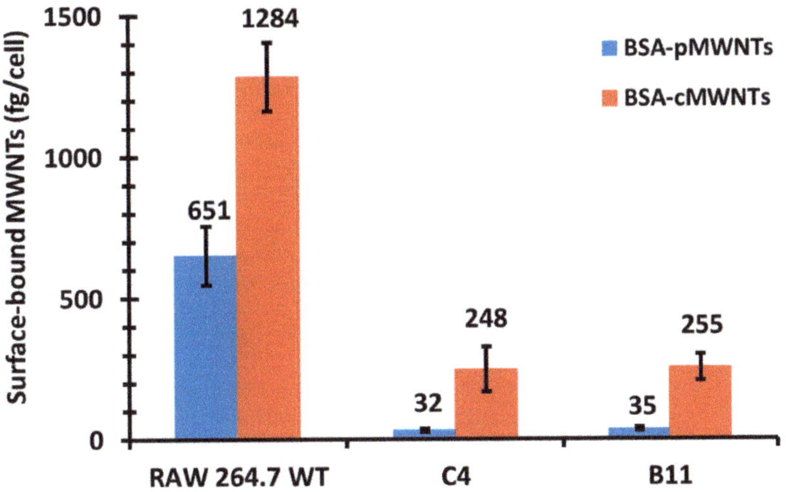

Figure 9. Surface binding of BSA-MWNTs by WT and SR-A1 knockout RAW 264.7 cells at 4 °C. MWNTs suspended in a 0.10 mg/mL BSA working solution were mixed with an equal volume of 2X-concentrated serum- and sodium bicarbonate-free medium to produce MWNT concentrations of 100 μg/mL. Equivalent numbers of WT and SR-A1 knockout RAW 264.7 cells were seeded in 6-well plates and incubated at 37 °C under standard cell culture conditions for 24 h prior to the experiment. Next, the cells were pre-incubated with serum-free medium (in the absence of BSA-MWNTs) for 2 h at 37 °C to deplete the serum in the cells. The cells were then pre-chilled to 4 °C and incubated at 4 °C for 1 h in serum- and sodium bicarbonate-free medium that contained either BSA-pMWNTs (blue bars) or BSA-cMWNTs (red bars). After incubation, surface-bound MWNTs were extracted and quantified by the SDS-PAGE method. Numbers above the data points are the mean femtograms of MWNTs/cell. Data are the mean of $\geq$3 independent experiments $\pm$ SD.

4. Discussion

WT RAW 264.7 cells accumulated both BSA-cMWNTs and BSA-pMWNTs as a function of concentration after a 24 h exposure at 37 °C, although BSA-coated cMWNTs were accumulated to almost twice the amount of pMWNTs at each concentration tested. Uptake for both was near linear up to 100 μg/mL, after which the rate of accumulation was reduced. The break in the uptake curve at 100 μg/mL suggests a saturable receptor could be involved in the uptake process; however, accumulation depends not only on uptake, but also on potential loss of the MWNTs from cells by either recycling or degradation, or a loss of surface receptors that are internalized from the cell surface but not replaced. To focus on the initial interaction of MWNTs with cells, binding experiments were performed at 4 °C where internalization is inhibited. Moreover, serum proteins other than BSA that might confound the interpretation of the results were absent from the binding medium. Under these conditions, the binding of BSA-coated cMWNTs or pMWNTs to RAW 264.7 cells was near linear up to 100 μg/mL and then began to plateau, suggesting a saturable receptor-mediated binding event. There were two notable observations in comparing the binding of BSA-coated MWNTs to that we previously described for PF108-coated MWNTs. First, BSA-pMWNTs bound to cells, whereas previous studies showed that PF108-coated pMWNTs did not [12,21]. This indicates that the BSA corona confers the ability of pMWNTs to bind cells. Second, the cells bound more BSA-cMWNTs than BSA-pMWNTs, evidence that there remains a difference in binding capacity between the two MWNT types. Differences between BSA-cMWNTs and BSA-pMWNTs were also seen in their kinetics of dissociation from cells: BSA-pMWNTs dissociated very slowly, whereas BSA-cMWNTs had a faster dissociating component followed by a slowly dissociating component.

One model to explain the difference in the binding of BSA-cMWNTs and BSA-pMWNTs to cells is that there are two independent receptors—one for each type of MWNT. If there are two receptors interacting independently with two ligands, then exposing cells simultaneously to both ligands should result in an amount bound that is the sum of both when added separately. However, this was not observed. The amount bound after simultaneous exposure to both BSA-cMWNTs and BSA-pMWNTs never exceed the amount bound to cells when BSA-cMWNTs were added alone, which is not a simple additive result. To further explore this issue, sequential binding experiments were undertaken. The level of cell-associated MWNTs when BSA-cMWNTs were added first, followed by BSA-pMWNTs, was equal to the amount of MWNTs bound when BSA-cMWNTs were added alone, which is not additive. However, when the order was reversed and BSA-pMWNTs were added first followed by BSA-cMWNTs, there was more binding than observed when BSA-pMWNTs were added alone, and the amount was again equal to the increased binding seen with BSA-cMWNTs alone, an additive result. Altogether, the results of the binding experiments suggest a semi-additive model: BSA-cMWNTs can occupy all the binding sites available to BSA-pMWNTs, plus additional sites not available to BSA-pMWNTs. Thus, when BSA-cMWNTs are added first, no binding of BSA-pMWNTs occurs because the sites are occupied by BSA-cMWNTs. However, when BSA-pMWNTs are added first, there remain sites available for BSA-cMWNTs to which BSA-pMWNTs cannot bind.

The semi-additive data are compatible with a two-receptor model and also with a model where a single receptor has two binding sites. In the two-receptor model, one receptor would bind both cMWNTs and pMWNTs, and the other receptor would bind only cMWNTs. To help address the question of whether one or two receptors were involved in binding cMWNTs and pMWNTs, the accumulation and binding of BSA-coated MWNTs was studied with RAW 264.7 cells in which the SR-A1 gene had been knocked out. Two clones isolated from the knockout pool, which were shown to lack immunologically detectable SR-A1 on their surfaces, failed to accumulate either BSA-coated cMWNTs or pMWNTs at 37 °C. In binding studies at 4 °C, the binding of BSA-pMWNTs was negligible and the binding of BSA-cMWNTs was reduced by 80%. It is not clear what is responsible for the 20% of BSA-cMWNT binding in the knockout cells, but perhaps one or more minor receptors for BSA-cMWNTs are present at low levels, and their contributions are seen in SR-A1 knockout cells. Nevertheless, it appears that knocking out SR-A1 severely affects the accumulation and binding of both BSA-cMWNTs and BSA-pMWNTs.

The simplest explanation for the knockout results is that SR-A1 is a receptor for both BSA-cMWNTs and BSA-pMWNTs. However, an alternative explanation is that knocking out SR-A1 suppresses the expression of one or more other cell surface proteins that could be major receptors for BSA-coated MWNTs. Two lines of evidence argue against this possibility. One is that dextran sulfate, a known antagonist of ligand binding to SR-A1, at least partially inhibited the binding of both BSA-coated pMWNTs and cMWNTs to cells, supporting the idea that SR-A1 is a receptor for these ligands. Second, CHO-K1 cells that ectopically express SR-A1 accumulated significantly more BSA-coated cMWNTs and pMWNTs than normal CHO-K1 cells. It seems unlikely that a covert receptor is activated in CHO cells, a cell type very different than RAW 264.7 macrophages, upon expression of SR-A1. Altogether, the simplest interpretation of the evidence argues that SR-A1 binds both BSA-cMWNTs and BSA-pMWNTs.

Understanding what features of BSA-coated MWNTs interact with SR-A1 is an interesting challenge. Previous work established that PF108-coated cMWNTs bound to and were accumulated by macrophages that expressed SR-A1 in the absence of serum or serum proteins [12], whereas alveolar macrophages derived from mice knocked out for SR-A1 failed to accumulate the MWNTs [21]. PF108-coated pMWNTs were not bound or accumulated by either SR-A1 positive or negative macrophages [12,21]. Thus, no protein corona was necessary for SR-A1 to interact with cMWNTs. This suggested that one or more oxidized functionalities intrinsic to cMWNTs (carboxyl, hydroxyl, phenolic, etc.) are structural features potentially recognized by SR-A1. SR-A1 access to cMWNT surface features might occur at nanotube ends where the high curvature may not support coat binding and where oxidized functionalities are often located due to ring strain [37–40]. In addition, the residence time of BSA on MWNTs appears to be short and not all the surface is covered with protein at one time [41]. Thus, it is likely that SR-A1 would have access to oxidized groups intrinsic to the MWNT surface of BSA-coated cMWNTs.

It is understood now that while native BSA does not interact with SR-A1, conformational changes in BSA upon binding several types of nanoparticles uncover latent sites that do bind SR-A1 [34–36]. Moreover, BSA undergoes significant conformation changes upon binding to cMWNTs [42]. This leads to Binding Hypothesis 1 in Figure 10A, where BSA-coated cMWNTs present two sites that can interact with SR-A1—one for oxidized groups inherent to the nanotube and another for the coat of conformationally altered BSA protein. This model may explain why more BSA-cMWNTs bind cells than BSA-pMWNTs, and also is consistent with the semi-additive binding data: all binding sites are occupied by BSA-cMWNTs, whereas only the BSA binding sites are occupied by BSA-pMWNTs. The model is also consistent with the differences in dissociation of the two MWNT types from cells assuming BSA-cMWNTs and BSA-pMWNTs bound to SR-A1 at BSA binding sites dissociate slowly and that BSA-cMWNTs bound to oxidized functionalities dissociates more rapidly.

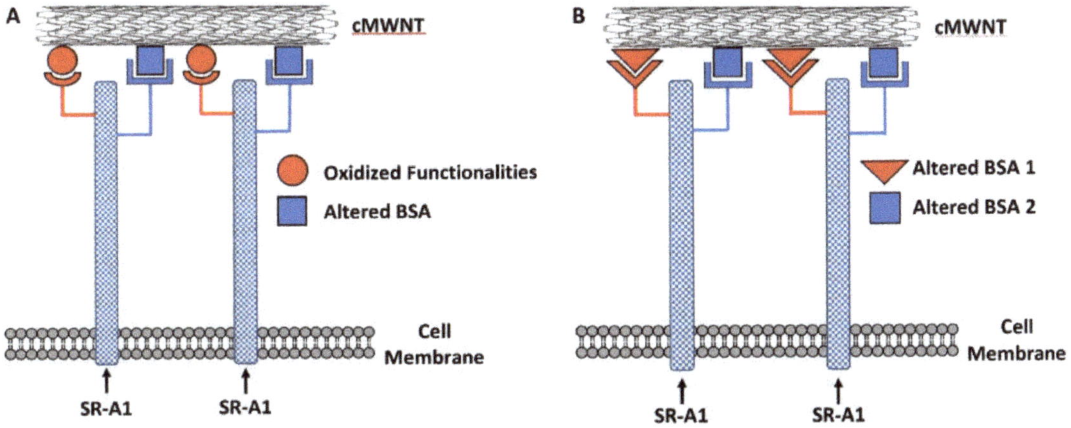

Figure 10. Models for the binding of cMWNTs to SR-A1. (**A**) Model where one site on SR-A1 interacts with altered binding sites on a BSA conformer and another site interacts with oxidized functionalities on cMWNTs. (**B**) Model where one site on SR-A1 interacts with altered binding sites on BSA Conformer 1 and another site interacts with altered binding sites on BSA Conformer 2.

An alternative model is one in which all the oxidized binding sites on cMWNTs are unavailable because they are covered by BSA, and that binding of BSA to cMWNTs exposes additional latent SR-A1 binding sites that are not exposed when BSA binds to pMWNTs; hence, cells bind more BSA-cMWNTs than BSA-pMWNTs. A model of this type shown in Figure 10B cannot be ruled out with the available data.

SR-A1 is a homotrimer and each monomer comprises an N-terminal cytoplasmic tail, a transmembrane domain, a spacer region, an α-helical coiled coil domain, a collagenous domain, and a C-terminal scavenger receptor cysteine rich (SRCR) domain [15,30,43]. Depending on the ligand, either the collagenous domain, the SRCR, or both, may be involved in ligand binding of various scavenger receptors, but the details are not well understood and appear to depend on the structural context within each receptor type. For example, there is evidence from mutational studies with SR-A1 that positively charged residues in the collagenous domain are important for binding oxidized LDL [31,44]. Further, SR-A1.1, an alternatively spliced variant of SR-A1 lacking the SRCR domain, still binds oxidized LDL, suggesting that the collagenous domain is the major binding site for this ligand, although this does not rule out that the SRCR domain of SR-A1 may also interact with oxidized LDL or other protein ligands. Indeed, recent work suggests that the SR-A1 SRCR domain binds spectrin [45] and ferritin [46]. The SRCR domain is involved in the ligand binding by MARCO, a member of the class A scavenger receptors that shares the highly conserved SRCR domain with SR-A1 [47–49]. The functional unit of many scavenger receptor family members is a trimer, including SR-A1, and the potential for three ligand binding sites per trimer is believed to enhance binding avidity to larger ligands, such as intact bacteria, and which would presumably include large ENPs such as MWNTs [33]. This feature is not explicitly shown in the models of Figure 10, but could be accommodated. Nevertheless, given the intricacies of how different domains in scavenger receptors interact with ligands, it is difficult to parse which SR-A1 domains interact with what features of BSA-coated MWNTs.

Additional complexities in scavenger receptor interaction with ligands arise from evidence that scavenger receptors, including SR-A1, may form complexes with other pattern recognition receptors, termed co-receptors, that also interact with the same ligand. The resulting complexes can then recruit components to form "Signalosomes" that contain two or more receptors bound to the same ligand plus associated signaling components that may activate cell signaling pathways [32,33,50]. For example, there is evidence from computational work [51] and from molecular docking studies that SWNTs may bind toll-like receptor 4 (TLR4) [52]. It would be interesting to know whether the ~20% of cMWNT binding to RAW 264.7 cells lacking SR-A1 seen in Figure 9 is due to TLR4. Thus, the simple models in Figure 10 may not capture the range of possibilities for how MWNTs interact with SR-A1 and other cell components via co-receptors. Nevertheless, SR-A1 is a key player evidenced by the major loss of binding in SR-A1 knockout cells and the gain of binding in CHO cells that ectopically express SR-A1.

5. Conclusions

From previous work, PF108-coated pMWNTs fail to bind to macrophages but BSA-coated pMWNTs do bind, suggesting that a BSA corona confers the ability of pMWNTs to bind to cells. Therefore, in this article we studied the interaction of BSA-MWNTs with macrophages using a direct binding assay under highly controlled conditions where the influence of nanotube functionalization and protein coronas could be controlled. The results demonstrated that the binding of both BSA-cMWNTs and BSA-pMWNTs to the cell surface was a dose-dependent and saturable function of the applied MWNT concentration. Both MWNT types bound and were accumulated by RAW 264.7 cells; however, the cells bound and accumulated two times more BSA-cMWNTs than BSA-pMWNTs, suggesting that there are more binding sites on the cell surface for BSA-cMWNTs than BSA-pMWNTs. The binding of BSA-coated cMWNTs and pMWNTs to RAW 264.7 cells was semi-additive, suggesting that a single receptor with two distinct binding sites could explain the data. SR-A1 knockout RAW 264.7 cells had significantly reduced binding and accumulation of both BSA-pMWNTs and cMWNTs and CHO cells that ectopically expressed SR-A1 accumulated both MWNT types, whereas WT CHO cells did not, suggesting that SR-A1 is the key receptor for both MWNT types. Models consistent with the data are proposed where SR-A1 has two binding sites that interact with BSA-coated MWNTs differently depending on the presence of a BSA corona and on the presence or absence of oxidized groups on the MWNTs. The approaches and observations in this study may contribute to the rational design of nanotoxicity remediation efforts and biomedical applications of engineered carbon nanoparticles.

Author Contributions: Conceptualization, M.T.H., C.M., P.P. and R.D.; methodology, M.T.H. and C.M.; investigation, M.T.H. and C.M.; writing—original draft preparation, M.T.H., C.M. and R.D.; writing—review and editing, M.T.H., C.M., P.P. and R.D.; supervision, C.M., P.P., and R.D.; funding acquisition, M.T.H., P.P. and R.D. All authors have read and agreed to the published version of the manuscript.

Funding: This research was funded by the Graduate Research Fellowship Program of the National Science Foundation (M.T.H.), the Eugene McDermott Graduate Fellows Program of The University of Texas at Dallas (M.T.H.), and Research Enhancement Funds from the University of Texas at Dallas (R.D.).

Data Availability Statement: The data presented in this study are available in Huynh, M.T.; Mikoryak, C.; Pantano, P.; Draper, R. Scavenger Receptor A1 Mediates the Uptake of Carboxylated and Pristine Multi-Walled Carbon Nanotubes Coated with Bovine Serum Albumin. *Nanomaterials* 2021, 11, 539, doi:10.3390/nano11020539.

Acknowledgments: The authors thank R. Wang and K. Kinghorn for contributions prior to the herein presented work.

Conflicts of Interest: The authors declare no conflict of interest.

Author Contributions: A companion paper has also been published in the Nanomaterials Special Issue "Nanoparticle-Macrophage Interactions: Implications for Nanosafety and Nanomedicine": Wang, R.; Lohray, R.; Chow, E.; Gangupantula, P.; Smith, L.; Draper, R. Selective Uptake of Carboxylated Multi-Walled Carbon Nanotubes by Class A Type 1 Scavenger Receptors and Impaired Phagocytosis in Alveolar Macrophages. *Nanomaterials (Basel)* **2020**, *10*, 2417. doi:10.3390/nano10122417.

References

1. Walczyk, D.; Bombelli, F.B.; Monopoli, M.P.; Lynch, I.; Dawson, K.A. What the Cell "Sees" in Bionanoscience. *J. Am. Chem. Soc.* **2010**, *132*, 5761–5768. [CrossRef] [PubMed]
2. Monopoli, M.P.; Walczyk, D.; Campbell, A.; Elia, G.; Lynch, I.; Baldelli Bombelli, F.; Dawson, K.A. Physical−Chemical Aspects of Protein Corona: Relevance to in Vitro and in Vivo Biological Impacts of Nanoparticles. *J. Am. Chem. Soc.* **2011**, *133*, 2525–2534. [CrossRef] [PubMed]
3. Westmeier, D.; Stauber, R.H.; Docter, D. The concept of bio-corona in modulating the toxicity of engineered nanomaterials (ENM). *Toxicol. Appl. Pharmacol.* **2016**, *299*, 53–57. [CrossRef]
4. Alberg, I.; Kramer, S.; Schinnerer, M.; Hu, Q.; Seidl, C.; Leps, C.; Drude, N.; Möckel, D.; Rijcken, C.; Lammers, T.; et al. Polymeric Nanoparticles with Neglectable Protein Corona. *Small* **2020**, *16*, 1907574. [CrossRef]
5. Schnorr, J.M.; Swager, T.M. Emerging Applications of Carbon Nanotubes†. *Chem. Mater.* **2011**, *23*, 646–657. [CrossRef]
6. De Volder, M.F.L.; Tawfick, S.H.; Baughman, R.H.; Hart, A.J. Carbon Nanotubes: Present and Future Commercial Applications. *Science* **2013**, *339*, 535–539. [CrossRef]
7. Sehrawat, P.; Julien, C.; Islam, S.S. Carbon nanotubes in Li-ion batteries: A review. *Mater. Sci. Eng. B* **2016**, *213*, 12–40. [CrossRef]
8. Rao, R.; Pint, C.L.; Islam, A.E.; Weatherup, R.S.; Hofmann, S.; Meshot, E.R.; Wu, F.; Zhou, C.; Dee, N.; Amama, P.B.; et al. Carbon Nanotubes and Related Nanomaterials: Critical Advances and Challenges for Synthesis toward Mainstream Commercial Applications. *ACS Nano* **2018**, *12*, 11756–11784. [CrossRef]
9. Petersen, E.J.; Zhang, L.; Mattison, N.T.; O'Carroll, D.M.; Whelton, A.J.; Uddin, N.; Nguyen, T.; Huang, Q.; Henry, T.B.; Holbrook, R.D.; et al. Potential release pathways, environmental fate, and ecological risks of carbon nanotubes. *Environ. Sci. Technol.* **2011**, *45*, 9837–9856. [CrossRef]
10. Sweeney, S.; Grandolfo, D.; Ruenraroengsak, P.; Tetley, T.D. Functional consequences for primary human alveolar macrophages following treatment with long, but not short, multiwalled carbon nanotubes. *Int. J. Nanomed.* **2015**, *10*, 3115–3129.
11. Allegri, M.; Perivoliotis, D.K.; Bianchi, M.G.; Chiu, M.; Pagliaro, A.; Koklioti, M.A.; Trompeta, A.-F.A.; Bergamaschi, E.; Bussolati, O.; Charitidis, C.A. Toxicity determinants of multi-walled carbon nanotubes: The relationship between functionalization and agglomeration. *Toxicol. Rep.* **2016**, *3*, 230–243. [CrossRef]
12. Wang, R.; Lee, M.; Kinghorn, K.; Hughes, T.; Chuckaree, I.; Lohray, R.; Chow, E.; Pantano, P.; Draper, R. Quantitation of cell-associated carbon nanotubes: Selective binding and accumulation of carboxylated carbon nanotubes by macrophages. *Nanotoxicology* **2018**, *12*, 677–690. [CrossRef]
13. Brown, M.S.; Goldstein, J.L. Lipoprotein Metabolism in the Macrophage: Implications for Cholesterol Deposition in Atherosclerosis. *Annu. Rev. Biochem.* **1983**, *52*, 223–261. [CrossRef]
14. Kingsley, D.M.; Krieger, M. Receptor-mediated endocytosis of low density lipoprotein: Somatic cell mutants define multiple genes required for expression of surface-receptor activity. *Proc. Natl. Acad. Sci. USA* **1984**, *81*, 5454–5458. [CrossRef]
15. PrabhuDas, M.R.; Baldwin, C.L.; Bollyky, P.L.; Bowdish, D.M.E.; Drickamer, K.; Febbraio, M.; Herz, J.; Kobzik, L.; Krieger, M.; Loike, J.; et al. A Consensus Definitive Classification of Scavenger Receptors and Their Roles in Health and Disease. *J. Immunol.* **2017**, *198*, 3775–3789. [CrossRef]
16. Dutta, D.; Sundaram, S.K.; Teeguarden, J.G.; Riley, B.J.; Fifield, L.S.; Jacobs, J.M.; Addleman, S.R.; Kaysen, G.A.; Moudgil, B.M.; Weber, T.J. Adsorbed proteins influence the biological activity and molecular targeting of nanomaterials. *Toxicol. Sci.* **2007**, *100*, 303–315. [CrossRef]
17. Singh, R.P.; Das, M.; Thakare, V.; Jain, S. Functionalization density dependent toxicity of oxidized multiwalled carbon nanotubes in a murine macrophage cell line. *Chem. Res. Toxicol.* **2012**, *25*, 2127–2137. [CrossRef]

18. Wang, X.; Guo, J.; Chen, T.; Nie, H.; Wang, H.; Zang, J.; Cui, X.; Jia, G. Multi-walled carbon nanotubes induce apoptosis via mitochondrial pathway and scavenger receptor. *Toxicol. In Vitro* **2012**, *26*, 799–806. [CrossRef]
19. Gao, N.; Zhang, Q.; Mu, Q.; Bai, Y.; Li, L.; Zhou, H.; Butch, E.R.; Powell, T.B.; Snyder, S.E.; Jiang, G.; et al. Steering carbon nanotubes to scavenger receptor recognition by nanotube surface chemistry modification partially alleviates NFκB activation and reduces its immunotoxicity. *ACS Nano* **2011**, *5*, 4581–4591. [CrossRef]
20. Hirano, S.; Fujitani, Y.; Furuyama, A.; Kanno, S. Macrophage receptor with collagenous structure (MARCO) is a dynamic adhesive molecule that enhances uptake of carbon nanotubes by CHO-K1 Cells. *Toxicol. Appl. Pharmacol.* **2012**, *259*, 96–103. [CrossRef]
21. Wang, R.; Lohray, R.; Chow, E.; Gangupantula, P.; Smith, L.; Draper, R. Selective Uptake of Carboxylated Multi-Walled Carbon Nanotubes by Class A Type 1 Scavenger Receptors and Impaired Phagocytosis in Alveolar Macrophages. *Nanomaterials* **2020**, *10*, 2417. [CrossRef]
22. Braun, E.I.; Pantano, P. The importance of an extensive elemental analysis of single-walled carbon nanotube soot. *Carbon* **2014**, *77*, 912–919. [CrossRef] [PubMed]
23. Huynh, M.T.; Veyan, J.F.; Pham, H.; Rahman, R.; Yousuf, S.; Brown, A.; Lin, J.; Balkus, K.J., Jr.; Diwakara, S.D.; Smaldone, R.A.; et al. The Importance of Evaluating the Lot-to-Lot Batch Consistency of Commercial Multi-Walled Carbon Nanotube Products. *Nanomaterials* **2020**, *10*, 1930. [CrossRef] [PubMed]
24. Ashkenas, J.; Penman, M.; Vasile, E.; Acton, S.; Freeman, M.; Krieger, M. Structures and high and low affinity ligand binding properties of murine type I and type II macrophage scavenger receptors. *J. Lipid Res.* **1993**, *34*, 983–1000. [CrossRef]
25. Wang, R.; Meredith, N.A.; Lee Jr., M.; Deutsch, D.; Miadzvedskaya, L.; Braun, E.; Pantano, P.; Harper, S.; Draper, R. Toxicity assessment and bioaccumulation in zebrafish embryos exposed to carbon nanotubes suspended in Pluronic® F-108. *Nanotoxicology* **2016**, *10*, 689–698. [CrossRef]
26. Nakata, T. Destruction of challenged endotoxin in a dry heat oven. *PDA J. Pharm. Sci. Technol.* **1994**, *48*, 59–63.
27. Wang, R.; Hughes, T.; Beck, S.; Vakil, S.; Li, S.; Pantano, P.; Draper, R.K. Generation of toxic degradation products by sonication of Pluronic® dispersants: Implications for nanotoxicity testing. *Nanotoxicology* **2013**, *7*, 1272–1281. [CrossRef]
28. Wang, R.; Mikoryak, C.; Li, S.; Bushdiecker 2nd, D.; Musselman, I.H.; Pantano, P.; Draper, R.K. Cytotoxicity screening of single-walled carbon nanotubes: Detection and removal of cytotoxic contaminants from carboxylated carbon nanotubes. *Mol. Pharm.* **2011**, *8*, 1351–1361. [CrossRef]
29. Wang, R.; Mikoryak, C.; Chen, E.; Li, S.; Pantano, P.; Draper, R.K. Gel electrophoresis method to measure the concentration of single-walled carbon nanotubes extracted from biological tissue. *Anal. Chem.* **2009**, *81*, 2944–2952. [CrossRef]
30. Krieger, M.; Herz, J. Structures and functions of multiligand lipoprotein receptors: Macrophage scavenger receptors and LDL receptor-related protein (LRP). *Annu. Rev. Biochem.* **1994**, *63*, 601–637. [CrossRef]
31. Andersson, L.; Freeman, M.W. Functional Changes in Scavenger Receptor Binding Conformation Are Induced by Charge Mutants Spanning the Entire Collagen Domain. *J. Biol. Chem.* **1998**, *273*, 19592–19601. [CrossRef] [PubMed]
32. Martínez, V.G.; Moestrup, S.K.; Holmskov, U.; Mollenhauer, J.; Lozano, F. The Conserved Scavenger Receptor Cysteine-Rich Superfamily in Therapy and Diagnosis. *Pharmacol. Rev.* **2011**, *63*, 967–1000. [CrossRef] [PubMed]
33. Canton, J.; Neculai, D.; Grinstein, S. Scavenger receptors in homeostasis and immunity. *Nat. Rev. Immunol.* **2013**, *13*, 621–634. [CrossRef]
34. Fleischer, C.C.; Payne, C.K. Nanoparticle–Cell Interactions: Molecular Structure of the Protein Corona and Cellular Outcomes. *Acc. Chem. Res.* **2014**, *47*, 2651–2659. [CrossRef] [PubMed]
35. Fleischer, C.C.; Payne, C.K. Secondary Structure of Corona Proteins Determines the Cell Surface Receptors Used by Nanoparticles. *J. Phys. Chem. B* **2014**, *118*, 14017–14026. [CrossRef] [PubMed]
36. Mortimer, G.M.; Butcher, N.J.; Musumeci, A.W.; Deng, Z.J.; Martin, D.J.; Minchin, R.F. Cryptic Epitopes of Albumin Determine Mononuclear Phagocyte System Clearance of Nanomaterials. *ACS Nano* **2014**, *8*, 3357–3366. [CrossRef]
37. Wong, S.S.; Joselevich, E.; Woolley, A.T.; Cheung, C.L.; Lieber, C.M. Covalently functionalized nanotubes as nanometre-sized probes in chemistry and biology. *Nature* **1998**, *394*, 52–55. [CrossRef]
38. Chen, J.; Hamon, M.A.; Hu, H.; Chen, Y.; Rao, A.M.; Eklund, P.C.; Haddon, R.C. Solution properties of single-walled carbon nanotubes. *Science* **1998**, *282*, 95–98. [CrossRef]
39. Sun, Y.P.; Fu, K.; Lin, Y.; Huang, W. Functionalized carbon nanotubes: Properties and applications. *Acc. Chem. Res.* **2002**, *35*, 1096–1104. [CrossRef] [PubMed]
40. Zhang, J.; Zou, H.; Qing, Q.; Yang, Y.; Li, Q.; Liu, Z.; Guo, X.; Du, Z. Effect of chemical oxidation on the structure of single-walled carbon nanotubes. *J. Phys. Chem. B* **2003**, *107*, 3712–3718. [CrossRef]
41. Frise, A.E.; Edri, E.; Furó, I.; Regev, O. Protein Dispersant Binding on Nanotubes Studied by NMR Self-Diffusion and Cryo-TEM Techniques. *J. Phys. Chem. Lett.* **2010**, *1*, 1414–1419. [CrossRef]
42. Lou, K.; Zhu, Z.; Zhang, H.; Wang, Y.; Wang, X.; Cao, J. Comprehensive studies on the nature of interaction between carboxylated multi-walled carbon nanotubes and bovine serum albumin. *Chem.-Biol. Interact.* **2016**, *243*, 54–61. [CrossRef] [PubMed]
43. Zani, I.; Stephen, S.; Mughal, N.; Russell, D.; Homer-Vanniasinkam, S.; Wheatcroft, S.; Ponnambalam, S. Scavenger receptor structure and function in health and disease. *Cells* **2015**, *4*, 178. [CrossRef]
44. Doi, T.; Higashino, K.; Kurihara, Y.; Wada, Y.; Miyazaki, T.; Nakamura, H.; Uesugi, S.; Imanishi, T.; Kawabe, Y.; Itakura, H. Charged collagen structure mediates the recognition of negatively charged macromolecules by macrophage scavenger receptors. *J. Biol. Chem.* **1993**, *268*, 2126–2133. [CrossRef]

45. Cheng, C.; Hu, Z.; Cao, L.; Peng, C.; He, Y. The scavenger receptor SCARA1 (CD204) recognizes dead cells through spectrin. *J. Biol. Chem.* **2019**, *294*, 18881–18897. [CrossRef] [PubMed]
46. Yu, B.; Cheng, C.; Wu, Y.; Guo, L.; Kong, D.; Zhang, Z.; Wang, Y.; Zheng, E.; Liu, Y.; He, Y. Interactions of ferritin with scavenger receptor class A members. *J. Biol. Chem.* **2020**, *295*, 15727–15741. [CrossRef] [PubMed]
47. Chen, Y.; Sankala, M.; Ojala, J.R.M.; Sun, Y.; Tuuttila, A.; Isenman, D.E.; Tryggvason, K.; Pikkarainen, T. A Phage Display Screen and Binding Studies with Acetylated Low Density Lipoprotein Provide Evidence for the Importance of the Scavenger Receptor Cysteine-rich (SRCR) Domain in the Ligand-binding Function of MARCO. *J. Biol. Chem.* **2006**, *281*, 12767–12775. [CrossRef] [PubMed]
48. Whelan, F.J.; Meehan, C.J.; Golding, G.B.; McConkey, B.J.; E Bowdish, D.M. The evolution of the class A scavenger receptors. *BMC Evol. Biol.* **2012**, *12*, 227. [CrossRef]
49. Ojala, J.R.M.; Pikkarainen, T.; Tuuttila, A.; Sandalova, T.; Tryggvason, K. Crystal Structure of the Cysteine-rich Domain of Scavenger Receptor MARCO Reveals the Presence of a Basic and an Acidic Cluster That Both Contribute to Ligand Recognition. *J. Biol. Chem.* **2007**, *282*, 16654–16666. [CrossRef]
50. Heit, B.; Kim, H.; Cosío, G.; Castaño, D.; Collins, R.; Lowell, C.A.; Kain, K.C.; Trimble, W.S.; Grinstein, S. Multimolecular Signaling Complexes Enable Syk-Mediated Signaling of CD36 Internalization. *Dev. Cell* **2013**, *24*, 372–383. [CrossRef]
51. Turabekova, M.; Rasulev, B.; Theodore, M.; Jackman, J.; Leszczynska, D.; Leszczynski, J. Immunotoxicity of nanoparticles: A computational study suggests that CNTs and C60 fullerenes might be recognized as pathogens by Toll-like receptors. *Nanoscale* **2014**, *6*, 3488–3495. [CrossRef] [PubMed]
52. Mukherjee, S.P.; Bondarenko, O.; Kohonen, P.; Andón, F.T.; Brzicová, T.; Gessner, I.; Mathur, S.; Bottini, M.; Calligari, P.; Stella, L.; et al. Macrophage sensing of single-walled carbon nanotubes via Toll-like receptors. *Sci. Rep.* **2018**, *8*, 1115. [CrossRef] [PubMed]

nanomaterials

Article

Interaction between Macrophages and Nanoparticles: In Vitro 3D Cultures for the Realistic Assessment of Inflammatory Activation and Modulation of Innate Memory

Benjamin J. Swartzwelter [1,†], Alessandro Verde [1], Laura Rehak [2], Mariusz Madej [1,‡], Victor. F. Puntes [3], Anna Chiara De Luca [1], Diana Boraschi [1,4,*] and Paola Italiani [1,4,*]

1 Institute of Biochemistry and Cell Biology, National Research Council, 80131 Napoli, Italy; swartzwe@colorado.edu (B.J.S.); alessandro.verde@ibbc.cnr.it (A.V.); mariusz.madej@ocello.nl (M.M.); annachiara.deluca@ibbc.cnr.it (A.C.D.L.)
2 Athena Biomedical Innovations, 00100 Roma, Italy; laurarehak@gmail.com
3 Institut Català de Nanociència i Nanotecnologia (ICN2), CSIC and The Barcelona Institute of Science and Technology (BIST), Campus UAB, 08193 Bellaterra, Barcelona, Spain; victor.puntes@icn2.cat
4 Stazione Zoologica Anton Dohrn, 80121 Napoli, Italy
* Correspondence: diana.boraschi@ibbc.cnr.it (D.B.); paola.italiani@ibbc.cnr.it (P.I.)
† Current address: Department of Microbiology, Immunology and Pathology, Colorado State University, Fort Collins, CO 80521, USA.
‡ Current address: OcellO B.V., 2333 CH Leiden, The Netherlands.

Abstract: Understanding the modes of interaction between human monocytes/macrophages and engineered nanoparticles is the basis for assessing particle safety, in terms of activation of innate/inflammatory reactions, and their possible exploitation for medical applications. In vitro assessment of nanoparticle-macrophage interaction allows for examining the response of primary human cells, but the conventional 2D cultures do not reproduce the three-dimensional spacing of a tissue and the interaction of macrophages with the extracellular tissue matrix, conditions that shape macrophage recognition capacity and reactivity. Here, we have compared traditional 2D cultures with cultures on a 3D collagen matrix for evaluating the capacity gold nanoparticles to induce monocyte activation and subsequent innate memory in human blood monocytes in comparison to bacterial LPS. Results show that monocytes react to stimuli almost in the same way in 2D and 3D cultures in terms of production of TNFα and IL-6, but that notable differences are found when IL-8 and IL-1Ra are examined, in particular in the recall/memory response of primed cells to a second stimulation, with the 3D cultures showing cell activation and memory effects of nanoparticles better. In addition, the response variations in monocytes/macrophages from different donors point towards a personalized assessment of the nanoparticle effects on macrophage activation.

Keywords: monocytes; macrophages; gold nanoparticles; in vitro models; innate immunity; inflammation; innate memory; 2D cultures; 3D cultures

Citation: Swartzwelter, B.J.; Verde, A.; Rehak, L.; Madej, M.; Puntes, V.F.; De Luca, A.C.; Boraschi, D.; Italiani, P. Interaction between Macrophages and Nanoparticles: In Vitro 3D Cultures for the Realistic Assessment of Inflammatory Activation and Modulation of Innate Memory. *Nanomaterials* **2021**, *11*, 207. https://doi.org/10.3390/nano11010207

Received: 22 December 2020
Accepted: 13 January 2021
Published: 15 January 2021

1. Introduction

The interaction of engineered nanoparticles (NPs) with the immune system is a key element both in the assessment of nanotoxicity and in the development of nanomedicines and nanomedical devices [1,2]. Possible changes in immune functions upon interaction with NPs may affect the defensive capability of exposed organisms, thereby increasing their susceptibility to infections and diseases. The immune mechanisms that are principally involved in the interaction with NPs are those of innate immunity, the ancient highly conserved defensive system shared by all organisms, from plants to humans [3]. In humans, innate immunity is mainly based on the surveillance action of a number of cell types, in particular the mononuclear phagocytes (monocytes and macrophages) that populate every tissue in the body with the task of recognizing and eliminating possible threats [4].

Macrophages are resident in tissues and are deputed to phagocytosis and efferocytosis, being a little reactive to stimulation (e.g., with bacteria) to avoid mounting a potentially destructive inflammatory reaction [5,6]. On the other hand, when a potential danger is identified, macrophages and other tissue cells produce chemotactic factors that attract effector cells from the blood. Monocytes are among these cells, and participate in the effector phase of inflammation/innate defence by efficiently reacting to foreign agents to produce a number of inflammation-related factors, including both inflammatory cytokines such as TNFα and anti-inflammatory agents able to turn off the reaction when the danger is eliminated [6,7]. Many studies have addressed the possible inflammatory/toxic effects of engineered NPs by examining their interaction with monocytes and macrophages. These studies yielded variable results, and their relevance in predicting effects in human beings is unclear. Many studies have been performed with NPs that were not tested for the presence of endotoxin, a ubiquitous bacterial contaminant that cannot be eliminated by sterilization and that is among the most effective activators of monocytes/macrophages [8], a fact that may lead to misinterpretation of the NP inflammatory effect results. In vivo studies are generally performed in the mouse, an animal that, like human beings, possesses both innate and adaptive immunity but that presents a number of important immune-related differences from humans [9,10]. In vitro studies are largely based on transformed macrophage-like cell lines, which ensure repeatability of results but do not reproduce the behaviour of normal non-tumour cells. Studies with human primary monocytes and monocyte-derived macrophages can mimic several of the conditions of real life, although in many cases they miss the important interaction of these cells with their tissue microenvironment. We have previously established a complex kinetic in vitro model that reproduces the entire course of an inflammatory reaction, as it is experienced by human monocytes that enter an inflamed tissue [11]. With this model, we have described the lack of toxicity/direct inflammatory effect of a number of engineered NPs (Au, Ag, Fe_xO_y), used at realistic concentrations, tested for the lack of endotoxin contamination and coated with a biocorona of human serum, as it would happen to NPs entering a human tissue [12,13]. The fact that NPs do not have a direct effect on monocytes/macrophages in inducing inflammation does not exclude that they could have other much subtler effects in modulating their functions. It is known that innate immune cells can develop memory, i.e., reprogram their responses to challenges based on their previous exposure experience [14–17]. Innate memory aims at making monocytes/macrophages better able to cope with subsequent challenges after an initial exposure and is the most important immune defensive mechanism in plants and invertebrates [18–20]. In some cases, however, innate memory can lead to a pathological exacerbation of secondary reactions [21–23]. While our understanding of innate memory is still largely incomplete, it is tempting to speculate that engineered NPs might be used for a targeted reprogramming of innate immunity for preventive and therapeutic scopes, such as in vaccination and immunotherapy [24–27]. Few recent studies show that indeed NPs may prime human monocytes and vertebrate/invertebrate macrophages and induce a modification of their response to a subsequent inflammatory challenge [28–32]. In this study, we have examined the memory-inducing capacity of AuNPs on human primary monocytes to define the most suitable conditions for a realistic evaluation. The choice of AuNPs is based on the fact that they are considered inert and harmless and are therefore largely used in many different clinical applications, raising our interest in examining the possibility that they may nevertheless display immunomodulatory effects. Thus, we have assessed the individual response of cells from six individual donors, to assess the impact of the "immunobiography", i.e., the previous history of exposure, on monocyte reactivity and memory [33]. We have measured the production of four different types of inflammation-related factors to better understand their mutual balance in the overall response; these are two inflammatory factors (TNFα and IL-6), an alarmin (the chemokine IL-8) and an anti-inflammatory cytokine (IL-1Ra). Lastly, we have compared the cell functions (primary activation, induction of memory, memory response) of monocytes/macrophages cultured in conventional 2D plates with those of cells seeded in a 3D collagen matrix that represents the architecture of a tissue (skin in this case) and its components. The results show that the production of inflammatory factors is not substantially different in cells cultured in 2D vs. 3D, whereas there is a more abundant production of the alarmin and the anti-inflammatory factor in 3D cultures. The results also show the capacity of AuNPs to induce innate memory was evident in 3D cultures, with the effects being strongly donor-dependent.

2. Materials and Methods

2.1. Synthesis and Characterization of AuNP

2.1.1. AuNP Synthesis and Purification

Synthesis of AuNPs was conducted using wet chemistry methods as previously described [34]. Briefly, 1 mL of 25 mM $HAuCl_4$ was rapidly added to 150 mL of a boiling aqueous solution of sodium citrate 2.2 mM. The formation of AuNPs (~10 nm) occurred in a few minutes, and was followed by growth-inducing steps, consisting of the addition of $HAuCl_4$ until reaching the desired NP size. Au NPs of 12 nm diameter were used in this study. Sodium citrate tribasic dihydrate (≥99% purity), gold (III) chloride trihydrate $HAuCl_4{\cdot}3H_2O$ (99.9% purity) were from Sigma-Aldrich, Inc. (St. Louis, MO, USA). All reagents were used as received without further purification, and all glass material was sterilized and dehydrogenated in an oven prior to use. Pyrogen-free milli-Q water was used in the preparation of all solutions. AuNPs were purified by centrifugation to discard byproducts and contaminants, then NPs were resuspended in a solution of 2.2 mM sodium citrate (final pH = 6.4) and stored at 4 °C in the dark.

2.1.2. Nanoparticle Characterization

NP characterisation was performed as previously described [34]. Briefly, STEM (scanning transmission electron microscopy) images were acquired with an FEI Magellan XHR scanning electron microscope (SEM) (FEI, Hillsboro, OR, USA), operated in transmission mode at 20 kV. UV-Vis spectra of AuNPs in sodium citrate were acquired at room temperature using a Shimadzu UV-2400 spectrophotometer (SSI; Kyoto, Japan), reading a spectral range from 300 to 750 nm. The NP hydrodynamic diameter and Z-potential were acquired by dynamic light scattering and laser doppler velocimetry, using a Malvern Zetasizer Nano ZS instrument (Malvern Panalytical Ltd., Malvern, UK) equipped with a light source wavelength of 632.8 nm and a fixed scattering angle of 173°.

2.2. LAL Assay

The endotoxin contamination of the NPs was assessed using the chromogenic Pyrochrome LAL assay (Associates of Cape Cod, Inc.; East Falmouth, MA, USA), according to an optimized protocol that included a number of interference controls [35]. The endotoxin contamination in the AuNPs used in this study was 9.0 EU/mg, which excluded the possibility that endotoxin could activate monocytes in the culture at the NP concentration used (1 µg/mL, corresponding to an endotoxin contamination of 0.009 EU/mL, and 10 µg/mL, corresponding to an endotoxin contamination of 0.09 EU/mL, with monocyte activation detectable above 0.1 EU/mL) [36].

2.3. Human Monocyte Isolation and Culture

Blood was obtained from healthy donors, upon informed consent and in agreement with the Declaration of Helsinki. The protocol was approved by the Regional Ethics Committee for Clinical Experimentation of the Tuscany Region (Ethics Committee Register n. 14,914 of 16 May 2019). Donors were between 25 and 35 years of age, healthy, non-obese, no smokers, not taking medications. Donors 5 and 6 were female, donors 1 and 3 were of Indo-Aryan ethnicity, and donors 2 and 4–6 were of Caucasian ethnicity. Monocytes were isolated by CD14 positive selection with magnetic microbeads (Miltenyi Biotec, Bergisch Gladbach, Germany) from peripheral blood mononuclear cells (PBMC), obtained by Ficoll-Paque gradient density separation (GE Healthcare, Bio-Sciences AB, Uppsala, Sweden).

Monocyte preparations used in the experiments were >95% viable and >95% pure (assessed by trypan blue exclusion and cytosmears).

Monocytes were cultured in culture medium (RPMI 1640 + Glutamax-I; GIBCO by Life Technologies, Paisley, UK) supplemented with 50 µg/mL gentamicin sulfate (GIBCO) and 5% heat-inactivated human AB serum (Sigma-Aldrich, Inc.). Cells (5×10^5) were seeded in a final volume of 0.5 mL in control wells of 24-well flat-bottom plates (well internal diameter 15.6 mm; Corning® Costar®; Corning Inc. Life Sciences, Oneonta, NY, USA), or in wells that contained a round clipping of a 3D collagen matrix (diameter 15.4 mm; stabilized collagen type I from decellularized bovine skin, pore size around 100 µm, thickness 2 mm; clinically used for dermal regeneration; Nevelia®, Symathese Biomateriaux, Chaponost, France), obtained with a puncheon tool. Characterisation of monocytes in 3D cultures showed that they can undergo differentiation into macrophages (both spontaneous and CSF-1 mediated) as expected, and express all the phenotypic and functional markers of resting, M1 and M2 macrophages, depending on the applied stimuli (data not shown).

2.4. Cell Activation and Induction of Innate Memory

After overnight resting, monocytes were exposed for 24 h to AuNPs (1 µg/mL) or LPS (1 ng/mL; from *E. coli* O55:B5; Sigma-Aldrich, Inc.) or left untreated (control). AuNPs were pre-incubated in 50% human AB serum for 60 min at 37 °C, before addition to monocyte cultures. This procedure allowed for the formation of a physiologically relevant biocorona that prevented particle aggregation in the culture medium [37]. Ion release and reduction of NP size were not detectable after 24 h in culture medium without monocytes, thereby excluding particle dissolution (data not shown) [38]. After supernatant collection, cells were washed and cultured with fresh culture medium for an additional 6 days (one medium change) to allow the extinction of the activation induced by the previous stimulation. After the resting phase, the supernatant was collected, and cells were challenged for an additional 24 h with fresh medium alone or containing a ten-fold higher concentration of LPS (10 ng/mL). All supernatants (after the first stimulation, after the resting phase and after the challenge phase) were frozen at −20 °C for subsequent cytokine analysis. By visual inspection, cell viability and cell number did not substantially change in response to the different treatments.

2.5. Cytokine Analysis

The levels of the inflammatory cytokines TNFα and IL-6, of the chemokine IL-8 and of the anti-inflammatory factor IL-1Ra were assessed by ELISA (R&D Systems, Minneapolis, MN, USA). The absorbance of the assay wavelength was measured at 450 nm (subtracting background present at 550 nm) using a Cytation 3 imaging reader (BioTek, Winooski, VT, USA).

2.6. Statistical Analysis

Data from cytokine measurements have been analysed using the GraphPad Prism9 software (GraphPad Inc., La Jolla, CA, USA), and are presented in terms of ng/10^6 plated monocytes. Results are reported as mean ± SD of values from 2–8 replicates from the same donor or as median ± quartiles of values from different donors. The statistical significance of differences is indicated by p values, calculated using a paired one-tailed non-parametric Wilcoxon signed-rank test.

3. Results

3.1. Gold Nanoparticle Characterisation

Gold nanoparticles (AuNPs) used in this study were synthesized in endotoxin-free conditions and characterized as described in Materials and Methods. The master batch contained 6×10^{12} monodispersed particles/mL of sodium citrate 2.2 mM (in endotoxin-free water) at pH 6.4, corresponding to 0.5 mM Au (0.1 mg/mL) and to a total surface area of 2.6×10^{15} nm^2/mL. AuNPs showed a diameter of 11.8 ± 0.8 nm by STEM, a hydrodynamic diameter of 15.1 ± 3.7 nm by DSL, an absorption peak at 516 nm by UV-VIS, a conductivity of 0.793 mS/cm and a Z-potential of −47.0 ± 5.0 mV. The main NP characteristics are shown in Figure 1.

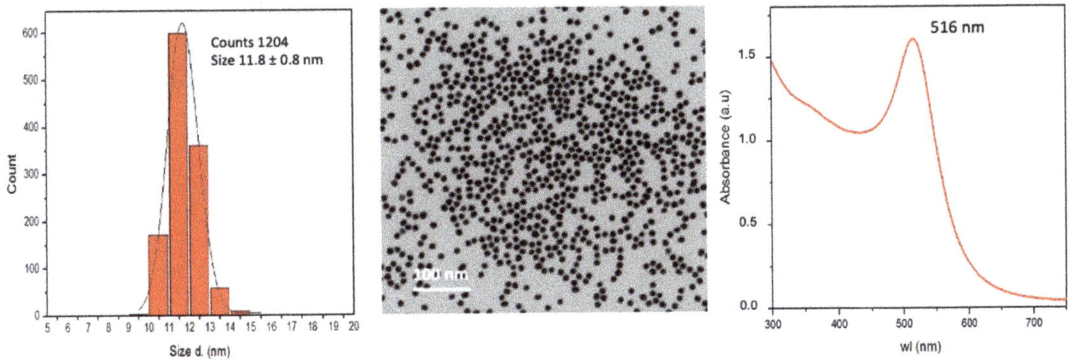

Figure 1. Main characteristics of AuNPs. (**Left**): size distribution by STEM; (**Centre**): STEM image; (**Right**): absorbance peak via UV-VIS.

Evaluation of the endotoxin contamination of AuNPs showed limited contamination (9.0 EU/mg). Since endotoxin could directly activate human monocytes in vitro at concentrations above 0.1 EU/mL [36,39], we used AuNP concentrations with endotoxin contamination below such threshold. After preliminary experiments, we selected 1 μg/mL AuNPs as priming concentration (containing 0.009 EU/mL endotoxin) and the 10-fold higher concentration of 10 μg/mL as challenge (containing 0.09 EU/mL endotoxin). Particles were pre-incubated for 60 min in 50% heat-inactivated human AB serum at 37 °C before being added to cells in culture to allow for the formation of a coating reproducing the naturally occurring biocorona when NPs come in contact with biological fluids. This procedure did not cause particle agglomeration, but instead it promoted monodispersity when added to the culture medium [37,40].

3.2. *In Vitro Development of Macrophage Innate Memory in 2D vs. 3D Cultures*

Purified human blood monocytes were placed in culture either in regular 2D plates or on top of a 3D collagen matrix, as described in Materials and Methods. Cells were either left untreated or exposed for 24 h to LPS or AuNPs. The primary cell activation was measured in terms of production, in the 24 h supernatant, of the inflammatory cytokines TNFα and IL-6, of the chemokine IL-8, and of the anti-inflammatory cytokine IL-1Ra. After supernatant removal and elimination of stimuli, cells were incubated in fresh medium for 6 days, to allow for return to baseline conditions. The 6-day supernatant was removed, and cells were exposed to either fresh medium (control) or LPS for an additional 24 h to assess memory responses, again in terms of cytokine production.

Cells from six donors were individually tested in parallel in 2D and 3D cultures for their primary and memory responses. SEM images in Figure 2 show the morphology of cells in 3D cultures after 24 h-stimulation with LPS (strong activation; upper right) as compared to cells exposed to medium or AuNPs (upper left) and to unprimed and LPS-primed cells after 6 days of culture (return to quiescent-like morphology; lower panels).

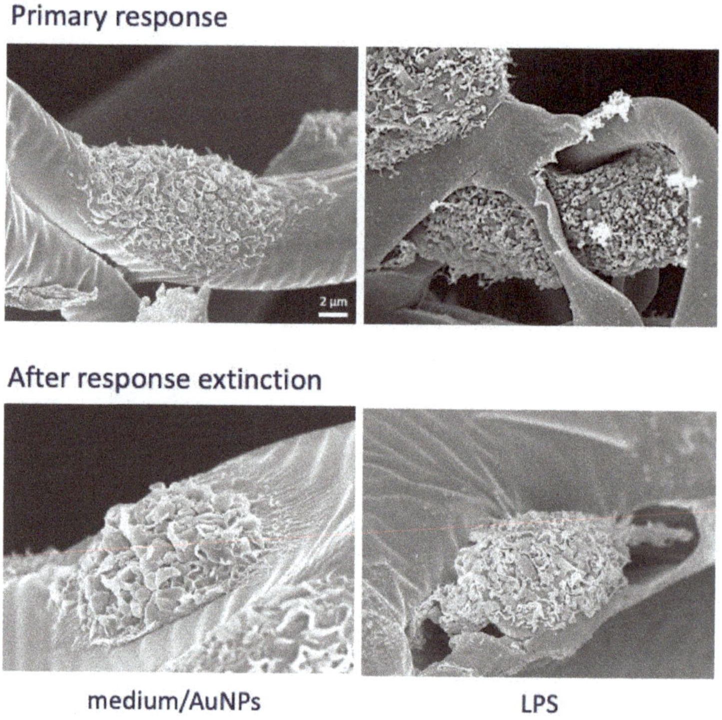

Figure 2. SEM images of monocytes in 3D culture. Upper panels: monocytes exposed for 24 h to culture medium alone or containing AuNPs (showing identical morphology; (**left**)) or LPS (**right**). Lower panels: monocytes primed with either culture medium alone or containing AuNPs (**left**) or LPS (**right**) observed after 6 days of resting in the absence of stimuli.

3.3. *Differences in the Primary Monocyte Reactivity in 2D vs. 3D Cultures*

When assessing the capacity of fresh monocytes to react to LPS and AuNPs in terms of cytokine production, no meaningful differences were in general observed between cells in 2D vs. 3D cultures, with some variability observed from donor to donor. Data in Figure 3 show that LPS significantly activates the production of the inflammatory cytokines TNFα and IL-6 and of the chemokine IL-8, while the levels of the anti-inflammatory factor IL-1Ra are already high in unstimulated cells and not substantially changed by LPS stimulation. AuNPs do not show direct activating capacity, in agreement with previous observations [12,28,39]. The individual donors' data are reported in Table S1.

3.4. *Extinction of Inflammatory Activation in Macrophages Six Days after Priming*

After the primary stimulation, monocytes were washed to eliminate the residual stimuli and cultured for an additional six days in fresh medium to allow for the extinction of their activation state and return to a quiescent condition. During this period, cells differentiate to macrophages. Their activation state at the end of the resting period was assessed by measuring the spontaneous production of cytokines. As shown in Table S2, the production of the inflammatory cytokines TNFα and IL-6 is essentially zero both in 2D and 3D cultures, independently of the previous priming of cells (with medium, LPS or AuNPs), suggesting that these cells are not any longer in an inflammatory activation state. The production of the chemokine IL-8 is, however, detectable in 3D (but not in 2D cultures) in unprimed/AuNP-primed cells from 4/6 donors and in LPS-primed cells of all donors. LPS-primed cells displayed a generally higher spontaneous IL-8 production as compared to unprimed cells, while AuNP priming did not have substantial effects. Regarding the anti-inflammatory cytokine IL-1Ra, this was detectable at low levels in 2D cultures, while it was easily detectable in all 3D samples. IL-1Ra production was measurable in the unprimed macrophages from all donors at significant levels. Priming with either LPS or AuNPs variably but not substantially modulated the spontaneous production of the anti-inflammatory factor in each donor.

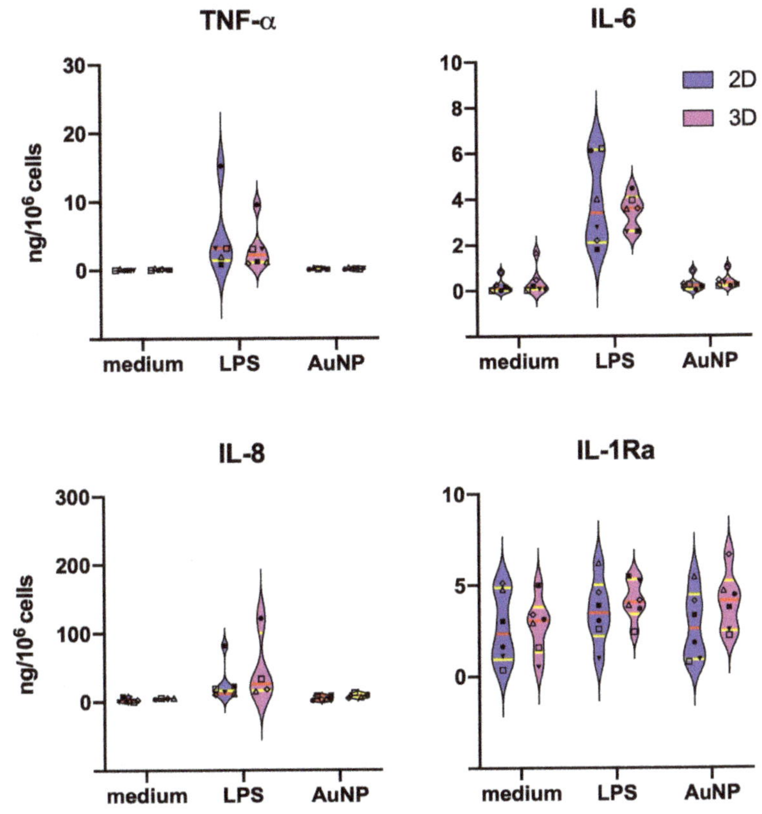

Figure 3. Primary cytokine production by monocytes in 2D vs. 3D culture. Production of the inflammatory cytokines TNFα and IL-6 (**upper panels**), of the chemokine IL-8 (**lower left panel**) and of the anti-inflammatory cytokine IL-1Ra (**lower right panel**) by monocytes of six individual donors stimulated for 24 h with culture medium alone (medium) or containing 1 ng/mL LPS (LPS) or 1 µg/mL AuNPs (AuNP). Parallel 2D (blue) and 3D (purple) cultures were established. Results are expressed in ng/10^6 cells. The violin plots represent the distribution of the individual donors' values in each experimental condition. The red line indicates the median value, and the yellow lines the first and third quartiles. Individual donors are represented with different symbols: ◇ donor 1; ■ donor 2; Δ donor 3; ▼ donor 4; □ donor 5; • donor 6. Statistical significance was assessed with the paired one-tailed non-parametric Wilcoxon signed-rank test. LPS stimulation induced a significant increase ($p < 0.05$) of TNFα, IL-6 and IL-8 vs. medium controls. All other differences, including the 2D vs. 3D comparisons, were not significant.

3.5. Secondary Response of Unprimed Macrophages

The memory response of macrophages that were previously exposed to culture medium alone (unprimed control), LPS or AuNP was examined, after six days of resting, upon a challenge with LPS. Challenge with AuNP was initially assessed as well (data not shown), but it turned out to be ineffective (no activation induced by AuNPs, as already observed in the primary response and in previous studies) [12,28,39], and therefore it was not further pursued. LPS challenge in unprimed control macrophages induced significant production of TNFα, IL-6, and IL-8, which was generally more pronounced in the 3D cultures (Figure 4). Again, the production of IL-1Ra was very low in 2D, while well measurable in 3D cultures. It is notable that, as in the primary response, LPS stimulation had relatively little effect on IL-1Ra production (Figure 4); however, with some donor-dependent variability (compare Tables S2 and S3 for individual data).

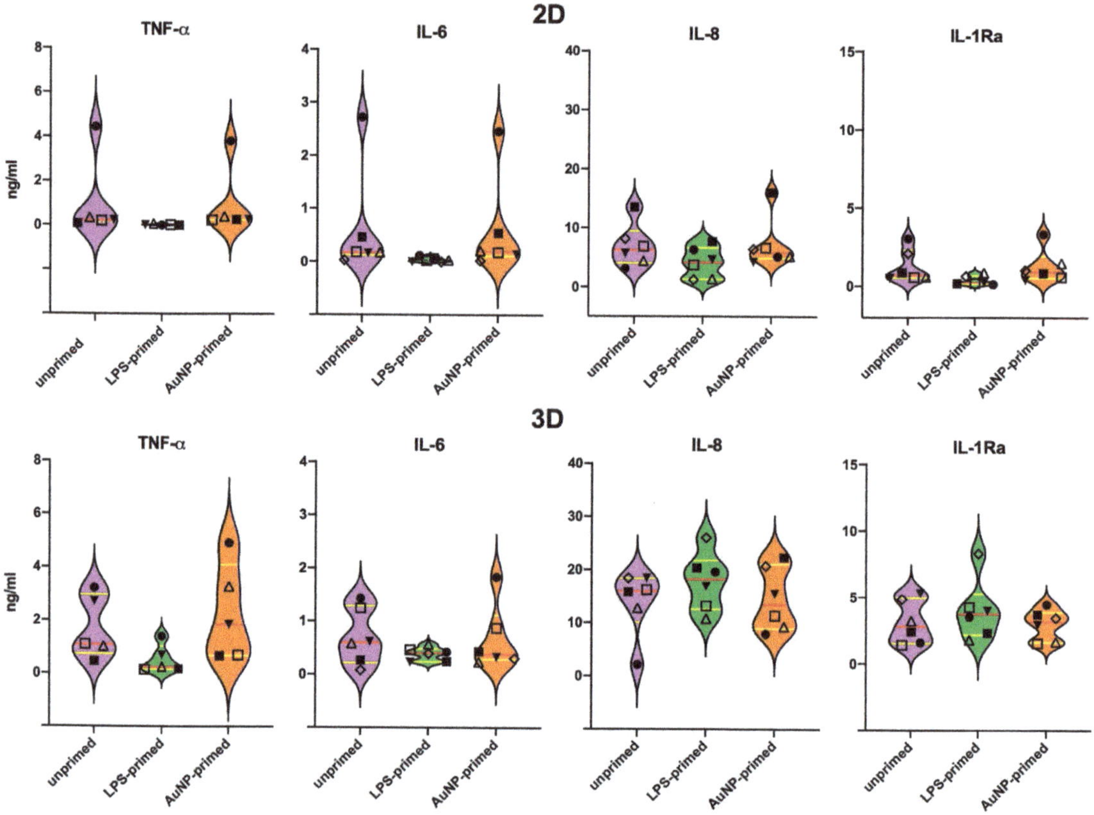

Figure 4. Secondary cytokine production by primed monocytes challenged with LPS in 2D vs. 3D culture. Production of the inflammatory cytokines TNFα and IL-6, the chemokine IL-8 and of the anti-inflammatory cytokine IL-1Ra by monocytes of six donors previously primed in vitro with culture medium alone (unprimed), LPS (LPS-primed) or AuNPs (AuNP-primed). After 24 h priming, cells were rested in culture for 6 days and then challenged with 10 ng/mL LPS for 24 h. Results obtained in 2D cultures are reported in the upper panels, while data from 3D cultures are reported in the lower panels. The violin plots represent the distribution of the individual donors' values in each experimental condition. The red line indicates the median value, and the yellow lines the first and third quartiles. Individual donors are represented with different symbols: ◇ donor 1; ■ donor 2; Δ donor 3; ▼ donor 4; □ donor 5; • donor 6. Statistical significance was assessed with the paired one-tailed non-parametric Wilcoxon signed-rank test, and show significant differences ($p < 0.05$) between unprimed and LPS-primed production of TNFα (2D and 3D), IL-6 (2D) and IL-1Ra (2D), while the differences between 2D and 3D were significant for IL-8 and IL-1Ra.

It should be noted that the response of macrophages to LPS, in terms of inflammatory cytokine production, is substantially less abundant compared to monocytes, whereas the quantitative response in terms of IL-8 and IL-1Ra was quite similar between macrophages and monocytes (Figure 4, Tables S1 and S3).

3.6. Memory Response of LPS-Primed Macrophages

Compared to unprimed cells, in LPS-primed macrophages, the production of TNFα in response to LPS was significantly decreased both in 2D and 3D cultures, in line with the expected tolerance effect of LPS priming (Figure 4). When looking at the individual data (Table S3), for IL-6 production, tolerance was detectable in 3/6 donors in 3D and in all six in 2D cultures, the overall difference being statistically significant only in the latter case (Figure 4). In the case of the chemokine IL-8, LPS priming did not induce a significant overall effect either in 2D or in 3D (Figure 4), although the individual reactivity varied between donors (Table S3). In 2D cultures, a partial decrease was observed in 2 donors and an increase was detectable in one, while in 3D samples LPS priming had no effect in 5/6 donors and increased the response to challenge in one (donor 6, the same as in 2D cultures) (Table S3). The memory response in terms of the production of the anti-inflammatory cytokine IL-1Ra could be better assessed in 3D cultures (as the IL-1Ra production in 2D cultures was very low) and was donor-dependent, with a partial potentiation in 2 donors, and a decrease in other two. Overall, LPS priming did not induce a significant change in IL-1Ra production (Figure 4). A notable difference between 2D and 3D cultures is in the quantitative production of IL-8 and IL-1Ra, substantially more abundant in 3D cultures, while the production of the inflammatory cytokines TNFα and IL-6 was only slightly higher in 3D cultures.

3.7. Memory Response of AuNP-Primed Macrophages

In AuNP-primed macrophages (Figure 4, Table S3), the challenge-induced TNFα production is modulated in a donor-specific fashion, with a difference between 2D and 3D cultures. Thus, while in 2D it seems that AuNP priming does not substantially influence the response to challenge, in 3D cultures a partial decrease of response is evident in 3 donors. A very similar picture can be observed for the production of the other inflammatory cytokine, IL-6, with a general lack of effect in 2D samples, whereas in 3D cultures two donors show partial potentiation and one partial tolerance. In the case of the chemokine IL-8, the results in 2D and 3D cultures were superimposable, with no substantial effect due to AuNP priming except for one donor (donor 6), in which priming induced a clear potentiation of the memory response. For the anti-inflammatory factor IL-1Ra, better detectable in 3D, AuNP priming could induce a partial tolerance response in one donor, a potentiated response in another one, and no significant changes in the others. Again, the memory effect seems to strongly depend on the donor.

4. Discussion

This study aimed at assessing whether human monocyte/macrophage reactivity in vitro can differ depending on the culture conditions. In particular, we compared conventional 2D cultures on flat plastic surfaces to 3D cultures in a biological matrix of collagen, derived from decellularized bovine skin and providing a mesh of collagen fibrils with pores around 100 µm. This matrix is used in clinical settings as dermal/epidermal substitute for repairing ulcers and was reportedly able to promote M2/healing macrophage phenotype, i.e., the default phenotype of resident macrophages in homeostatic conditions [40]. Cells seeded in the 3D matrix survived and differentiated as expected, and their sensitivity to activation stimuli was evident also from the morphological point of view (Figure 2). We used the two culture systems in comparison to assess the reactivity of human monocytes/macrophages to AuNPs, using the bacterial LPS as an activation benchmark and examining two important innate immune functions, i.e., the immediate inflammation-related response to the stimulation of fresh monocytes and the secondary reaction of monocyte-derived macrophages after previous priming (innate memory response). The results show that the primary response is not significantly different between 2D and 3D cultures (Figure 3) and that, in agreement with previous results [12,28,39], AuNPs do not induce a significant cell activation, opposite to the substantial induction of TNFα, IL-6 and IL-8 production in response to LPS. On the other hand, the production of the anti-inflammatory factor IL-1Ra is detectable at measurable levels in unstimulated cells and is not significantly varied in cells exposed to LPS or AuNPs. It is known that LPS can induce IL-1Ra production at later times as a feedback mechanism to shut down inflammation. Our data show a slight tendency towards increased IL-1Ra production to LPS, and also to AuNPs in 3D cultures, which, however, did not reach statistical significance due to the substantial donor-to-donor variability. Indeed, monocytes from some donors showed a clear increase while others did not, implying different response kinetics depending on the individual conditions.

While it is now clear that many NPs do not have the capacity for activating human monocytes if they are endotoxin-free [12,13,35,36,39], some data point to the possibility that they can prime monocytes and induce innate memory, which then changes the secondary reaction of cells to a subsequent stimulation [28–32]. We have examined the capacity of AuNPs to induce innate memory in monocytes from six different donors in 2D and 3D cultures. Innate memory is an important phenomenon of immune reprogramming that allows innate cells to react is a more efficient way to a challenge if previously exposed to foreign/dangerous agents [14–20]. The results show that AuNPs do not have a significant capacity to induce memory in 2D cultures, with unprimed vs. AuNP-primed cells from all donors showing a comparable response to LPS (Figure 4, Table S3). In 3D cultures, although the global response is never different between unprimed and AuNP-primed cells, when examining the response of individual donors, it is possible to see memory effects, as for instance for Donor 3 that shows an AuNP priming-dependent decrease in TNFα, IL-6, and IL-1Ra production, which is not evident in 2D cultures, or for Donor 6 that shows an AuNP priming-dependent increase in IL-8 and IL-1Ra that was undetectable in 2D cultures.

Two important notions should be underlined here. First, the unstimulated production of IL-8 and IL-1Ra is detectable at higher levels in unprimed/primed macrophages in 3D cultures compared to the 2D cultures, whereas the production of the inflammatory cytokines TNFα and IL-6 is essentially undetectable in both conditions (Table S2). This implies that the 3D cultures provide a more physiological microenvironment, which promotes the homeostatic tissue-like functions of macrophages, characterised by lack of production of inflammatory factors and abundant production of anti-inflammatory factors [7,8,41]. The significant production of IL-8 goes in the same direction, as this chemokine is involved in ensuring the appropriate homeostatic trafficking of neutrophils and other cells in non-inflammatory conditions [42–44]. Thus, in 3D cultures monocytes developed in the direction of M2/healing macrophages by adopting a classical tissue resident-like anti-inflammatory and homeostatic functional phenotype. Notably, IL-1Ra is detectable at significantly lower levels in macrophage 2D cultures, a finding that supports the suitability of 3D cultures for a more realistic assessment of macrophage reactivity. However, it should be noted that we could not find significant qualitative differences in the innate memory activities between cells cultured in 2D vs. 3D conditions. On the other hand, as already mentioned, there is no substantial qualitative and quantitative difference in the reactivity of fresh monocytes in 2D vs. 3D cultures, suggesting that 2D cultures are fully suitable for evaluating acute innate responses.

The second important finding is that the memory response to AuNPs is strongly dependent on donors. While memory responses induced by priming with LPS (a very strong stimulus) are clearer, with exposure to AuNPs (a stimulus that does not induce a detectable primary response) it becomes evident that the priming capacity substantially depends on the donor. Thus, as an example, the 3D memory response in terms of IL-6 is increased production in two donors, a decrease in another two, and no change in the last two donors. This is fully in line with previous preliminary observations [28,30] and underlines the importance of 'immunobiography", i.e., the history of exposure and challenges experienced by the immune system, which is unique for each of us and that can significantly bias our capacity to react appropriately to new challenges [33]. Although the number of donors in this study is limited (six donors), they are quite homogeneous in terms of age and health status (young, healthy, no medications, non-smokers). They encompass individual of both sexes and of two different ethnic groups, but neither parameter is associated with a defined type of response, further suggesting that the individual history of exposure may be at the basis of response variability.

These findings suggest some important issues in directing future research: the need for adopting suitable models for our in vitro studies of human innate memory, and the importance of performing individual assessments (precision medicine, precision diagnosis, precision toxicology), since it is not possible to generalize findings of efficacy or toxicity to a population that is widely different also in terms of immune history.

Supplementary Materials: The following are available online at https://www.mdpi.com/2079-4991/11/1/207/s1, Table S1: Primary cytokine production by monocytes in 2D vs. 3D cultures; Table S2: Baseline cytokine production by unprimed and primed monocytes after 6-day resting in 2D vs. 3D cultures; Table S3: Secondary cytokine production by unprimed and primed monocytes challenged with LPS after 6-day resting in 2D vs. 3D cultures.

Author Contributions: B.J.S. designed and performed the experiments; A.V. analysed the data and performed the statistical analysis; L.R. provided information of the collagen matrix and contributed to data analysis and discussion; M.M. participated to experimental work and data analysis; V.F.P. synthesized and characterized the AuNPs; A.C.D.L. analysed and discussed the results; D.B. analysed and discussed the data and wrote the manuscript; P.I. analysed and discussed the data, prepared the figures and wrote the manuscript. All authors have read and agreed to the published version of the manuscript.

Funding: This research was funded by the European Commission FP7 project HUMUNITY (GA 316383), the Horizon 2020 projects PANDORA (GA 671881) and ENDONANO (GA 812661), the Italian MIUR Flagship InterOmics project MEMORAT and the PRIN project 20173ZECCM.

Institutional Review Board Statement: The study was conducted according to the guidelines of the Declaration of Helsinki, and the protocol was approved by the Regional Ethics Committee for Clinical Experimentation of the Tuscany Region (Ethics Committee Register n. 14,914 of 16 May 2019).

Informed Consent Statement: Informed consent was obtained from all subjects involved in the study.

Data Availability Statement: The data presented in this study are available in this article and its supplementary material.

Acknowledgments: The authors wish to thank Paola Migliorini (University of Pisa, Italy) for her help in the coordination and ethical monitoring of the study, and the Morpho-Functional Analysis and Bioimaging Unit of the Stazione Zoologica Anton Dohrn for providing technical assistance for SEM images.

Conflicts of Interest: The authors declare no conflict of interest.

References

1. Dobrovolskaia, M.A.; Shurin, M.; Shvedova, A.A. Current understanding of interactions between nanoparticles and the immune system. *Toxicol. Appl. Pharmacol.* **2016**, *299*, 78–89. [CrossRef]
2. Fadeel, B. Hide and seek: Nanomaterial interactions with the immune system. *Front. Immunol.* **2019**, *10*, 133. [CrossRef]
3. Boraschi, D.; Italiani, P.; Palomba, R.; Decuzzi, P.; Duschl, A.; Fadeel, B.; Moghimi, S.M. Nanoparticles and innate immunity: New perspectives on host defence. *Sem. Immunol.* **2017**, *34*, 33–51. [CrossRef]
4. Medzhitov, R.; Janeway, C.A. Innate immunity: The virtues of a non-clonal system of recognition. *Cell* **1997**, *91*, 295–298. [CrossRef]
5. Carta, S.; Yassi, S.; Pettinati, I.; Delfino, L.; Dinarello, C.A.; Rubartelli, A. The rate of IL-1β secretion in different myeloid cells varies with the extent of redox response to TLR triggering. *J. Biol. Chem.* **2011**, *286*, 27069–27080. [CrossRef]
6. Italiani, P.; Boraschi, D. From monocytes to M1/M2 macrophages: Phenotypical vs. functional differentiation. *Front. Immunol.* **2014**, *5*, 514. [CrossRef]
7. Mills, C.D.; Lenz, L.L.; Ley, K. *M1/M2 Macrophages: The Arginine Fork in the Road to Health and Disease*; Frontiers Media: Lausanne, Switzerland, 2015; p. 280. [CrossRef]
8. Holst, O.; Ulmer, A.J.; Brade, H.; Flad, H.D.; Rietschel, E.T. 1996. Biochemistry and cell biology of bacterial endotoxins. *FEMS Immunol. Med. Microbiol.* **1996**, *16*, 83–104. [CrossRef] [PubMed]
9. Mestas, J.; Hughues, C.C.W. Of mice and not men: Differences between mouse and human immunology. *J. Immunol.* **2004**, *172*, 2731–2738. [CrossRef] [PubMed]

10. Davis, M.M. A prescription for human immunology. *Immunity* **2008**, *29*, 835–838. [CrossRef] [PubMed]
11. Italiani, P.; Mazza, E.M.C.; Lucchesi, D.; Cifola, I.; Gemelli, C.; Grande, A.; Battaglia, C.; Bicciato, S.; Boraschi, D. Transcriptomic profiling of the development of the inflammatory response in human monocytes in vitro. *PLoS ONE* **2014**, *9*, e87680. [CrossRef]
12. Li, Y.; Italiani, P.; Casals, E.; Valkenborg, D.; Mertens, I.; Baggerman, G.; Nelissen, I.; Puntes, V.; Boraschi, D. Assessing the immunosafety of engineered nanoparticles with a novel in vitro model based on human primary monocytes. *ACS Appl. Mater. Interfaces* **2016**, *8*, 28437–28447. [CrossRef] [PubMed]
13. Ferretti, A.M.; Usseglio, S.; Mondini, S.; Drago, C.; La Mattina, R.; Chini, B.; Verderio, C.; Leonzino, M.; Cagnoli, C.; Joshi, P.; et al. Towards bio-compatible magnetic nanoparticles: Immune-related effects, in vitro internalization, and in vivo bio-distribution of zwitterionic ferrite nanoparticles with unexpected renal clearance. *J. Colloid Interface Sci.* **2020**, *582*, 678–700. [CrossRef] [PubMed]
14. Beeson, P.B. Development of tolerance to typhoid bacterial pyrogen and its abolition by reticulo-endothelial blockade. *Proc. Soc. Exp. Biol. Med.* **1946**, *61*, 248–250. [CrossRef] [PubMed]
15. Howard, J.G.; Biozzi, G.; Halpern, B.N.; Stiffel, C.; Mouton, D. The effect of *Mycobacterium tuberculosis* (BCG) infection on the resistance of mice to bacterial endotoxin and *Salmonella enteritidis* infection. *Br. J. Exp. Pathol.* **1959**, *40*, 281–290. [PubMed]
16. Bistoni, F.; Vecchiarelli, A.; Cenci, E.; Puccetti, P.; Marconi, P.; Cassone, A. Evidence for macrophage-mediated protection against lethal *Candida albicans* infection. *Infect. Immun.* **1986**, *51*, 668–674. [CrossRef]
17. Netea, M.G.; Quintin, J.; van der Meer, J.W.M. Trained immunity: A memory for innate host defense. *Cell Host Microbe* **2011**, *9*, 355–361. [CrossRef]
18. Milutinovi'c, B.; Kurtz, J. Immune memory in invertebrates. *Sem. Immunol.* **2016**, *28*, 328–342. [CrossRef]
19. Cooper, D.; Eleftherianos, I. Memory and specificity in the insect immune system: Current perspectives and future challenges. *Front. Immunol.* **2017**, *8*, 539. [CrossRef]
20. Gourbal, B.; Pinaud, S.; Beckers, G.J.M.; Van Der Meer, J.W.M.; Conrath, U.; Netea, M.G. Innate immune memory: An evolutionary perspective. *Immunol. Rev.* **2018**, *283*, 21–40. [CrossRef]
21. Arts, R.J.W.; Joosten, L.A.B.; Netea, M.G. The potential role of trained immunity in autoimmune and autoinflammatory disorders. *Front. Immunol.* **2018**, *9*, 298. [CrossRef]
22. Salam, A.P.; Borsini, A.; Zunszain, P.A. Trained innate immunity: A salient factor in the pathogenesis of neuroimmune psychiatric disorders. *Mol. Psychiatry* **2018**, *23*, 170–176. [CrossRef] [PubMed]
23. Salani, F.; Sterbini, V.; Sacchinelli, E.; Garramone, M.; Bossu, P. Is innate memory a double-edge sword in Alzheimer's Disease? A reappraisal of new concepts and old data. *Front. Immunol.* **2019**, *10*, 1768. [CrossRef] [PubMed]
24. Töpfer, E.; Boraschi, D.; Italiani, P. Innate immune memory: The latest frontier of adjuvanticity. *J. Immunol. Res.* **2015**, *2015*, 478408. [CrossRef] [PubMed]
25. Xing, Z.; Afkhami, S.; Bavananthasivam, J.; Fritz, D.K.; D'Agostino, M.R.; Vaseghi-Shanjani, M.; Yao, Y.; Jeyanathan, M. Innate immune memory of tissue-resident macrophages and trained innate immunity: Re-vamping vaccine concept and strategies. *J. Leukocyte Biol.* **2020**, *108*, 825–834. [CrossRef]
26. Sánchez-Ramón, S.; Conejero, L.; Netea, M.G.; Sancho, D.; Palomares, Ó.; Subiza, J.L. Trained immunity-based vaccines: A new paradigm for the development of broad-spectrum anti-infectious formulations. *Front. Immunol.* **2018**, *9*, 2936. [CrossRef] [PubMed]
27. Mulder, W.J.M.; Ochando, J.; Joosten, L.A.B.; Fayad, Z.A.; Netea, M.G. Therapeutic targeting of trained immunity. *Nat. Rev. Drug Discov.* **2019**, *18*, 553–566. [CrossRef]
28. Italiani, P.; Boraschi, D. Induction of innate immune memory by engineered nanoparticles: A hypothesis that may become true. *Front. Immunol.* **2017**, *8*, 734. [CrossRef]
29. Lebre, F.; Boland, J.B.; Gouveia, P.; Gorman, A.; Lundahl, M.; O'Brien, F.J.; Coleman, J.; Lavelle, E.C. Pristine graphene induces innate immune training. *Nanoscale* **2020**, *12*, 11192–11200. [CrossRef]
30. Swartzwelter, B.J.; Barbero, F.; Verde, A.; Mangini, M.; Pirozzi, M.; De Luca, A.C.; Puntes, V.F.; Leite, L.C.C.; Italiani, P.; Boraschi, D. Gold nanoparticles modulate BCG-induced innate iummune memory in nhuman monocytes by shifting the memory response towards tolerance. *Cells* **2020**, *9*, 284. [CrossRef]
31. Auguste, M.; Balbi, T.; Ciacci, C.; Canonico, B.; Papa, S.; Borello, A.; Vezzulli, L.; Canesi, L. Shift in immune parameters after repeated exposure to nanoplastics in the Marine Bivalve *Mytilus*. *Front. Immunol.* **2020**, *11*, 426. [CrossRef]
32. Italiani, P.; Della Camera, G.; Boraschi, D. Induction of innate immune memory by engineered nanoparticles in monocytes/macrophages: From hypothesis to reality. *Front. Immunol.* **2020**, *11*, 566309. [CrossRef]
33. Franceschi, C.; Salvioli, S.; Garagnani, P.; de Eguileor, M.; Monti, D.; Capri, M. Immunobiography and the heterogeneity of immune responses in the elderly: A focus on inflammaging and trained immunity. *Front. Immunol.* **2017**, *8*, 982. [CrossRef]
34. Ojea-Jiménez, I.; Bastús, N.G.; Puntes, V. Influence of the sequence of the reagents addition in the citrate-mediated synthesis of gold nanoparticles. *J. Phys. Chem. C* **2011**, *115*, 15752–15757. [CrossRef]
35. Li, Y.; Italiani, P.; Casals, E.; Tran, N.; Puntes, V.F.; Boraschi, D. Optimising the use of commercial LAL assays for the analysis of endotoxin contamination in metal colloids and metal oxide nanoparticles. *Nanotoxicology* **2015**, *9*, 462–473. [CrossRef]
36. Oostingh, G.J.; Casals, E.; Italiani, P.; Colognato, R.; Stritzinger, R.; Ponti, J.; Pfaller, T.; Kohl, Y.; Ooms, D.; Favilli, F.; et al. Problems and challenges in the development and validation of human cell-based assays to determine nanoparticle-induced immunomodulatory effects. *Particle Fibre Toxicol.* **2011**, *8*, 8. [CrossRef]

37. Piella, J.; Bastús, N.G.; Puntes, V. Size-dependent protein-nanoparticle interaction in citrate-stabilized gold nanoparticles: The emergence of the protein corona. *Bioconj. Chem.* **2017**, *28*, 88–97. [CrossRef]
38. Comenge, J.; Sotelo, C.; Romero, F.; Gallego, O.; Barnadas, A.; Garcia-Caballero Parada, T.; Dominguez, F.; Puntes, V.F. Detoxifying antitumoral drugs via nanoconjugation: The case of gold nanoparticles and cisplatin. *PLoS ONE* **2012**, *7*, e47562. [CrossRef]
39. Li, Y.; Shi, Z.; Radauer-Preiml, I.; Andosch, A.; Casals, E.; Luetz-Meidl, U.; Cobaleda, M.; Lin, Z.; Jaberi-Douraki, M.; Italiani, P.; et al. Bacterial endotoxin (LPS) binds to the surface of gold nanoparticles, interferes with biocorona formation and induces human monocyte inflammatory activation. *Nanotoxicology* **2017**, *11*, 1157–1175. [CrossRef]
40. Montanaro, M.; Meloni, M.; Anemona, L.; Giurato, L.; Scimeca, M.; Izzo, V.; Servadei, F.; Smirnov, A.; Candi, E.; Mauriello, A.; et al. Macrophage activation and M2 polarization in wound bed of diabetic patients treated by dermal/epidermal substitute Nevelia. *Int. J. Lower Extr. Wounds* **2020**. online ahead of print. [CrossRef]
41. Röszer, T. Understanding the misterious M2 macrophage through activation markers and effector mechanisms. *Med. Inflamm.* **2015**, *2015*, 816460. [CrossRef]
42. Sherwood, J.; Bertrand, J.; Nalesso, G.; Poulet, B.; Pitsillides, A.; Brandolini, L.; Karystinou, A.; De Bari, C.; Luyten, F.P.; Pitzalis, C.; et al. A homeostatic function of CXCR2 signalling in articular cartilage. *Ann. Rheum. Dis.* **2015**, *74*, 2207–2215. [CrossRef]
43. Nicolás-Ávila, J.A.; Adrover, J.M.; Hidalgo, A. Neutrophils in homeostasis, immunity and cancer. *Immunity* **2017**, *46*, 15–28. [CrossRef]
44. Pekalski, M.L.; Rubio Garcia, A.; Ferreira, R.C.; Rainbow, D.B.; Smyth, D.J.; Mashar, M.; Brady, J.; Savinykh, N.; Castro Dopico, X.; Mahmood, S.; et al. Neonatal and adult recent thymic emigrants produce IL-8 and express complement receptors CR1 and CR2. *JCI Insight* **2017**, *2*, e93739. [CrossRef]

nanomaterials

MDPI

Article

Selective Uptake of Carboxylated Multi-Walled Carbon Nanotubes by Class A Type 1 Scavenger Receptors and Impaired Phagocytosis in Alveolar Macrophages

Ruhung Wang [1,2], Rishabh Lohray [1,†], Erik Chow [3,‡], Pratima Gangupantula [1], Loren Smith [2] and Rockford Draper [1,2,*]

1. Department of Biological Sciences, The University of Texas at Dallas, 800 West Campbell Road, Richardson, TX 75080, USA; ruhung.wang@utdallas.edu (R.W.); Rishabh.Lohray@bcm.edu (R.L.); Pratima.Gangupantula@utdallas.edu (P.G.)
2. Department of Chemistry & Biochemistry, The University of Texas at Dallas, 800 West Campbell Road, Richardson, TX 75080, USA; Loren@utdallas.edu
3. Department of Bioengineering, The University of Texas at Dallas, 800 West Campbell Road, Richardson, TX 75080, USA; ec829@cornell.edu

* Correspondence: draper@utdallas.edu

† Present Affiliation: Baylor College of Medicine, School of Medicine, Houston, TX 77030, USA.

‡ Present Affiliation: Meinig School of Biomedical Engineering, Cornell University, Ithaca, NY 14850, USA.

Received: 19 October 2020; Accepted: 27 November 2020; Published: 3 December 2020

Abstract: The production and applications of multi-walled carbon nanotubes (MWNTs) have increased despite evidence that MWNTs can be toxic. Recently, we reported that the binding of Pluronic® F-108 (PF108)-coated carboxylated MWNTs (C-MWNTs) to macrophages is inhibited by class A scavenger receptors (SR-As) antagonists (R. Wang et al., 2018. Nanotoxicology 12:677–690). The current study investigates the uptake of PF108-coated MWNTs by macrophages lacking SR-A1 and by CHO cells that ectopically express SR-A1. Macrophages without SR-A1 failed to take up C-MWNTs and CHO cells that expressed SR-A1 did take up C-MWNTs, but not pristine MWNTs (P-MWNTs) or amino-functionalized MWNTs (N-MWNTs). The dependence of C-MWNT uptake on SR-A1 is strong evidence that SR-A1 is a receptor for C-MWNTs. The consequences of SR-A1-dependent C-MWNT accumulation on cell viability and phagocytic activity in macrophages were also studied. C-MWNTs were more toxic than P-MWNTs and N-MWNTs in cell proliferation and colony formation tests. C-MWNTs reduced surface SR-A1 levels in RAW 264.7 cells and impaired phagocytic uptake of three known SR-A1 ligands, polystyrene beads, heat-killed *E. coli*, and oxLDL. Altogether, results of this study confirmed that SR-A1 receptors are important for the selective uptake of PF108-coated C-MWNTs and that accumulation of the C-MWNTs impairs phagocytic activity and cell viability in macrophages.

Keywords: nanomaterials; macrophages; class A type 1 scavenger receptors; cytotoxicity; macrophage–nanoparticle interaction

1. Introduction

Carbon nanotubes (CNTs) are graphene sheets rolled into cylindrical tubes. Single-walled carbon nanotubes (SWNTs) contain a single graphene tube while multi-walled carbon nanotubes (MWNTs) contain multiple tubes concentrically nested inside each other. The light weight, strength, electrical and thermal conductivity of CNTs make them suited for applications in diverse fields including flexible electronics, medicine, reinforced composites, sensors, and Li-ion batteries [1–3]. The production of various CNT types is expected to exceed 15 kilotons/year by 2020 [3]. The increased production and use of CNTs raises the risk of unwanted exposure and subsequent toxicity. Sustained exposure has been shown to cause pulmonary inflammation [4,5], fibrosis [6], gene damage [7], and even mesothelioma [8] in lab animals. A better understanding of the pathology of CNT exposure is important to facilitate the design of less toxic CNT forms and to develop rational strategies for treating persons who may be accidentally exposed.

The surfaces of CNTs are often chemically functionalized, for example, by addition of carboxyl or amino groups, to tune their properties for increased dispersibility in aqueous solution, for decreased toxicity, or for higher drug load and targeting specificity in advanced drug delivery options. In nanomedicine, specific CNT functionalizations have been shown to facilitate the delivery of anticancer agents and biomolecules to target tissues for cancer therapy, thermal ablation therapy, gene therapy, immunotherapy, and for diagnostic applications [9]. However, these applications encounter a common significant challenge, where 30–99% of nanoparticles administered in vivo are sequestered by liver macrophages [10], and the mechanisms underlying the interaction between CNTs and macrophages remain poorly understood.

Recently, we reported that both human and mouse alveolar macrophages accumulated far more Pluronic® F-108 (PF108)-coated carboxylated MWNTs (C-MWNTs) and carboxylated SWNTs (C-SWNTs) at 37 °C than the non-functionalized pristine MWNTs (P-MWNTs) and SWNTs (P-SWNTs) [11]. In addition, more C-MWNTs than P-MWNTs bound to macrophages in direct binding assays at 4 °C [11]. These data suggested that there were cell surface receptors that bound C-MWNTs but not P-MWNTs. Since the binding of C-MWNTs and C-SWNTs to macrophages was inhibited by known antagonists of class A scavenger receptors [11], members of this receptor class may be involved in the specific uptake of carboxylated CNTs in macrophages.

Class A scavenger receptors (SR-As) are pattern recognition receptors expressed by various cell types including macrophages, endothelial cells, and dendritic cells [12–14]. There are six types of SR-As, classified by a consensus nomenclature, which all contain a collagenous domain believed to bind a wide variety of polyanionic ligands, including modified low density lipoproteins, polysaccharides, nucleic acids, and various bacteria [14]. Since C-MWNTs are polyanions, it is possible that they could be SR-A ligands. Dextran sulfate and fucoidan are known antagonists of SR-A ligands, and in previous work we noted that both of these compounds partially blocked the binding of C-MWNTs to RAW 264.7 macrophages [11]. In addition, RAW 264.7 cells express high levels of scavenger receptor A1 (SR-A1) [15], leading to the hypothesis that SR-A1 might be a receptor for C-MWNTs. However, polyanionic inhibitors may affect more than one type of SR-A and it is difficult to pinpoint which type may be interacting with C-MWNTs. One main objective of the present paper was to test the hypothesis that SR-A1 is a receptor for C-MWNTs by measuring C-MWNT accumulation by macrophages that lack SR-A1 and by Chinese Hamster Ovary K1 cell (CHO-K1) clones that have been transfected with mouse SR-A1 cDNA. SR-A1 deficient macrophages and wild type CHO-K1 that do not normally express SR-A1 failed to accumulate significant amounts of C-MWNTs, whereas SR-A1 expressing CHO-K1 clones did accumulate C-MWNTs, strong evidence that SR-A1 is a C-MWNT receptor.

Possible physiological consequences of C-MWNT accumulation on cell viability and SR-A1 function were also explored in the current study. RAW 264.7 cell proliferation and colony formation efficiency were impaired in a dose and time dependent manner after exposure to C-MWNTs. In addition, exposure of RAW 264.7 cells to C-MWNTs reduced the level of SR-A1 on their surface and reduced the uptake of three known SR-A1 ligands: polystyrene beads, heat-killed *E. coli*, and oxidized low density lipoprotein (oxLDL).

2. Materials and Methods

2.1. MWNTs and other Materials

Three different research grade MWNT powders were used in this work, all purchased from NanoCyl (NanoCyl SA, Sambreville, Belgium). (1) Non-functionalized pristine MWNTs (P-MWNTs, NC3150™); (2) Carboxyl-functionalized MWNTs (C-MWNTs, NC3151™); and (3) Amino-functionalized MWNTs (N-MWNTs, NC3152™). The MWNTs were produced by the catalytic chemical vapor deposition process to an average outside diameter of ~9.5 nm, purified to >95 wt.% carbon content and shortened to an average length of <1.0 µm, according to the product specifications provided by the manufacturer. Proprietary surface modification methods were used by the manufacturer to introduce <8.0 wt.% content of -COOH groups in the C-MWNT product and <0.6 wt.% of -NH_2 groups in the N-MWNT product. Additional physicochemical properties of these and other MWNT products, including bulk metal catalysts composition by energy dispersive X-ray spectroscopy (EDX) and surface chemical compositions by X-ray photoelectron spectroscopy (XPS), are available from previous work in the literature [16,17]. Caution: a fine particulate respirator and other appropriate personal protective equipment should be worn when handling dry MWNT powders.

Pluronic® F-108 (PF108) (cat. No. 542342), G418 disulfate salt solution (cat. No. G8168), IgG from mouse serum (cat. No. I5381), and Trypan Blue solution (cat. No. T8154) were purchased from Sigma Aldrich (St. Louis, MO, USA). Mouse SR-AI/MSR Alexa Fluor® 488-conjugated antibody (cat. No. FAB1797G), rat IgG2b Alexa Fluor® 488-conjugated isotype control antibody (cat. No. IC013G), mouse MARCO allophycocyanin (APC)-conjugated antibody (cat. No. FAB2956A), rat IgG1 APC-conjugated isotype control antibody (cat. No. IC005A), and flow cytometry (FCyt) staining buffer (cat. No. FC001) were purchased from R&D Systems, Inc. (Minneapolis, MN, USA) and used as received. Non-functionalized fluorescent polystyrene beads with a nominal diameter of 1 µm were acquired from Bangs Laboratories Inc. (cat. No. FSDG004, Fishers, Indiana). According to the manufacturer, the beads were produced by an emulsion polymerization technique resulting in a net negative surface charge. They were internally labeled with Dragon Green Dye (Ex: 480 nm, Em: 520 nm), using a solvent swelling/dye entrapment technique. Annexin V-FITC apoptosis detection kit (Invitrogen™ cat. No. V13242), heat-killed Alexa Fluor® 488 conjugated *Escherichia coli* (K-12 strain) BioParticles™ (Invitrogen™ cat. No. E13231), and oxidized low density lipoprotein from human plasma (Invitrogen™ cat. No. L34357) were purchased from Thermo Fisher Scientific (Waltham, MA, USA). Oxidized LDL uptake assay kit was purchased from Cayman Chemical (cat. No. 601180, Ann Arbor, MI, USA).

2.2. Preparation and Characterization of PF108 MWNT Dispersions

Pluronic® F-108 (PF108) is a non-ionic triblock copolymer, also known as poloxamer 338. PF108 and related poloxamers have been used as effective surfactants to prepare aqueous dispersions of hydrophobic nanomaterials, including MWNTs and SWNTs, for nanotoxicity studies [11,18,19]. A stock PF108 solution at 5 mM concentration was prepared by dissolving PF108 powder in DI water purified using a Milli-Q system (Billerica, MA, USA), filtered through a 0.22 µm membrane, and stored at 4 °C in the dark. All MWNT dispersions were prepared with a freshly diluted and filtered 0.2 mM PF108 solution. To reduce potential endotoxin contaminants that could lead to ambiguous toxicity results, all MWNT powders were baked at 200 °C for 2 h [20] before PF108 solution was added. The sonication, centrifugation, and dialysis protocols described in our previous work [18,19] were used to prepare PF108-coated MWNT dispersions. Note that the dialysis step is crucial to remove toxic PF108 products generated by sonication [18,21]. The prepared dispersions of P-, N-, and C-MWNTs in PF108 solution were denoted as PMPF, NMPF, and CMPF dispersions, respectively.

The concentration of MWNTs in each prepared dispersion was measured using the absorbance at 500 nm. Dynamic light scattering (DLS) and zeta potential (ZP) analyses were used as part of a quality control routine for the preparation of all MWNT dispersions [18,19]. In addition, zeta potentials of all

MWNT dispersions diluted to ~50 μg/mL in water and in cell culture medium with 10% fetal bovine serum (FBS) were acquired at 25 °C and 37 °C, respectively.

The physicochemical properties of the three MWNT powders provided by the manufacturer and the properties of PF108-coated MWNT dispersions prepared for this study are shown in Table 1. Note that the zeta potentials for C-MWNTs were slightly more negative than those for P- and N-MWNTs in water. Also, the zeta potential values were less negative for all MWNT types in medium with serum than in water, as expected due to the increase in salt and serum protein concentrations, and the C-MWNTs still had slightly more negative zeta potentials than P- or N-MWNTs.

2.3. Cell Lines and Cell Culture

Dulbecco's modified Eagle medium (DMEM) was purchased from Gibco (Grand Island, NY, USA). Ham's F-12K (ATCC® 30-2004) and RPMI 1640 (ATCC® 30-2001) media were purchased from the American Type Culture Collection (ATCC, Manassas, VA, USA). FBS was purchased from Atlanta Biologicals (Flowery Branch, GA, USA). Penicillin-streptomycin solution (100 U penicillin/0.1 mg streptomycin per mL) was purchased from Sigma Aldrich and used only in terminal cultures. Gibco™ PBS-based enzyme-free cell dissociation buffer (cat. No. 13151-014), Accumax™ (cat. No. 00-4666-56), Accutase™ (cat. No. A1110501), and 10× concentrated phosphate buffered saline (cat. No. BP399-1) were purchased from Thermo Fisher Scientific (Waltham, MA, USA).

Abelson murine leukemia virus transformed macrophage RAW 264.7 cells (ATCC® TIB-71) and Chinese Hamster Ovary CHO-K1 cells (ATCC® CCL-61) were purchased from ATCC. Two immortalized alveolar macrophage cell lines, B6 and ZK, were kindly provided by Prof. L. Kobzik (retired, Harvard TH Chan School of Public Health, Boston, MA, USA). B6 cells were derived from wild type (WT) C57BL/6 mice and ZK cells were derived from MARCO and SR-AI/II deficient ($MS^{-/-}$) mice [22]. RAW 264.7 cells were cultured in DMEM base medium and WT B6 and $MS^{-/-}$ ZK cells were cultured in RPMI 1640 base medium. CHO cells stably transfected with full length mouse SR-A1 cDNA, termed CHO[mSR-AI] cells [23], were kindly provided by Prof. M. Krieger (Massachusetts Institute of Technology, Boston, MA, USA). As received CHO[mSR-AI] cells were cultured in selective medium containing 0.5 mg/mL of geneticin (G418) and single colonies were isolated by dilution plating. The surviving colonies were screened for high surface SR-A1 receptor expression by immuno-fluorescent FCyt, from which three sub-clones, termed CHO + mSRA1.A, CHO + mSRA1.B, and CHO + mSRA1.C were selected. CHO-K1 and transfected CHO + mSRA1.A, CHO + mSRA1.B, and CHO + mSRA1.C cells were cultured in F-12K base medium. All regular culture media were supplemented with 1.5 mg/mL sodium bicarbonate, 10% (*v*/*v*) FBS, and 10 mM HEPES buffer at pH 7.4 for cells cultured in a 37 °C incubator with 95% air and 5% CO_2. For cells incubated in a 4 °C incubator without CO_2 supplement, no sodium bicarbonate was added to the media to maintain proper pH.

Table 1. Properties of pristine- (P-), amino-functionalized- (N-), and carboxylated-multi-walled carbon nanotubes (C-MWNT) powders and prepared Pluronic® F108-coated MWNT dispersions.

	MWNT Product Specification Provided by NanoCyl								MWNT Particles in Pluronic® F-108 Dispersions			
									Particle Size		Zeta Potential (mV)	
MWNT Product	**Batch No.**	**Carbon Purity (wt.%)**	**Surface Modification**	**NH_2 COOH (wt.%)**	**Metal Oxide (wt.%)**	**Average Length (μm)**	**Average Diameter (nm)**	**MWNT-PF108 Dispersion**	**HDD (nm)**	**PDI**	**Water 25 °C**	**Medium +10% FBS 37 °C**
NC3150™ Pristine **(P-MWNT)**	100426	>95	-	-	<5.0	<1.0	9.5	**PMPF**	114 ± 1.0	0.22	−22.2 ± 2.6	−1.2 ± 0.3
NC31520™ Amino-functionalized **(N-MWNT)**	MEL 160125	>95	$-NH_2$	<0.6	<5.0	<1.0	9.5	**NMPF**	108 ± 0.2	0.22	−20.9 ± 0.7	−1.2 ± 0.3
NC31510™ Carboxyl-functionalized **(C-MWNT)**	120828	>95	-COOH	<8.0	<5.0	<1.0	9.5	**CMPF**	86 ± 1.0	0.23	−26.8 ± 1.0	−4.8 ± 0.6

2.4. Surface Expression of Class A Type 1 Scavenger Receptors SR-A1 and MARCO

Macrophage cell surface expression of SR-A1 and MARCO receptors was determined by a direct immunofluorescence FCyt assay. Macrophages cultured in 6-well plates at 37 °C were washed three times with warm PBS to remove serum components present in the media and detached from the plate with gentle pipetting in enzyme-free PBS. Cells in suspension were washed twice with cold PBS and aliquots of ~1×10^6 cells/100 µL in cold PBS were prepared. Macrophages often express Fc receptors on their surface that can bind to the Fc portion of a fluorescent reporter antibody. To block Fc receptors, 10 µg of unlabeled mouse IgG was added and incubated with the cells for 15 min at 4 °C. For immunostaining of surface SR-A1, 1 µg of rat anti-mouse mSR-AI/MSR Alexa Fluor® 488-conjugated monoclonal antibody (R&D Systems cat. No. FAB1797G) was added and incubated with the cells for 30 min at 4 °C in the dark. A duplicate cell aliquot was incubated with an isotype control rat IgG2b Alexa Fluor® 488-conjugated monoclonal antibody (R&D Systems cat. No. IC013G) to assess possible off-target staining by the anti-SR-A1 antibody. For immunostaining of surface MARCO receptors, a similar procedure was used but with a rat anti-mouse MARCO APC-conjugated monoclonal antibody (R&D Systems cat. No. FAB2956A) and the corresponding APC-conjugated rat IgG1 isotype control antibody (R&D Systems cat. No. IC005A). After incubation, unbound antibodies were washed away by centrifugation twice with 1 mL of cold FCyt staining buffer (R&D Systems cat. No. FC001) at $1000 \times g$ for 8 min. The washed cells were re-suspended in cold buffer and stored on ice in the dark. Flow cytometric analysis of 20,000 counts per sample was used to determine the presence or absence of specific fluorescent antibodies bound to SR-A1 or MARCO receptors on the cell surface. Cells with fluorescence intensity greater than the background isotype control were considered positive for the receptors.

2.5. Accumulation of MWNTs in RAW 264.7, B6, ZK Macrophages and CHO Cell Lines

The sodium dodecyl sulfate polyacrylamide gel electrophoresis (SDS-PAGE) procedure described in our previous work [11,18,19] was used to determine the amount of MWNTs accumulated by cells after a 24 h exposure at 37 °C. Briefly, cells were seeded in 6-well plates in regular culture media overnight before incubating in either control media that contained no MWNTs or test media with 100 µg/mL of P-, N-, or C-MWNTs for 24 h at 37 °C. After incubation, cells were washed extensively with fresh medium and PBS and detached from culture plates with Accutase™ cell dissociation buffer. Cell numbers were determined using a Coulter Particle Counter, and MWNTs were extracted from cells and quantified using the SDS-PAGE method. The average amount of P-, N-, or C-MWNTs accumulated by the cell over a 24 h period was expressed as fg MWNT per cell.

2.6. Apoptosis Assay

The induction of apoptosis in RAW 264.7 cells was assessed after a 24 h incubation with media containing either 0.1 mM PF108 alone, or 100 µg/mL of P-, N-, or C-MWNTs using an apoptosis detection kit (Invitrogen™ cat. No. V13242) with FITC-conjugated annexin V and propidium iodide (PI) duo fluorescent markers for FCyt analysis. A total of 3×10^4 RAW 264.7 cells/well were seeded in 24-well plates and incubated at 37 °C overnight before the regular culture medium was replaced with freshly prepared control or test media and incubated for 24 h. Untreated cells provided a negative control and cells treated with 100 nM camptothecin (CPT) were used as a positive control for apoptosis. After the incubation, cells were washed 3 times with fresh medium and twice with PBS, then detached from culture plate by incubating in a PBS-based enzyme-free buffer for 5 min at 37 °C. Cells in suspension were washed, kept on ice, and stained with FITC-conjugated annexin V and PI for 15 min in the dark, according to the protocol provided by the kit. The externalization of phosphatidylserine in apoptotic cells was detected using green fluorescent-conjugated recombinant annexin V and the nuclei of dead or necrotic cells were detected using red fluorescent PI. After treatment with annexin V and PI, 10,000 cell counts per sample were analyzed using an FCyt cell analyzer (BD Accuri™ C6 Plus flow cytometer) where binding of annexin V was recorded in the green fluorescent channel and the binding of PI in the red fluorescent channel. Data were presented as dot plots, where green fluorescence for annexin V-FITC was plotted on the *X*-axis with a threshold set to 2×10^4, and red fluorescence for PI was plotted on the *Y*-axis with a threshold set to 1×10^4. In general, apoptotic cells show higher green fluorescence, necrotic cells show both higher green and higher red fluorescent signals, dead cells show high red but not green fluorescence, and viable cells show little or no fluorescence higher than background levels. The fractions of viable, apoptotic, necrotic, and dead cells in 10,000 counts analyzed per measurement were recorded.

2.7. Crystal Violet Cell Proliferation Assay

A standardized cytotoxicity assay based on cell proliferation described previously in our MWNT toxicity work [11,18] was used for cytotoxicity assessments with RAW 264.7 cells exposed to various MWNT types, doses, and exposure times. Briefly, 4×10^4 RAW 264.7 cells/well were seeded in 48-well plates and incubated at 37 °C overnight before the regular cell culture media was replaced with freshly prepared control or test media for a 24 h exposure. 1×10^4 and 5×10^3 cells/well were seeded for longer exposures of 48 h and 72 h, respectively. At the end of the incubation, cells were washed 3 times with fresh media, 2 times with PBS, and air-dried to fix the cells on the plate. Cell proliferation was determined using a crystal violet assay, as described in our previous work where it was also demonstrated that cell-associated CNTs do not interfere with the assay [24]. The proliferation of the untreated control cells was set to 100%. IC50 values were estimated from a linear regression dose-effect trend line where the concentration of MWNT is needed to inhibit cell proliferation by 50%.

2.8. Colony Formation Efficiency (CFE) Assay

A well-established CFE assay based on the ability of a cell to grow into a colony under the test condition [25] was used to assess the viability of RAW 264.7 cells exposed to different MWNT types and doses continuously for 8 day. 300 RAW 264.7 cells per well were seeded in 6-well plates, filled with 5 mL/well of control regular culture medium or test media that contained either P-, N-, or C-MWNTs at a final MWNTs concentration of 25, 50, or 100 μg/mL, and incubated at 37 °C without disturbance to allow colony formation. At the end of the 8 day incubation, colonies were washed gently twice with fresh medium and twice with PBS, fixed to the plate by air-drying at room temperature, and stained with crystal violet (0.1% *w*/*v* in 10% ethanol) for 15 min at room temperature. Excess unbound dye was removed by rinsing the plate with tap water gently. Images of the wells with stained colonies were acquired using a stereomicroscope (NikonSMZ745T with Nikon DS-Fi2 camera) with a 0.5× objective lens magnification. The number of colonies in a well was counted and colony formation efficiency (CFE) was defined as the ratio of the number of colonies formed over the number of cells seeded in the well. The CFE of the untreated control was set to 100% and the IC50 value was estimated from a linear regression dose-effect trend line where the concentration of MWNT is needed to inhibit CFE by 50%.

2.9. Detection of Surface SR-A1 on RAW 264.7 Cells by Laser Scanning Confocal Fluorescence Microscopy (LSCFM)

A total of 2×10^4 RAW 264.7 cells/well were seeded on glass coverslips in 4-well plates in regular culture media supplemented with 10% FBS for 24 h at 37 °C. The culture medium was replaced with freshly prepared control medium that contained no MWNTs or test media containing 100 μg/mL of P-, N-, or C-MWNTs and incubated for 24 h at 37 °C. After incubation, control and test media were removed, cells were washed extensively, and chilled to 4 °C in media that contained no sodium bicarbonate. To block surface Fc receptors, 10 μg of mouse IgG was added and incubated with the cells for 15 min at 4 °C. For immunostaining of surface SR-A1, 1 μg of rat anti-mouse mSR-AI/MSR Alexa Fluor® 488-conjugated monoclonal antibody (R&D Systems cat. No. FAB1797G) was added and incubated with the cells for 30 min at 4 °C in the dark. After incubation, cells were washed to remove unbound antibodies and fixed with 4% *w*/*v* paraformaldehyde in PBS at room temperature for

15 min. The nuclei were stained with Hoechst 33342 in PBS at room temperature for 5 min in the dark. The cells were then washed with PBS twice to remove excess Hoechst dye, rinsed in Milli-Q water, and the coverslips were mounted on glass slides in Fluoromount G.

Confocal fluorescence images were acquired at the Imaging and Histology Core Facility at UT Dallas using LSCFM (Olympus FV3000RS) with a 100× magnification UPLSAPO objective lens (NA 1.35) immersed in silicone oil. Blue fluorescence in the images denotes nuclei stained with Hoechst dye and was detected with Ex. 405 nm and Em. 430–470 nm wavelengths. Green fluorescence denoting surface SR-A1 was detected with Ex. 488 nm and Em. 500–600 nm wavelengths. At least 30 confocal stacks were acquired per field and Z-projected images were overlaid using *ImageJ* software. 3D rendering of cells was reconstructed from ~30 confocal images along the Z-axis and 360° rotating images were recorded as video clips using *ImageJ* software.

2.10. Phagocytosis of Polystyrene Beads Assessed by LSCFM, FCyt, and LSCRM

A total of 2×10^4 cells/well were seeded in 4-well plates for FCyt analysis in regular culture media (DMEM for RAW 264.7 cells and RPMI 1640 for B6 and ZK cells) supplemented with 10% FBS for 24 h at 37 °C. For LSCFM analysis, glass coverslips were inserted in the wells before 2×10^4 cells/well were seeded. The culture medium was replaced with either freshly prepared test media containing 100 µg/mL of P-, N-, or C-MWNTs or control medium containing no MWNTs and incubated for 20 h at 37 °C. After incubation, control and test media were removed and cells were washed extensively with fresh medium and followed by a 1 h chase period in fresh culture medium at 37 °C. The medium was then replaced with fresh medium containing fluorescent polystyrene beads (10 µg/mL for RAW 264.7 cells and 25 µg/mL for the B6 or ZK cells). The cells were exposed to the beads for 2 h at 37 °C. After the 2 h exposure, cells were washed extensively to remove excess beads in the media and chased in fresh medium at 37 °C for phagocytosis of surface-bound but not yet internalized beads.

For LSCFM analysis, cells on coverslips were washed extensively, fixed with 4% *w/v* paraformaldehyde in PBS at room temperature for 15 min, and washed twice with PBS. The nuclei were stained with Hoechst 33342 in PBS at room temperature for 5 min in the dark. The cells were washed with PBS twice to remove excess Hoechst dye, rinsed in Milli-Q water, and the coverslips were mounted on glass slides in Fluoromount G. The acquisition and processing of confocal fluorescence images of the cells were the same as those described in the previous section.

For FCyt analysis, cells were washed, detached from the well with Accumax™, and re-suspended in PBS. The cells in suspension were washed again with PBS and kept on ice in the dark. 10,000–20,000 cells per sample were analyzed using a flow cytometer where the green fluorescence intensity correlates to the number of phagocytosed beads in a cell. Cells with a green fluorescence intensity greater than the background auto-fluorescence intensity are considered positive for phagocytosed beads. The mean fluorescence index (MFI) of a sample, obtained by multiplying the % of positive cells with phagocytosed beads and the mean fluorescence intensity, represents the phagocytic activity of the cells to take up polystyrene beads under the experimental conditions.

For laser scanning confocal Raman microscopy (LSCRM) analysis, RAW 264.7 cells were cultured on glass coverslips, incubated in control culture medium or in test medium containing 100 µg/mL C-MWNT for 2 h at 37 °C, washed extensively, chased in fresh culture for 30 min, prior to exposure to 25 µg/mL of non-fluorescence and non-functionalized polystyrene beads for 2 h at 37 °C, washed again, then air-dried to prepare for Raman microscopy scanning. The polystyrene beads and C-MWNTs phagocytosed by the control or C-MWNT treated cells were detected using a WITec 500R LSCRM system and the acquired Raman scan images were processed using *WITec Project 4 plus* software (see further details in the SI Methods).

2.11. Phagocytosis of Heat-Killed Fluorescent Bacteria Assessed by FCyt

A total of 4×10^5 RAW 264.7 cells/well were seeded in 6-well plates in regular culture media supplemented with 10% FBS for 24 h at 37 °C. The culture medium was replaced with freshly prepared test media containing either 0.1 mM PF108 alone, 100 µg/mL of P-, N-, or C-MWNTs, or control medium that contained no PF108 or MWNTs and incubated for 24 h at 37 °C. After incubation, control and test media were removed and cells were washed extensively with fresh medium and followed by a 1-h chase period in fresh culture medium at 37 °C. Cells were chilled to 4 °C and exposed to heat killed, Alexa Fluor® 488-conjugated *E. coli* particles, at 30 *E. coli* particles per cell in fresh cold medium for 1 h at 4 °C in the dark. After the 1h exposure, cells were washed extensively to remove unbound *E. coli*, chased in fresh medium at either 37 °C or 4 °C for 1 h, washed, and detached from the plate in enzyme-free buffer. Cells in suspension were washed twice in cold PBS and 20,000 cell counts per measurement were analyzed using a flow cytometer where the green fluorescence intensity correlates to the number of *E. coli* associated with a cell. Cells with a fluorescence intensity greater than the background auto-fluorescence intensity are considered positive for phagocytosed (for cells chased at 37 °C) or surface-bound (for cells kept at 4 °C) *E. coli*.

2.12. Distinguishing Extracellular from Internalized Florescent Markers by Trypan Blue Quenching

A common fluorescence quenching technique with trypan blue (TB) [26,27] was used to distinguish internalized fluorescent-labeled particles from those attached to the cell surface, such as the Alexa Fluor® 488-conjugated monoclonal antibody specific for SR-A1 or the heat killed *E. coli* particles used in the current study. Since trypan blue dye does not penetrate cell membranes, it may quench the green fluorescence of extracellular, i.e., free and surface-bound fluorescent-labeled particles, but has no effect on the fluorescence of particles internalized by the cell. To quantify the extent of fluorescence quenching by trypan blue, flow cytometric measurements of a sample were acquired as usual, in the absence of trypan blue, followed immediately by consecutive analysis in the presence of 0.1% trypan blue dye. The fluorescence intensity quenched by trypan blue is defined as the difference in fluorescence intensities measured in the absence (−TB) and presence (+TB) of the dye. The percent quenching by trypan blue was calculated as [(−TB)−(+TB)]/(−TB), where the fluorescence intensity in the absence of dye was set to 100%. A sample with high trypan blue quenching implies that the fluorescent markers reside on the cell surface. On the contrary, a sample with no fluorescence quenching by trypan blue suggests that the fluorescent markers were internalized by the cells.

2.13. Uptake of Fluorescent and Non-Fluorescent OxLDL Assessed by FM, FCyt and Oil Red O (ORO) Stain

A total of 2×10^4 cells/well were seeded in 4-well plates for FCyt analysis in regular culture media supplemented with 10% FBS for 24 h at 37 °C. For FM and ORO stain analysis, glass coverslips were inserted in the wells before cells were seeded. The culture medium was replaced with freshly prepared test media containing 0.1 mM PF108 alone, 100 µg/mL of P-, N-, or C-MWNTs, or with fresh control medium containing no PF108 nor MWNTs and incubated for 20–24 h at 37 °C. After incubation, control and test media were removed and cells were washed extensively with fresh serum-free medium supplemented with 3% *w/v* BSA (SF + BSA medium) and followed by a 4 h serum starvation period at 37 °C.

For fluorescent oxLDL uptake assays, cells were incubated with fresh serum free (SF) + BSA medium containing DyLight™ 488-conjugated oxLDL (1:20 dilution for FM and 1:40 dilution for FCyt) for 2 h at 37 °C. Cells were then washed extensively to remove excess oxLDL in the media. For FM analysis, cells on coverslips were fixed with 4% *w/v* paraformaldehyde in PBS at room temperature for 15 min, washed again with PBS, and the nuclei were stained with Hoechst 33342 in PBS at room temperature for 5 min in the dark before the coverslips were mounted on glass slides in Fluoromount G. Epi-fluorescence images were acquired using an inverted fluorescence microscope (Nikon Eclipse TE2000) with a 60× magnification oil immersion objective lens (NA 1.40). Blue color in the images denotes nuclei stained with Hoechst 33342 dye, detected with Ex. 365 nm and Em. 435–485 nm wavelengths. Green fluorescent oxLDL was detected with Ex. 475 nm and Em. 500–550 nm wavelengths. The Nikon *NIS-Elements AR* (v.4.40.00) software was used for image acquisition and includes a 2D deconvolution module used to reduce the imperfection of convolution on the fluorescence cell images. For FCyt analysis, cells were washed with PBS, detached from the well with Accumax^{TM}, washed again, and kept on ice in the dark. A total of 10,000 cells per sample were analyzed using a flow cytometer where the green fluorescence intensity correlates to the abundance of oxLDL in a cell. Cells with a green fluorescence intensity greater than the background auto-fluorescence intensity are considered positive for active oxLDL uptake. The mean fluorescence intensity of a sample represents the phagocytic activity of the cells to take up oxLDL under the experimental conditions.

To measure the uptake of non-fluorescent oxLDL using ORO staining, cells were incubated with fresh SF+BSA media with or without 25 μg/mL oxLDL for 16 h at 37 °C. After the incubation, cells were washed extensively and fixed with 4% *w*/*v* paraformaldehyde in PBS at room temperature for 15 min. The oil droplets present in cells were stained with a freshly prepared 0.3% *w*/*v* ORO solution in 60% isopropanol for 15 min at room temperature. The ORO working solution was prepared by diluting a stock 0.5% *w*/*v* ORO in isopropanol solution (Sigma, cat. No. O1391) with MilliQ H_2O at a 3:2 ratio. The solution was mixed, set for 10 min, passed through a 0.22 μm PVDF membrane syringe filter unit (MillexGV by Millipore, cat. No. SLGV033RS), and used within 30 min. After staining with ORO, cells were washed extensively with water. To remove ORO stains on the glass coverslips and on the wells of culture plates, coverslips were removed from the wells carefully and dipped first in a beaker filled with clean water for 10 s, then dipped in a second beaker filled with 50% isopropanol for 10 s, quickly dipped in a third beaker filled with clean water for 10 s, and transferred to wells filled with PBS in new 4-well plates. Bright-field images were acquired using a digital inverted microscope cell imaging system (EVOS FL AMEFC-4300) with a 40× magnification objective lens (NA 0.65), illuminated with an LED transmitted light at 60% intensity, and saved as 24-bit color TIFF files. To quantitate the amount of ORO associated with cells, the dye was eluted in 200 μL/well of 100% isopropanol (Sigma, cat. No. C-2432). The plates were placed on an orbital shaker for 15 min at room temperature and 150 μL eluate from each well was transferred to a well in a 96-well plate. The absorbance at 510 nm, corresponding to the ORO absorbance peak, was measured using a BioTek Synergy 2 Multi-Mode microplate reader (Winooski, VT, USA).

3. Results

3.1. Surface SR-A1 and MARCO Receptor Expression in RAW 264.7, B6, and ZK Cells

The mouse alveolar macrophage-derived cell line RAW 264.7 and two immortalized alveolar macrophage cell lines, B6 and ZK, were studied to evaluate the participation of SR-A receptors in MWNT uptake. B6 cells are derived from wild type (WT) C57BL/6 mice and ZK cells are from MARCO and SR-AI/II deficient ($MS^{-/-}$) mice [22]. The expression of surface SR-A1 and MARCO (SR-A6) receptors on RAW 264.7, WT B6, and $MS^{-/-}$ ZK cells was detected by immunofluorescence staining and determined quantitatively using FCyt, as described in the Methods section. Representative histograms of surface SR-A1 and MARCO receptor expression with RAW 264.7, B6, and ZK cells are shown in Figure 1A. Fluorescent staining with respective isotype control mAbs was included as a negative control. Both RAW 264.7 and WT B6 cells express high levels of surface SR-A1 whereas $MS^{-/-}$ ZK cells do not (Figure 1A, left panel). No relevant amount of MARCO receptors were detected on the surface of RAW 264.7, WT B6, or $MS^{-/-}$ ZK cells (Figure 1A, right panel). For quantitative analysis, cells with fluorescence intensity greater than that of the isotype control are considered positive and the fraction of positive cells among 20,000 counts analyzed for each sample are plotted in Figure 1B. The results demonstrate that more than 90% of RAW 264.7 and WT B6 cells express surface SR-A1 and only 2% $MS^{-/-}$ ZK cells tested positive for surface SR-A1. The MFI is the average fluorescence signal from the cells analyzed and gives a quantitative comparison of the population fluorescence. The MFI for RAW 264.7 and WT B6 cells was $(102.4 \pm 4.2) \times 10^3$ and $(22.4 \pm 8.6) \times 10^3$, respectively. In contrast, $MS^{-/-}$ ZK cells express low surface SR-A1, evidenced by an MFI of $(1.6 \pm 1.5) \times 10^3$, barely exceeding the isotype control background level MFI of $(1.3 \pm 0.6) \times 10^3$. Unlike the SR-A1, the constitutive expression of the MARCO receptor appears to be low in all three alveolar macrophage cell lines tested (Figure 1B), with MFIs of (1.2 ± 0.7) × 10^3, (0.8 ± 0.3) × 10^3, and (0.7 ± 0.3) × 10^3 for RAW 264.7, WT B6, and $MS^{-/-}$ ZK mouse macrophages, respectively. This is consistent with prior studies indicating that RAW 264.7 cells express high levels of SR-A1 but not MARCO [15]. Note that the surface SR-A1 and MARCO receptor levels measured here using FCyt agree with PCR genotyping results reported previously by the Kobzik group [22]. Next, the amount of MWNTs accumulated by these cells was correlated with their expression of surface SR-A1 receptors.

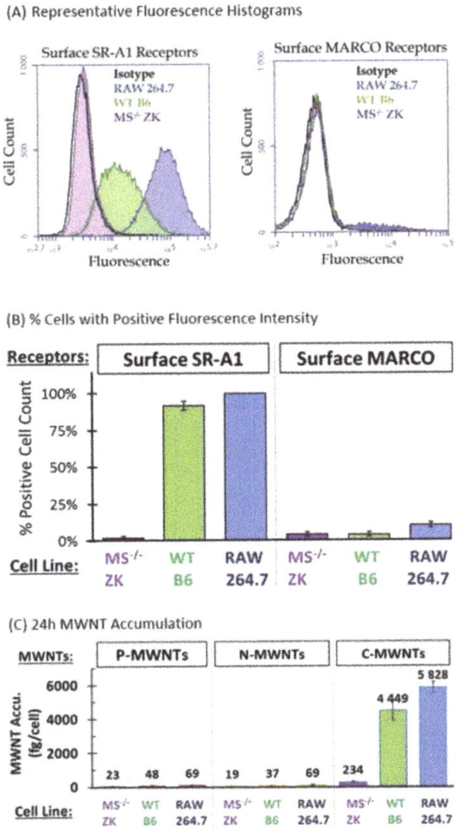

Figure 1. Surface SR-A1 receptor expression correlates with the accumulation of C-MWNTs by RAW 264.7, wild type (WT) B6, and MARCO and SR-AI/II deficient $(MS)^{-/-}$ ZK murine alveolar macrophages. (**A**,**B**) Cell surface expression of SR-A1 and MARCO receptors was determined by direct immunofluorescence FCyt assays. Cells were prepared for cytometry as described in Methods using Alexa Fluor® 488-conjugated monoclonal anti-mouse SR-A1 or APC-conjugated monoclonal anti-mouse MARCO antibody. Cells with fluorescence intensity greater than the background isotype control were considered positive. (**A**) Representative fluorescence histograms of cells stained with anti-mouse SR-A1 (left panel) or with anti-MARCO (right panel), and corresponding isotype control antibodies. Black, isotype control; blue, RAW 264.7 cells; green, WT B6 cells; purple, $MS^{-/-}$ ZK cells. (**B**) The fraction of positive cells out of a total 20,000 analyzed was expressed as the % of cells positive for surface SR-A1 (left panel) or for surface MARCO (right panel) receptors. (**C**) The accumulation of P-, N-, or C-MWNTs by RAW 264.7, WT B6, and $MS^{-/-}$ ZK cells was determined after exposing cells to media containing 100 µg/mL of either P-, N-, or C-MWNT for 24 h at 37 °C as described in Methods. Numbers above the bars are the average fg MWNTs per cell. Data in all panels of this figure are the average ± SD of ≥3 independent experiments.

3.2. *Accumulation of MWNTs by RAW 264.7, WT B6, and $MS^{-/-}$ ZK cells*

Results of our previous study on MWNT uptake by RAW 264.7 cells suggested that class A scavenger receptors might be involved in the 100-fold preferential uptake of C-MWNTs over P-MWNTs [11]. In the present study, in addition to P- and C-MWNTs, the interaction of N-MWNTs with macrophages was assessed to see if a surface functionalization other than oxidation affected uptake by cells. After a 24 h incubation in media containing 100 μg/mL of PF108-coated MWNTs, RAW 264.7 cells accumulated 69 ± 18 and 69 ± 22 fg/cell of P- and N-MWNTs, respectively, and accumulated ~85 fold more C-MWNTs at 5828 ± 325 fg/cell (Figure 1C). This is consistent with our previous results [11] and shows that N-MWNTs, like P-MWNTs, are not highly accumulated. Under the same experimental conditions as with RAW 264.7 cells, WT B6 cells also accumulated ~100 fold more C-MWNTs than P- or N-MWNTs, with an average of 48 ± 25, 37 ± 8, and 4,449 ± 591 fg/cell of P-, N-, and C-MWNTs, respectively (Figure 1C). Notably, $MS^{-/-}$ ZK cells that lack SR-A1 accumulated minimal P-, N-, or C-MWNTs (Figure 1C). Thus, high C-MWNT accumulation correlates with high expression of surface SR-A1. Moreover, since RAW 264.7 and WT B6 cells express minimal MARCO receptors on their surface (Figure 1A,B), MARCO receptors apparently cannot be responsible for the high C-MWNTs uptake in these cells (Figure 1C). To further investigate the effect of SR-A1 on the accumulation of MWNTs, transfected CHO cells that stably express mouse SR-A1 were studied next.

3.3. *Selective High Uptake of C-MWNTs in CHO Cells Expressing SR-A1*

CHO cells stably transfected with full length mouse class A type I scavenger receptor cDNA, termed CHO[mSR-AI] cells, were kindly provided by Prof. M. Krieger [23]. As received CHO[mSR-AI] cells were re-selected in medium containing 0.5 mg/mL of geneticin (G418, Gibco) and single colonies were isolated by dilution plating. The surviving colonies were screened for high surface SR-A1 expression by immunofluorescence FCyt, from which three sub-clones, termed CHO + mSRA1.A, CHO + mSRA1.B, and CHO + mSRA1.C, were selected and used to investigate the involvement of SR-A1 on the accumulation of P-, N-, and C-MWNTs by CHO cells.

Immunofluorescence FCyt showed that these sub-clones of CHO[mSR-AI] cells stably expressed transfected murine surface SR-A1 at various levels, all greater than the background level of the non-transfected wild type CHO-K1 cells (Figure 2A). MFI comparisons indicated that surface SR-A1 levels were increased significantly over wild type CHO-K1 cells, by ~7-fold for CHO + mSRA1.A and CHO + mSRA1.B cells, and by ~3-fold for CHO + mSRA1.C cells (Figure 2B).

To assess the contribution of SR-A1 to MWNT uptake, P-, N-, and C-MWNTs accumulated by wild type CHO-K1 and transfected CHO + mSRA1.A, CHO + mSRA1.B, and CHO + mSRA1.C cells were determined under the same experimental conditions as described in the previous section for macrophages. Data in Figure 2C demonstrate an increased C-MWNT uptake in all three CHO + mSR-A1 sub-clones, specifically, 358 ± 211, 812 ± 221, and 247 ± 159 fg/cell C-MWNT for CHO + mSRA1.A, CHO + mSRA1.B, and CHO + mSRA1.C, respectively, which corresponds to 6-, 14-, and 4-fold increases relative to the 59 ± 17 fg/cell for CHO-K1 cells. The uptake of P- or N-MWNTs, however, remained minimal for all three CHO+mSR-A1 sub-clones, despite the higher SR-A1 expression levels compared to wild type CHO-K1 cells. Thus, the amount of surface SR-A1 correlates with the selective uptake of C-MWNT, but not P- or N-MWNT in CHO clones expressing SR-A1.

Altogether, the low C-MWNT uptake by cells that lack SR-A1 ($MS^{-/-}$ ZK macrophages, Figure 1) and the high uptake of C-MWNT by cells that over-express SR-A1 (CHO + mSRA1 clones, Figure 2) provide strong evidence that SR-A1 underlies the selective uptake of C-MWNTs in macrophages. To determine the potential physiological consequences of high-level accumulation of C-MWNT by macrophages, the cytotoxicity of PF108 alone, P-, N-, and C-MWNTs in RAW 264.7 cells was compared next using three different assays.

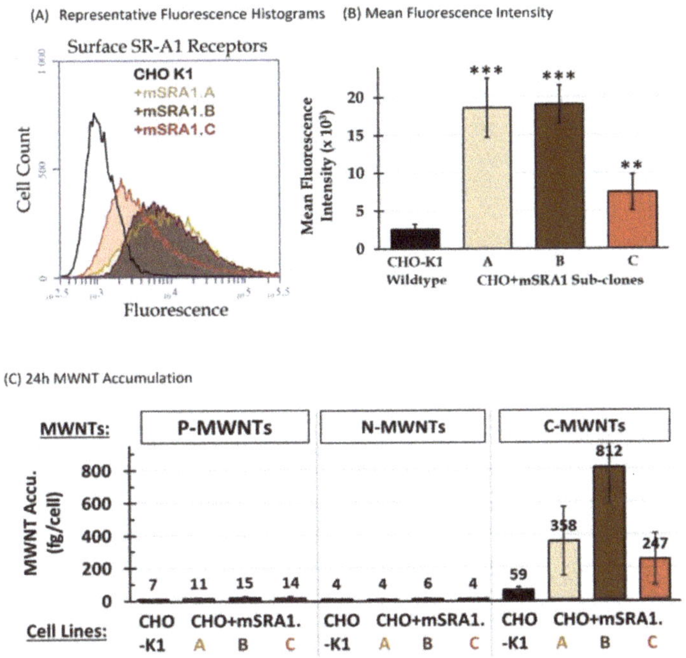

Figure 2. Surface SR-A1 receptor expression correlates with C-MWNT uptake by CHO-K1 and transfected CHO + mSRA1 clones. (**A**,**B**) Cell surface expression of SR-A1 receptors was determined by direct immunofluorescence FCyt assays. Cells detached from the culture vessel with enzyme-free buffer were incubated with mouse IgG to block Fc receptors before incubation with Alexa Fluor® 488-conjugated monoclonal anti-mouse mSR-A1 antibody. Alexa Fluor® 488-conjugated rat IgG2b was used as isotype control. Cells with fluorescence intensity greater than the background isotype control were considered positive. The mean fluorescence intensity represents the surface expression level of SR-A1 receptors by the 20,000 cells analyzed. (**A**) Representative fluorescence histograms of cells stained with anti-mSR-A1. Black, untransfected CHO-K1 cells; beige, brown, and red, transfected CHO + mSRA1 sub-clones A, B, and C, respectively. (**B**) The surface SR-A1 receptor expression level represented as the mean fluorescence intensity of 20,000 cells analyzed per sample. Data are the mean ± SD of triplicate measurements of each sample in ≥3 independent experiments. ** is for $p < 0.0005$ and *** is for $p < 0.00005$, compared to CHO-K1. (**C**) The accumulation of P-, N-, or C-MWNTs by untransfected CHO-K1 cells and transfected CHO + mSRA1 sub-clones A, B, and C was determined after exposing cells to media containing 100 µg/mL of P-, N-, or C-MWNT for 24 h at 37 °C. After incubation, the cells were washed, cell counts were determined using a Coulter Particle Counter, and MWNTs were extracted and quantified using the SDS-PAGE method. Numbers above the bars are the average fg MWNTs per cell. Data are the average ± SD of ≥3 independent experiments.

3.4. *The Effect of MWNT Accumulation on Apoptosis, Proliferation, and Colony Formation Efficiency*

The first set of experiments assessed the consequences of MWNT exposure on RAW 264.7 cell proliferation using a standardized crystal violet cell proliferation assay [11,24]. Specifically, the ability of cells to proliferate was determined as a function of P-, N-, or C-MWNT concentration in the media, from 25 up to 200 µg/mL, as well as a function of incubation time of 24, 48, or 72 h. Control cells were incubated in regular culture medium that contained no MWNTs or PF108 and their proliferation measured after incubation was set to 100%.

After a 24 h incubation (Figure 3A), there was no significant decline in RAW 264.7 cell proliferation for cells with either P- or N-MWNTs at concentrations up to 200 µg/mL, relative to the untreated controls.

A slight reduction in proliferation was detected only for cells with C-MWNTs at concentrations of 150 and 200 μg/mL. After a 48 h incubation (Figure 3B), again, no significant effects on cell proliferation were detected for cells with P- or N-MWNTs; however, a greater impact was observed for cells exposed to C-MWNTs, with an estimated IC50 of 120 μg/mL. A longer incubation of 72 h with C-MWNTs aggravated the adverse effect on cell proliferation (Figure 3C), indicated by an IC50 of 80 μg/mL. A 40–50% reduction in cell proliferation for cells with P- or N-MWNTs only became notable after a 72 h exposure and at 200 μg/mL, the highest P- or N-MWNT concentration tested. These data indicate that the IC50 values for exposure to C-MWNTs decrease significantly with time. Therefore, we also studied the effect of MWNTs on RAW 264.7 cells in long-term colony formation assays.

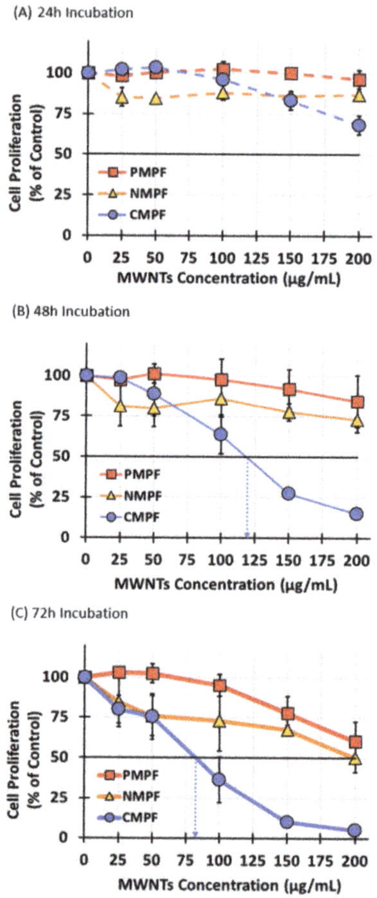

Figure 3. Effects of P-, N-, and C-MWNTs dose and exposure time on RAW 264.7 cell proliferation. RAW 264.7 cells in 48-well plates were incubated in media containing 25, 50, 100, 150, or 200 μg/mL of P-, N-, or C-MWNTs at 37 °C. Cells incubated in regular culture medium in the absence of MWNTs was the untreated control. IC50 values were estimated from a linear regression dose-effect trend line as the concentration of MWNTs needed to inhibit cell proliferation by 50%. Cell proliferation after a (**A**) 24 h, (**B**) 48 h, or (**C**) 72 h exposure to MWNTs was determined by the crystal violet assay where the proliferation of control cells was set to 100%. Dotted arrows indicate estimated IC50 values of 120 and 80 μg/mL for cells treated with C-MWNTs for 48 and 72 h, respectively. Data are the average of quadruplicate measurements per sample in ≥3 independent experiments ± SEM.

Colony formation assays (CFA), were performed next to assess the impact of various MWNTs on RAW 264.7 cells' survival upon long-term exposure. This assay tests the ability of single cells to proliferate and form a visible colony under the test condition [25] and has been previously used in studies with CNTs [28,29]. A total of 300 RAW 264.7 cells/well were seeded in a control of regular culture medium or in test media that contained either P-, N-, or C-MWNTs at various MWNT concentrations up to 100 μg/mL, and incubated without disturbance for 8 day to allow colony formation. Colonies were fixed, stained with crystal violet, imaged using a stereomicroscope, and counted.

Representative images of colonies of the untreated control group and cells incubated with 100 μg/mL P-, N-, or C-MWNTs are shown in Figure 4A. A total of 46 ± 13% of seeded control RAW 264.7 cells formed colonies in 8 day whereas fewer colonies were produced from cells exposed to 100 μg/mL of P- or N-MWNTs. The efficiency of colony formation was near zero for C-MWNT-treated cells. The % colony formation efficiency (CFE) was calculated for each sample, relative to the number of colonies produced by the untreated control set to 100%. A dose-effect curve was plotted for each MWNT type in Figure 4B and demonstrates a dose-dependent decline for CFE. The IC50 values for cells exposed continuously to P-, N-, and C-MWNTs for 8 day were 79, 77, and 29 μg/mL, respectively. The IC50 of 29 μg/mL for the effect of C-MWNT on viability suggests that even lower concentrations could have some adverse effects on cells after long-term exposure.

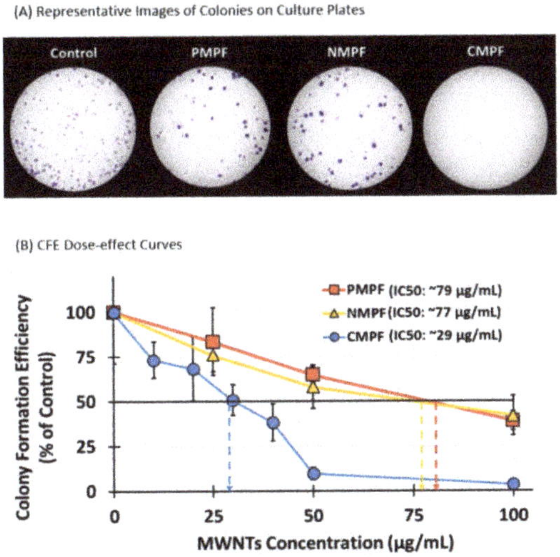

Figure 4. Colony formation efficiency (CFE) of RAW 264.7 cells after 8d of continuous exposure to P-, N-, or C-MWNTs at various concentrations up to 100 μg/mL. 300 RAW 264.7 cells were seeded in 35 mm culture plates with media containing various concentrations of P-, N-, or C-MWNTs up to 100 μg/mL and incubated at 37 °C in a 5% CO_2 incubator without disturbance for 8 day, then stained as described in Methods. CFE was defined as the ratio of the colony count over the seeded cell count in a plate. The concentration of MWNTs required to inhibit CFE by 50% (IC50) value was estimated from a linear regression dose-effect trend line. (**A**) Representative images of stained colonies in plates with control or cells treated with 100 μg/mL of P-, N-, or C-MWNTs. (**B**) CFE of RAW 264.7 cells incubated in media containing P-, N-, or C-MWNTs for 8 day at 37 °C, relative to untreated control where the CFE was set to 100%. Dotted arrows indicate estimated IC50 values. Data are the average of 6 replicate plates per sample in ≥3 independent experiments ± SD.

Apoptosis was also assessed after a 24 h incubation with media containing either 0.1 mM PF108 alone, or 100 μg/mL of P-, N-, or C-MWNTs. Untreated cells provided a negative control and cells treated with 100 nM CPT, a known DNA topoisomerase I inhibitor that causes DNA double-strand breaks [30], were used as positive controls for apoptosis. After the treatments, apoptotic, necrotic, and dead cells were detected using an apoptosis/dead cell detection kit with Annexin V-FITC and PI, according to the manufacturer's instruction. The % of viable, apoptotic, necrotic, and dead cell fractions in 10,000 cell counts analyzed per sample were acquired using an FCyt cell analyzer. There was negligible necrosis and a background of 4% apoptosis in negative control cells. In CPT treated positive control cells, almost 53% of the cells were apoptotic while necrosis was still low (Figure S1A). Only a low level of apoptosis (11.4–18.0%) was detected in cells exposed to PF108 surfactant alone or to the various MWNTs. The mean % apoptotic cell fractions are plotted as bar graphs in SI Figure S1B to further illustrate that regardless of high accumulation, C-MWNTs had only a mild apoptotic effect on cells in the first 24 h exposure. We next looked at what consequences C-MWNT accumulation via SR-A1 receptors might have on functions related to this receptor.

3.5. *Treatment of Cells with C-MWNTs, but Not P- or N-MWNTs, Depletes Surface SR-A1*

Phagocytosis is important for alveolar macrophages to remove foreign particles such as invading pathogens and dust from the lung. The interaction of C-MWNTs with SR-A1 receptors, and subsequent accumulation in cells, could impair macrophage phagocytic activity. The experiments described in the following sections address: (1) whether the accumulation of C-MWNTs via SR-A1 depletes this important receptor from the cell surface; and (2) whether C-MWNT accumulation impairs the ability of cells to phagocytose ligands, such as polystyrene beads, *E. coli*, and oxidized LDL (oxLDL) that are known to interact with SR-A1 [22,31–34].

Two approaches were used to assess the effects of MWNTs on surface SR-A1 levels in RAW 264.7 cells, a qualitative immunofluorescence microscopy (IFM) assay and a quantitative FCyt assay. The timeline schematic in Figure 5A presents the key steps used to prepare samples for the IFM and FCyt experiments (full details described in the Methods section). Briefly, RAW 264.7 cells were incubated in control medium that contained no PF108 or MWNTs or in test media that contained 0.1 mM PF108 alone or 100 µg/mL of P-, N-, or C-MWNTs at 37 °C for 24 h, washed extensively, chased in fresh medium for 1 h at 37 °C, and then chilled to 4 °C. Half of the cells were incubated with a green Alexa Fluor® 488-conjugated mAb specific for mouse SR-A1 and the other half with an Alexa Fluor® 488-conjugated isotype control mAb as a negative control, at 4 °C for 30 min in the dark. The cells were then prepared either for IFM or FCyt as described in Methods.

Representative LSCFM images of cells stained with Alexa Fluor® 488-conjugated mAbs for SR-A1 and Hoechst dye for the nucleus are shown in Figure 5B. Green fluorescence marking surface SR-A1 was in punctate spots, noted previously and attributed to the localization of SR-A1 in lipid rafts on the cell surface [33]. After C-MWNT treatment, considerably fewer green punctate spots were observed and the spots appeared mainly at cell margins where the cell membrane was attached to the glass coverslip. The untreated control cells appeared to have abundant SR-A1 stains while cells treated with P- and N-MWNTs had slightly less SR-A1 on their surface (Figure 5B). See SI Figure S2 for 360° rotating video clips of representative control and C-MWNT-treated RAW 264.7 cells stained with green fluorescent mAbs against surface SR-A1. None of the cells stained with isotype control mAbs emitted detectable green fluorescence signal, which indicates negligible background fluorescence in this assay (data not shown). These data suggested that SR-A1 might be depleted from the cell surface in RAW 264.7 cells pre-exposed to C-MWNTs, and this was next tested by quantitative FCyt assay.

Cells with a green fluorescence intensity $>1 \times 10^4$ in the FCyt assay were considered positive for surface SR-A1. Results (Figure 5C, left panel) indicated that ≥97% of RAW 264.7 cells tested positive for surface SR-A1, regardless of any pre-treatment or not. However, as previously noticed in the LSCFM images (Figure 5B), not all SR-A1 positive cells express the same level of surface SR-A1 (Figure 5C right panel). Exposing cells to PF108 alone for 24 h had no effects on their surface SR-A1 expression. A mild reduction in surface SR-A1 expression, of 7% and 16%, was detected in cells pre-treated with either P- or N-MWNTs, respectively, compared to the untreated control cells. A 40% reduction of surface SR-A1 was detected in RAW 264.7 cells pre-treated with 100 µg/mL C-MWNTs for 24 h (Figure 5C, right panel). One interpretation of these data is that notable amounts of surface SR-A1 are depleted from the cell surface upon exposure to C-MWNTs over time. Alternatively, it is possible that cell-associated MWNTs interfere with quantifying surface SR-A1, by quenching the antibody fluorophore signal or by preventing the binding of the reporter antibody in the FCyt experiments. To assess the alternative possibilities, further control experiments were performed, as described next.

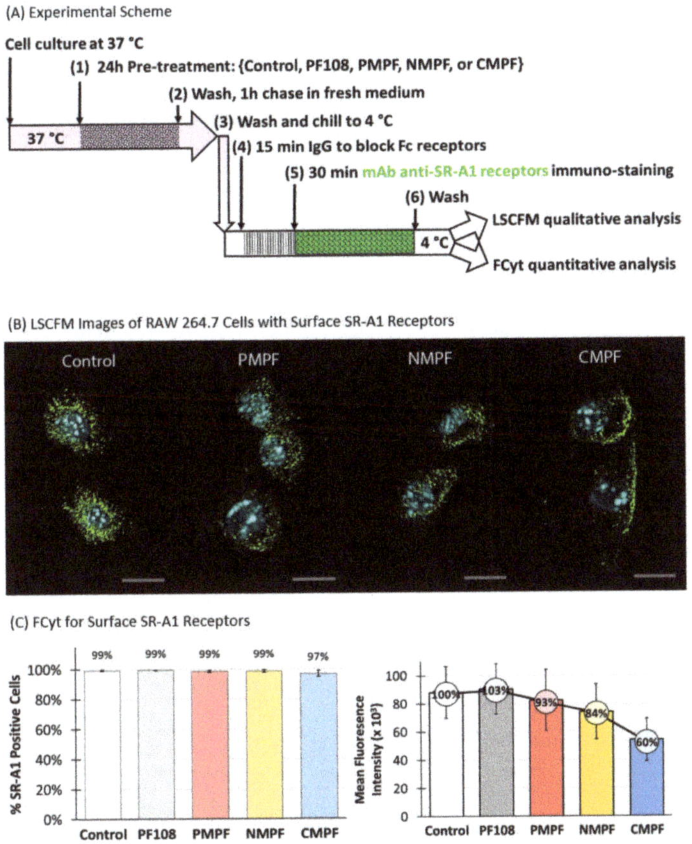

Figure 5. Effects of MWNT accumulation on surface SR-A1 receptor expression in RAW 264.7 cells. RAW 264.7 cells were incubated in media containing 0.1 mM PF108 alone or 100 μg/mL of P-, N-, or CMPF at 37 °C for 24 h. Cells incubated in regular culture medium in the absence of PF108 and MWNTs are the untreated control. Cells were washed and chased in fresh medium at 37 °C for 1 h to promote internalization of MWNTs that may have been on the cell surface. SR-A1 on the cell surface was immunologically detected by either FCyt or LSCFM as described in Methods. Briefly, cells were detached from culture plates with enzyme-free buffer, washed, chilled on ice, and appropriate antibodies were added to cells at 4 °C to prevent internalization of receptors or ligands. (**A**) The timeline scheme outlines the key experimental steps. (**B**) Representative Laser Scanning Confocal Fluorescence Microscopy (LSCFM) images of untreated control and MWNT-treated cells. Blue fluorescence is emitted from Hoechst 33342 stained nucleus and green fluorescence is from Alexa Fluor® 488-conjugated SR-A1 receptors. Scale bars are 10 μm. (**C**) The fraction of positive cells out of a total 20,000 analyzed by flow cytometry was expressed as the % of positive for surface SR-A1 (left panel). The surface SR-A1 receptor expression level is represented as the mean fluorescence intensity of 20,000 cells analyzed per sample (right panel). Percent values inside circles are the mean fluorescence intensity relative to untreated control where the surface SR-A1 receptor level was set to 100%. Data are the mean ± SD of triplicate measurements per sample in ≥3 independent experiments.

3.6. MWNTs Do Not Interfere with Immunofluorescence FCyt Assays for Surface SR-A1

To test whether surface-bound MWNTs interfered with the detection of SR-A1 receptors, RAW 264.7 cells were exposed to MWNTs at 4 °C for 1 h, washed to remove unbound MWNTs, and incubated in fresh medium for 1 h at 4 °C. Control cells were kept in medium in the absence of MWNTs at 4 °C. Cells were immuno-stained with fluorescent-conjugated monoclonal anti-SR-A1 antibodies and analyzed for the presence of surface-SR-A1 by FCyt (See SI Figure S3A for a timeline of the treatment). The fluorescent signal in cells treated with MWNTs at 4 °C was compared with the signal from untreated control cells. Interference would be indicated if the signal is attenuated by surface bound MWNTs in the MWNT-treated cells. There was no effect of exposing cells to any type of MWNT at 4 °C on the mean fluorescence intensity of the anti-SR-A1 antibody compared to the untreated control (SI Figure S3B, left side).

Furthermore, to determine whether internalized MWNTs could interfere with the detection of surface anti-SR-A1 immunofluorescence, cells were exposed to MWNTs at 4 °C for 1 h to allow binding, washed to remove unbound material, and then chased at 37 °C for 1 h to permit internalization (see SI Figure S3A). The results in SI Figure S3B, right side, indicate that the internalized MWNTs did not reduce the mean fluorescent signal of the anti-SR-A1 antibody compared to the control. Altogether, these data suggest that neither surface-bound nor internalized MWNTs block the binding of anti-SR-A1 antibody or quench the fluorescent signals of the antibody in the FCyt assay. Thus, the observed 40% reduction of surface SR-A1 in RAW 264.7 cells exposed to C-MWNTs for 24 h is most likely due to a depletion of the SR-A1 receptors from the cell surface over time.

Considering that the accumulation of C-MWNTs by RAW 264.7 cells appears to reduce the expression of SR-A1 on the cell surface, there should be a corresponding effect on the uptake of other SR-A1 receptor ligands. To test this, we next compared the uptake of polystyrene beads, *E. coli*, and oxLDL by untreated control and MWNT-treated RAW 264.7 cells.

3.7. Accumulation of C-MWNTs, but Not P- or N-MWNTs, Reduces Uptake of Polystyrene Beads

Polystyrene beads are negatively charged and are known to bind SR-A1 [22,33,34]. To check the phagocytic ability of RAW 264.7 cells after exposure to different MWNTs, polystyrene beads with internally bound green fluorophores and a nominal diameter of 0.9 μm were used as phagocytic markers. RAW 264.7 cells were pre-incubated with 100 μg/mL P-, N-, or C-MWNTs, or with 0.1 mM PF108 alone at 37 °C for 20 h, washed, and then exposed to 10 μg/mL fluorescent polystyrene beads for 2 h at 37 °C, followed by a 1-h chase at 37 °C in the dark (Figure 6A). The presence of the beads in cells was determined by qualitative assessment using LSCFM and by quantitative FCyt measurement. Representative confocal fluorescence images of untreated control cells and MWNT-treated cells (Figure 6B) visually demonstrate a reduced number of beads in C-MWNT-treated RAW 264.7 cells, whereas cells treated with P- or N-MWNTs have a sparingly reduced number of beads, relative to that of the control cells.

The quantitative results of FCyt analysis (Figure 6C) revealed that the untreated control and cells exposed to either PF108 alone, P-, or N-MWNTs all have high levels of phagocytosed beads, with MFIs of 2.6×10^6, 2.1×10^6, 2.0×10^6, and 2.1×10^6, respectively, indicative of robust phagocytic activity. On the contrary, cells treated with C-MWNTs displayed a significantly reduced level of phagocytosed polystyrene beads, evidenced by a low MFI of 1.0×10^6, ~40% that of the control cells (Figure 6C). These data are consistent with the qualitative observations with LSCFM (Figure 6B and SI Figure S4) and support the idea that the accumulation of C-MWNTs impairs the subsequent uptake of a SR-A1 receptor ligand. Note that in Figure 6B there appears to be fewer, but bright, beads within C-MWNT treated cells, suggesting that quenching is not responsible for the reduced fluorescence signal in cytometry experiments with C-MWNT treated cells.

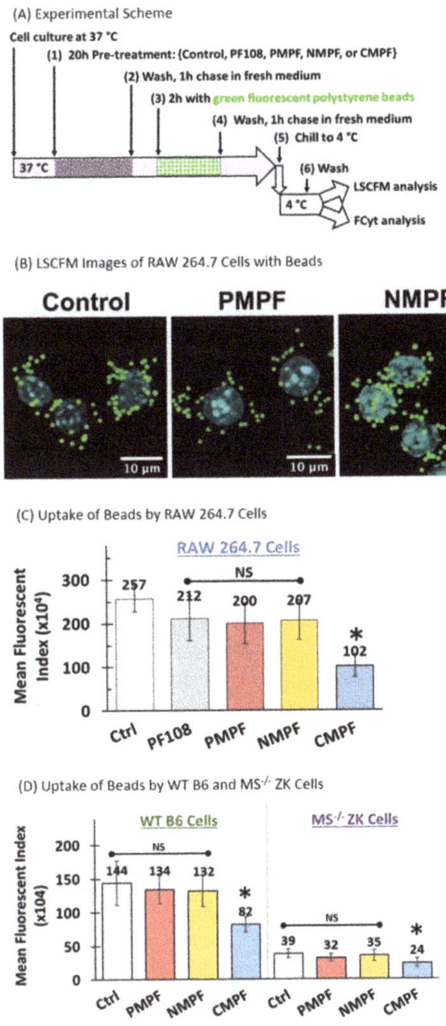

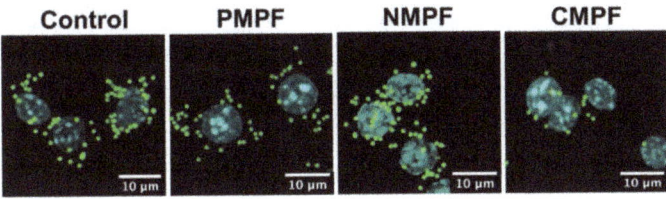

Figure 6. Effects of MWNT accumulation on subsequent phagocytosis of polystyrene beads in murine alveolar macrophage cell lines. RAW 264.7, wild type B6, and $MS^{-/-}$ ZK cells were incubated in media containing 100 μg/mL of P-, N-, or C-MWNTs at 37 °C for 20 h. Untreated control cells were incubated in regular culture medium in the absence of PF108 surfactant or MWNTs. Cells were prepared for LSCFM or FCyt as described in Methods. (**A**) The timeline scheme outlines the key experimental steps. (**B**) Representative LSCFM images of untreated control and MWNT-treated cells. Blue fluorescence is emitted from Hoechst 33342 stained nuclei and green fluorescence is from phagocytosed polystyrene beads. (**C**) Mean fluorescence index of RAW 264.7 control, cells pre-treated with 0.1 mM PF108 alone, or with 100 μg/mL of P-, N-, or C-MWNTs. (**D**) Mean fluorescence index of WT B6 (left panel) and $MS^{-/-}$ ZK (right panel) controls and cells pre-treated with 100 μg/mL of P-, N-, or C-MWNTs. Data are the mean ± SD of duplicate measurements per sample in ≥3 independent experiments. NS is for no significant differences ($p > 0.05$) among test groups, * is for $p < 0.0005$ against control.

The possibility that polystyrene beads and PF108-coated C-MWNTs are internalized by the same receptor predicts that they might sometimes both end up within the same phagolysosomes in cells exposed to both ligands. To test this prediction, we used LSCRM to determine whether the distinct

Raman signals of polystyrene beads and C-MWNTs co-localized. In LSCRM, a laser scans the cells attached on a coverslip and briefly pauses at each pixel to collect a complete Raman scattering spectrum of the sample, one spectrum per pixel. The scattering signals of C-MWNTs and polystyrene beads in different regions can be extracted, separated, assigned colors, and overlaid to see if they overlap. However, since our results suggest that C-MWNTs and polystyrene beads may use the same receptor, the cells were not simultaneously exposed to both to avoid competition; rather, they were first exposed to C-MWNTs for 2 h, washed, then exposed to beads for 2 h. The cells were then fixed and analyzed by LSCRM as described in the Supplemental Information methods. The Raman signal (red) of cells exposed to beads alone for 2 h mapped to the position of beads seen by bright field microscopy (SI Figure S6, top, left and right). In cells first treated with C-MWNTs for 2 h, washed, then exposed to beads for 2 h, the location of C-MWNTs (green) was visible, as were structures that were yellow, indicating colocalization of beads and C-MWNTs (SI Figure S6, bottom, left and right). The colocalization is partial, as expected because the cells were exposed to the two ligands at separate times. These data provide evidence independent of fluorescence methods that C-MWNTs are internalized and appear with beads in structures that have the expected perinuclear distribution of phagolysosomes.

The effect of MWNTs on the uptake of polystyrene beads was also tested with wild type B6 macrophages, which have SR-A1, and with $MS^{-/-}$ ZK cells, which lack SR-A1. Wild type B6 and $MS^{-/-}$ ZK cells pre-incubated with 100 μg/mL P-, N-, or C-MWNTs at 37 °C for 20 h were washed, chased in fresh medium for 1 h, incubated with 25 μg/mL fluorescent polystyrene beads for 2 h at 37 °C, and washed again prior to FCyt analysis for phagocytosed beads in the cells. Quantitative FCyt results (Figure 6D, left panel) showed that untreated control WT B6 cells and those treated with P- and N-MWNTs have similar phagocytic function and internalized a large number of beads within 2 h of exposure at 37 °C, indicated by their MFI values of 1.4×10^6, 1.3×10^6, and 1.3×10^6, respectively. WT B6 cells treated with C-MWNT, in contrast, displayed a 43% reduction in the uptake of polystyrene beads (MFI 8.2×10^5), compared to the control B6 cells, consistent with the idea that accumulation of C-MWNTs via SR-A1 impairs subsequent uptake of polystyrene beads by WT B6 cells. Unlike the RAW 264.7 or the WT B6 cells, untreated $MS^{-/-}$ ZK cells tested under the same experimental conditions show minimal uptake of polystyrene beads (MFI 3.9×10^5) by the untreated control ZK cells, verifying that SR-A1 are essential for the phagocytosis of polystyrene beads (Figure 6D, right panel). $MS^{-/-}$ ZK cells treated with P-, N-, or C-MWNTs also showed minimal uptake of polystyrene bead (MFIs 3.2×10^5, 3.5×10^5, and 2.4×10^5, respectively).

Replicate experiments of WT B6 and SR-A1-deficient $MS^{-/-}$ ZK cells were analyzed using LSCFM. SI Figure S4 displays representative confocal fluorescence images of B6 and ZK cells with phagocytosed green fluorescent beads and nuclei stained with blue fluorescent Hoechst 33342 dye. The qualitative visual assessment of WT B6 and $MS^{-/-}$ ZK cells using LSCFM (SI Figure S4) confirms the quantitative FCyt results (Figure 6D) for these cells under the same experimental conditions. Altogether, the attenuated uptake of an SR-A1 ligand by cells pre-treated with C-MWNTs correlates well with the observation that C-MWNT accumulation appears to deplete SR-A1 from the cell surface. This correlation was further tested using a bacterial SR-A1 ligand.

3.8. Accumulation of C-MWNTs, but Not P- or N-MWNTs, Impairs Subsequent E. coli Uptake

Alveolar macrophages play a key role in host defense against invading pathogens where SR-A1 is critical for bacteria clearance [31,35]. In the following experiments, the potential adverse impacts of C-MWNT accumulation in alveolar macrophage-derived RAW 264.7 cells on *E. coli* clearance were investigated. A schematic of the experimental approach is shown in Figure 7A. Briefly, RAW 264.7 cells were incubated with 100 μg/mL of the indicated MWNTs for 24 h at 37 °C, chased for 1 h at 37 °C and then exposed to heat-killed, green fluorescent-conjugated *E. coli* particles with a multiplicity of infection (MOI) of 30 at 4 °C for 1 h in the dark. Cells were washed to remove unbound *E. coli* particles, placed in fresh medium at 37 °C for 1 h to allow phagocytosis, washed, and analyzed for *E. coli* inside the cells by FCyt. To verify that the fluorescence measured under such conditions was from internalized *E. coli*, cells were treated with TB, which is known to quench extracellular fluorescent signals but has no effect on internalized fluorescence [26,27]. To confirm that TB was an effective quencher of fluorescent *E. coli*, the bacteria were directly exposed to TB in solution and the quenching was assessed by cytometry. The results of this control experiment indicated that the fluorescent signal was quenched by 94%, as shown in SI Figure S5.

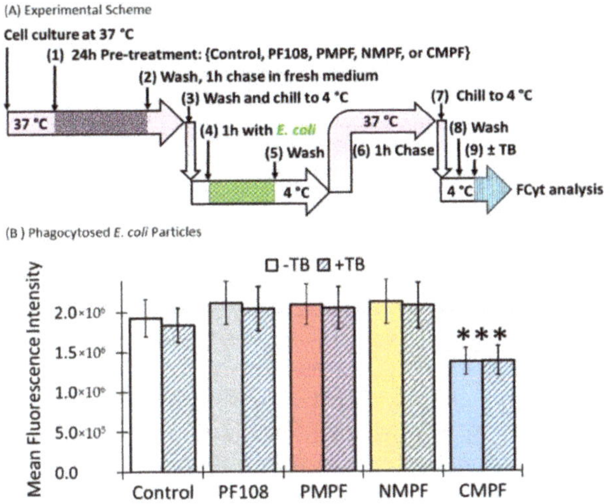

Figure 7. A 24 h exposure of RAW 264.7 cells to C-MWNTs, but not P- or N-MWNTs, impairs subsequent phagocytosis of *E. coli*. RAW 264.7 cells were incubated in media containing 100 µg/mL of P-, N-, or C-MWNTs, or 0.1 mM PF108 alone at 37 °C for 24 h. The cells were chilled to 4 °C and exposed to heat-killed Alexa Fluor® 488-conjugated *E. coli*, at 30 *E. coli* particles per cell, for 1 h at 4 °C, washed, chased for 1 h at 37 °C to allow phagocytosis, washed again, and analyzed by FCyt as described in Methods. Cells with a fluorescence intensity greater than the background auto-fluorescence were considered positive for phagocytosed *E. coli*. Flow cytometric measurements of a sample were followed immediately by consecutive analysis in the presence of 0.1% trypan blue dye, as described in Methods. (**A**) The timeline scheme outlines the key experimental steps. (**B**) *E. coli* phagocytosed by untreated control, PF108-treated, MWNT-treated cells. Mean fluorescence intensity was measured in the absence (−TB) and subsequent presence (+TB) of 0.1% trypan blue. *** is for $p < 0.0005$. Data are the mean ± SD of triplicate measurements per sample in ≥3 independent experiments.

The results in Figure 7B revealed that pre-treatment of cells with PF108, P-MWNTs, or N-MWNTs did not reduce their MFI compared to the control cells. In addition, the fluorescence was unaffected by TB, evidence that the fluorescence was from internalized *E. coli* in these cells. However, cells pre-treated with C-MWNTs had a 30% reduction in MFI, even though the fluorescence was, again, highly resistant to quenching by TB. These results support the idea that C-MWNT accumulation impairs *E. coli* clearance by macrophages. In addition, the resistance to TB quenching in the control and cells pre-treated with MWNTs also implies that the plasma membrane of the cells was intact.

3.9. Reduced OxLDL Uptake by RAW 264.7 Cells Pre-Exposed to C-MWNTs, but Not P- or N-MWNTs

SR-A1 is one of the three major SRs involved in the recognition and uptake of oxLDL by macrophages, in addition to CD36 and LOX-1 [36]. The uptake and the subsequent intracellular accumulation of oxLDL have been shown to promote the transformation of lipid-laden macrophages to foam cells with proatherogenic effects [36–38]. The effect of MWNTs on the uptake of oxLDL was tested with RAW 264.7 cells using the schematic experimental approach shown in Figure 8A. Cells were incubated in media containing either 0.1 mM PF108 alone, 100 µg/mL P-, N-, or C-MWNTs, or in control medium that contained no PF108 or MWNTs for 20 h at 37 °C. After this pre-treatment, the cells were washed and incubated in fresh serum-free medium for 4 h at 37 °C to remove lipid components in the culture medium and then exposed to Alexa Fluor® 488-conjugated oxLDL for 2 h at 37 °C in the dark. Cells were washed and assessed for phagocytosed oxLDL by epi-fluorescence microscopy (FM) and FCyt analysis. Representative fluorescence images of untreated control and MWNT-treated cells are shown in Figure 8B. Active uptake of fluorescent oxLDL was readily visible in untreated control and cells treated with P- or N-MWNTs, whereas green fluorescence was reduced in C-MWNT-treated cells, correlating C-MWNT accumulation with impaired oxLDL uptake by RAW 264.7 cells.

Quantitative results of FCyt analysis (Figure 8C) confirmed the qualitative FM observations shown in Figure 8B. The untreated control and cells exposed to either PF108 alone, P-, or N-MWNTs all had active oxLDL uptake, with mean fluorescence intensities of 2.5×10^5, 2.8×10^5, 3.0×10^5, and 3.1×10^5, respectively, indicative of robust phagocytic activities in these cells. On the contrary, cells with accumulated C-MWNTs displayed a significantly lower fluorescence intensity of 1.3×10^5, indicative of a reduced activity (by ~50%) for oxLDL uptake (Figure 8C). These data, again, support the idea that the accumulation of C-MWNTs impairs the subsequent uptake of SR-A1 receptor ligands.

The concern that C-MWNTs may have quenching effects on the internalized fluorescent oxLDL was addressed with independent oxLDL uptake experiments using non-fluorescent oxLDL. The development of oil droplets from oxLDL uptake by cells was detected visually and measured quantitatively based on an ORO staining assay [39–41], with optimization detailed in the Methods section. RAW 264.7 cells seeded on glass coverslips were pre-treated either with regular culture medium as control or with test media containing 100 µg/mL of P-, N-, or C-MWNTs at 37 °C for 24 h. After pre-treatment, cells were washed and serum-starved for 4 h before exposure to non-fluorescent oxLDL for 16 h. The uptake of oxLDL was detected as red oil droplets stained with ORO dye. The red stained oil droplets were readily visible under a bright-field microscope with LED transmitted light and a 40× magnification objective lens. In addition, the ORO stain was eluted in isopropanol and measured quantitatively as absorbance intensity at 510 nm.

Representative ORO stained images of control and MWNT-treated cells, with and without oxLDL exposure, are shown in SI Figure S7B. Without oxLDL exposure, no ORO stains were visible in either control or any of the MWNT-treated cells, indicating that endogenous oil droplets were successfully depleted during the serum starvation period. On the contrary, robust oxLDL uptake was evidenced by the red ORO stain in cells allowed to take up oxLDL present in the media. Notice that internalized MWNTs were clearly visible as dark gray vesicular structures inside cells pre-treated with C-MWNTs that may obstruct visual assessment of red oil droplets in these cells. Thus, cell-associated ORO was determined by extracting the dye from cells with isopropanol, and the eluent was then transferred to new plates and measured spectrophotometrically free of potential MWNT interference. Results of the quantitative oxLDL uptake assessment, represented by the relative ORO stain intensities of the untreated control and cells pre-treated with MWNTs, indicated that oxLDL uptake was reduced by ~30% in cells pre-treated with C-MWNTs, whereas P- or N-MWNTs had no effect on subsequent oxLDL uptake (SI Figure S7C). These results agree with data in Figure 8 using fluorescent oxLDL and validate the finding that accumulation of C-MWNTs in RAW 264.7 cells affects subsequent phagocytosis of oxLDL.

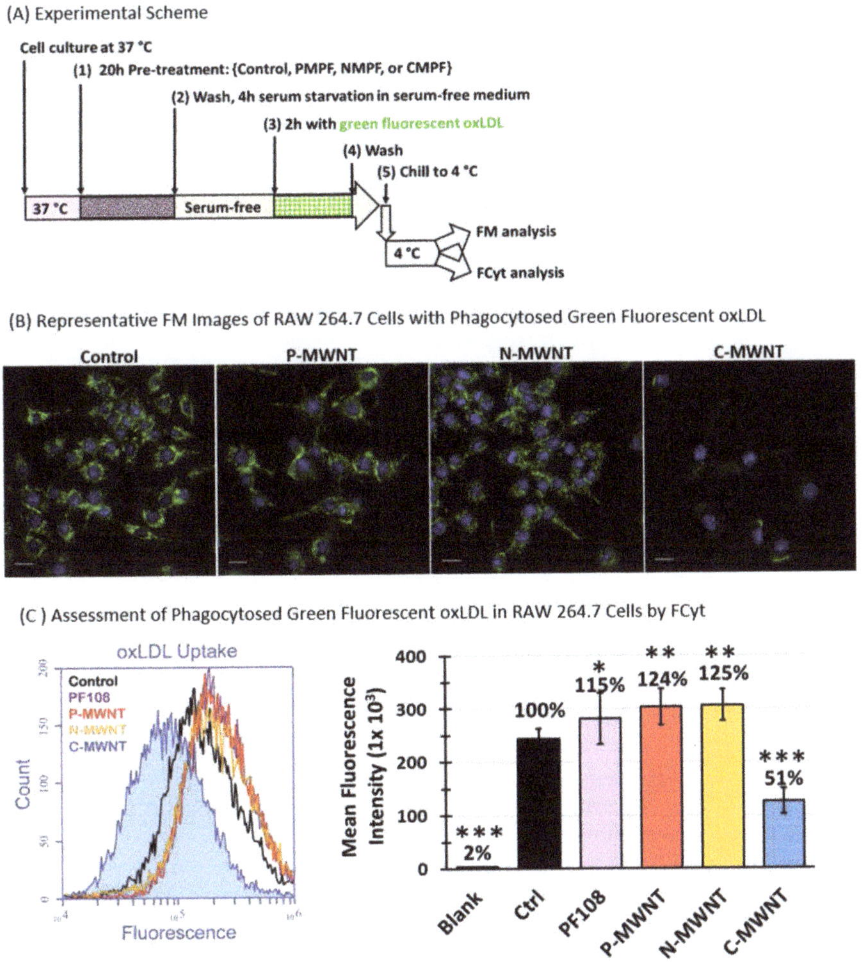

Figure 8. Reduced fluorescent oxLDL uptake by RAW 264.7 cells pre-treated with C-MWNTs, but not P- or N-MWNTs. RAW 264.7 cells were incubated in media containing either 0.1 mM PF108 alone or 100 µg/mL of P-, N-, or C-MWNTs at 37 °C for 24 h. Untreated control cells were incubated in regular culture medium in the absence of PF108 surfactant or MWNTs. After the pre-treatments, cells were washed and serum starved for 4 h in serum-free medium before incubation in fresh serum-free medium containing Alexa Fluor® 488-conjugated oxLDL (1:20 dilution for FM and 1:40 dilution for FCyt) for 2 h at 37 °C. Cells were washed again, chilled to 4 °C, and prepared for FM or FCyt as described in Methods. (**A**) The timeline schematic outlining the key experimental steps. (**B**) Representative epi-fluorescence images of the control and treated cells. Blue fluorescence is emitted from Hoechst 33342 stained nuclei and green fluorescence is from internalized Alexa Fluor® 488-conjugated oxLDL. (**C**) Representative fluorescence histograms of control cells (black), cells pre-treated with 0.1 mM PF108 (purple), 100 µg/mL of P-MWNTs (red), N-MWNTs (yellow), or C-MWNTs (blue) are plotted on the left. The internalized oxLDL is represented as the mean fluorescence intensity of a total of 10,000 cells analyzed per sample and plotted as a bar graph on the right. Data are the mean ± SD of triplicate samples in ≥4 independent experiments. Percent values shown above the bars indicate mean fluorescence intensity relative to untreated control cells where the level of oxLDL was set to 100%. * is for $p < 5.0 \times 10^{-2}$, ** is for $p < 5.0 \times 10^{-5}$, and *** is for $p < 5.0 \times 10^{-10}$ against control.

4. Discussion

Our present hypothesis for the selective interaction of PF108-coated C-MWNTs with macrophages is that the primary determinant of the interaction is oxidative functionalities on nanotubes, which could include carboxylation, hydroxylation, and other carbon-oxygen bonded groups. This idea is supported by our previous work comparing various physical properties of the carbon nanotubes that are highly accumulated by cells. Both carboxylated single-walled carbon nanotubes (C-SWNTs) as well as C-MWNTs are highly accumulated, but not their pristine counterparts, suggesting that neither nanotube diameter nor chirality are critical parameters for accumulation [11]. Moreover, both short and long C-MWNTs were accumulated, so length is apparently not a factor [11]. It is unlikely that the non-ionic Pluronic® coat on the nanotubes influences interactions with cells because both carboxylated and pristine nanotubes bear the same coat yet they bind and accumulate differently. It is also notable that a protein corona is not required for receptor interaction as binding to cells occurs at 4 °C in the absence of serum [11]. The zeta potentials of the carboxylated nanotubes are more negative than their pristine counterparts, as expected, and a negative charge is a common physical feature related to carboxylation shared by nanotubes that are highly accumulated. Members of Class A SRs interact with certain anionic ligands and polyanions such as dextran sulfate often antagonize this interaction. Dextran sulfate and similar compounds were previously noted to affect the response of cells to carbon nanotubes, suggesting that scavenger receptors may be involved [42–44]. In addition, Singh et al. observed that increased carboxylation of MWNTs correlated with MWNT accumulation at 37 °C by RAW 264.7 cells, and accumulation was inhibited by dextran sulfate [45]. We previously noted that dextran sulfate partially inhibits the binding of C-MWNTs to cells at 4 °C and accumulation at 37 °C, suggesting that SR-A members might be C-MWNT receptors [11]. However, data from inhibitor studies can be difficult to interpret when assigning a ligand interaction to a specific receptor, especially with scavenger receptors that often share similar binding domain structures. One main objective of the present study was to test the hypothesis that SR-A1 is a receptor for C-MWNTs using cell lines that either do or do not express SR-A1, a more informative approach than using inhibitors of ligand binding.

ZK alveolar macrophages, derived from SR-A1/MARCO deficient mice [22], were verified to lack SR-A1 and MARCO by FCyt. B6 cells, a wild type alveolar macrophage control, were positive for SR-A1, as was the established alveolar macrophage-derived cell line RAW 264.7. Both B6 and RAW 264.7 cells robustly accumulated C-MWNTs during a 24 h exposure, while ZK cells did not, thus correlating the presence of SR-A1 with the capacity to accumulate C-MWNTs. None of the cells expressed significant levels of MARCO making it unlikely that MARCO contributes to C-MWNT uptake by B6 and RAW 264.7 cells. However, this does not imply that MARCO cannot bind C-MWNTs because MARCO, like SR-A1, contains a collagenous domain believed to bind polyanionic ligands. In fact, it was observed that ectopic expression of MARCO in CHO cells enhanced the uptake of MWNTs [46]. Therefore, MARCO may be involved in C-MWNTs uptake by other cell types that express this scavenger receptor. N-MWNTs, like P-MWNTs, did not accumulate in any of the cells tested, consistent with the idea that the anionic carboxyl groups of C-MWNTs are a determinant of receptor-mediated uptake.

CHO[mSR-AI] cells that express SR-A1 were studied to determine whether SR-A1 expression caused a gain in the capacity to accumulate C-MWNTs. As received CHO[mSR-AI] cells were re-cloned and all three clones were positive for surface SR-A1 by FCyt compared to wild type CHO-K1 cells and all three clones accumulated C-MWNTs, but not P-MWNTs or N-MWNTs. In summary, cells that did not express SR-A1 did not accumulate C-MWNTs, while those that expressed SR-A1 did accumulate C-MWNTs, strong evidence that SR-A1 is a C-MWNT receptor and functions in the receptor-mediated uptake of C-MWNTs.

A corona of proteins derived from biological fluids is often believed to be a major determinant in the interaction of engineered nanoparticles with cells [47–50]. For C-MWNTs coated with Pluronic®, since binding and uptake can occur in the absence of serum, the major determinant of C-MWNT binding and accumulation appears to be the oxidized functionalities and not a protein corona on the MWNT surface; nevertheless, serum is a dose dependent inhibitor of binding [11]. This suggests that something in serum either interacts with C-MWNTs, with SR-A1, or both, to influence accumulation. Thus, although a protein corona derived from serum is not necessary for C-MWNTs to bind to cells, it may still affect interactions if present. Moreover, it should be possible to increase the complexity of the model system by adding a defined protein corona to C-MWNTs to determine whether carboxylation still contributes to the interaction of nanotubes with SR-A1 and whether the protein expands interactions to other receptors.

A second objective of this study was to assess the effects on cell viability of short- and long-term exposure of SR-A1-positive cells to MWNTs. Apoptosis was measured by flow cytometry using an apoptotic/dead cell kit after a 24 h exposure of RAW 264.7 cells to MWNTs (100 μg/mL), and there was no significant difference among cells treated with PF108 alone and cells treated with C-MWNTs, P-MWNTs and N-MWNTs, compared to a positive control of CPT treated cells where apoptosis was obvious. In previous work, we found that a 24 h exposure to C-MWNTs had little effect on cell proliferation [11], and here we compared cell proliferation as a function of MWNT concentration at 24, 48, and 72 h. Beyond 24 h, C-MWNTs more adversely affected proliferation than P-MWNTs and N-MWNTs. By 72 h, the IC50 for C-MWNTs was ~80 μg/mL whereas P-MWNTs had not reached an IC50 at 200 μg/mL and N-MWNTs had barely reached IC50 at 200 μg/mL, the highest MWNT concentration tested. Because exposure time was an important parameter in toxicity experiments, colony formation efficiency assays were done where cells were continuously exposed to different MWNT concentrations for 8 day. After an 8-d exposure to 100 μg/mL C-MWNTs, there were essentially no colonies formed whereas P-MWNTs and N-MWNTs had ~40% colony formation efficiency compared to the untreated control under the same condition. The IC50 for C-MWNTs was ~29 μg/mL, but there was a reduction in colony formation efficiency even in the range of a few μg/mL, which is important as it suggests that even low doses of C-MWNTs over time may accumulate and adversely affect cells. These data emphasize that C-MWNTs are more toxic than P-MWNTs or N-MWNTs, especially after longer exposures, which is not surprising considering that RAW 264.7 cells accumulate about 80–100 times more C-MWNTs than P-MWNTs or N-MWNTs in 24 h. However, it is also notable that for a given IC-50, the amount of C-MWNTs in the cell on a per cell basis is much higher than for P-MWNTs or N-MWNTs, indicating that on an MWNT weight basis per cell, C-MWNTs appear to be less toxic than P-MWNTs or N-MWNTs. Thus, long-term exposure to MWNTs at lower concentration, regardless of carboxylation, may affect cell viability.

A third objective of this study was to assess what might be the spectrum of physiological consequences to macrophage functions after exposure to MWNTs, specifically related to the interaction of C-MWNTs with SR-A1. One possibility is that internalization of surface SR-A1/C-MWNT complexes could deplete the plasma membrane of SR-A1 receptors. To assess this, cells were treated with MWNTs at 37 °C followed by immunofluorescence detection of surface SR-A1 with a specific antibody, using both qualitative IFM images and quantitative FCyt analysis. In untreated cells and those treated with P-MWNTs or N-MWNTs, SR-A1 was present in punctate spots that are believed to be receptors clustered in lipid rafts scattered over the cell surface [33]. However, after C-MWNT treatment, the overall surface SR-A1 signal was reduced and redistributed mainly to the cell margins. The reason for this abnormal distribution is not clear, but it might adversely affect SR-A1 function. In addition, the fluorescent signal from C-MWNT-treated cells by FCyt analysis was reduced by about 40% whereas the signal from P-MWNT- or N-MWNT-treated cells was much less affected. A concern in the interpretation of the FCyt results is that C-MWNTs might interfere with the fluorescence signal, even though the internalized C-MWNTs are mainly within intracellular vesicles and the fluorescent anti-SR-A1 is on the cell surface. To address this concern, cells were treated with MWNTs at 4 °C to allow binding, then chased for an hour at either 37 or 4 °C. The 37 °C chase was to allow surface MWNTs to be internalized and the 4 °C treatment was to keep them on the cell surface. Fluorescent monoclonal anti-SR-A1 was then added at 4 °C and the fluorescence signal was measured by FCyt. There was no attenuation of the surface fluorescence signal by C-MWNTs, suggesting that C-MWNTs have little influence on the signal of anti-SR-A1 antibody regardless of whether the MWNTs were internalized or on the cells surface.

These data are consistent with the idea that internalization of C-MWNTs via SR-A1 depletes the cell surface of this important receptor.

The ability of C-MWNT-treated RAW 264.7 cells to respond to several known SR-A1 ligands was also examined. The internalization of fluorescent polystyrene beads measured by FCyt was impaired by over 50% after C-MWNT treatment, but not markedly affected after P-MWNT or N-MWNT treatment. Note also that ZK cells lacking SR-A1 failed to accumulate beads when untreated with C-MWNTs, verifying that SR-A1 was a receptor for the beads. We previously reported that the uptake of non-fluorescent polystyrene beads by RAW 264.7 cells treated with C-MWNTs for 2 or 20 h was reduced by 2-fold and 6-fold, respectively, when assayed by directly counting the number of beads in cells [11]. This adds confidence that the decline in the fluorescence signal from internalized beads in C-MWNT-treated cells is not an artifact of fluorescence quenching by cell-associated C-MWNTs.

The uptake of heat-killed Alexa Fluor® 488-conjugated *E. coli* was measured as another model system to assess SR-A1 function after MWNT treatment. RAW 264.7 cells treated with or without MWNTs for 24 h were chilled and incubated with *E. coli* at 4 °C low temperature to load receptors, followed by incubation at 37 °C to permit internalization. Cells treated with P-MWNTs or N-MWNTs showed no decline in fluorescence signal whereas cells treated with C-MWNTs showed a 30% decline, evidence that the clearance of a physiologically relevant SR-A1 ligand is affected. In these experiments, the ability of trypan blue to quench Alexa Fluor® 488 was used to verify that the fluorescent *E. coli* were inside the cell sheltered from contact with trypan blue, which does not penetrate the plasma membrane of intact cells.

The final SR-A1 ligand studied was oxLDL. One assay measured the accumulation of fluorescent oxLDL by FCyt and another used a non-fluorescence-based approach to measure the development of fat droplets induced by oxLDL accumulation. Both assays revealed reduced oxLDL accumulation by cells treated with C-MWNTs but not with P-MWNTs or N-MWNTs, confirming that another important function of SR-A1, the clearance of oxLDL, was impaired.

In summary, the uptake of three different SR-A1 ligands was impaired in RAW 264.7 cells by C-MWNT accumulation. One major factor affecting the uptake is likely to be the reduced number of SR-A1 receptors on the cell surface. Impaired functionality related to one or more of these ligands could contribute to the observed reduced viability of C-MWNT-treated cells. Thus, there are likely related adverse consequences affecting other biological functions, in addition to impaired SR-A1 functions demonstrated here, resulting from selective C-MWNT uptake in macrophages.

5. Conclusions

The binding and accumulation of Pluronic®-coated MWNTs described here provides a model system where key experimental parameters of the interaction of carbon nanomaterials with cells can be controlled. One feature of the approach is the SDS-PAGE assay that quantitates nanotubes extracted from cells, enabling the direct measurement of nanotube binding and accumulation by cells. In addition, binding of MWNTs to cell surface receptors can be determined at 4 °C and in the absence of serum where other physiological activities, such as endocytosis, vesicle recycling, enzymatic degradation, or interaction influenced by serum proteins corona were curtailed. The approach permitted the direct observation that carboxylated nanotubes, but not pristine or amino-functionalized counterparts, could selectively bind to and be accumulated by cells, suggesting that there were receptors that recognized carboxylated nanotubes. The results of studies with cells that either over or under express SR-A1 strongly implicate SR-A1 as the key receptor for carboxylated nanotubes. Two lines of evidence also suggest that there are adverse consequences of nanotube accumulation related to SR-A1 functions. First, the uptake of three different SR-A1 ligands (polystyrene beads, *E. coli*, and oxLDL) was impaired in RAW 264.7 cells laden with C-MWNT, emphasizing that pathogen clearance and lipid homeostasis could be affected in macrophages exposed to C-MWNTs. Second, C-MWNT uptake via SR-A1 leads to a concentration and time dependent reduction in the viability of alveolar macrophages. The results of this study may have implications for other oxidized carbon nanomaterials and it would be interesting to know if graphene oxide and carbon-based quantum dots also bind SR-A1.

Supplementary Materials: The following are available online at http://www.mdpi.com/2079-4991/10/12/2417/s1, Figure S1: MWNTs induce mild apoptosis in RAW 264.7 cells. Figure S2: Representative 3D video clips of control and C-MWNT-treated RAW 264.7 cells immuno-fluorescent stained for surface SR-A1 receptors. Figure S3: Surface-bound or phagocytosed MWNTs do not interfere with immunofluorescence FCyt assays for surface SR-A1 receptors on RAW 264.7 cells. Figure S4: Effects of MWNT accumulation on subsequent phagocytosis of polystyrene beads in WT B6 and $MS^{-/-}$ ZK cells assessed by LSCFM. Figure S5: Fluorescence quenching of fluorescent-conjugated, heat killed *E. coli* particles by trypan blue dye. Figure S6: Laser scanning confocal Raman microscopy analysis of RAW 264.7 cells with phagocytosed polystyrene beads in the present or absence of C-MWNTs. Figure S7: Reduced oxLDL uptake by RAW 264.7 cells pre-treated with C-MWNTs, but not P- or N-MWNTs, assessed using ORO staining assays. (Directions to access the SI will be updated in the final version of the manuscript.)

Author Contributions: Conceptualization, R.W. and R.D.; methodology, R.W.; investigation, R.W., R.L., E.C., P.G. and L.S.; resources, R.D.; writing—original draft preparation, R.W. and R.D.; writing—review and editing, R.L., E.C., P.G., and L.S.; supervision, R.W. and R.D; funding acquisition, R.D. All authors have read and agreed to the published version of the manuscript.

Funding: This research was funded by Research Enhancement Funds from the University of Texas at Dallas provided to R.D., E.C. and P.G. were recipients of Undergraduate Research Scholar Awards from the University of Texas at Dallas.

Acknowledgments: The authors are grateful to the Undergraduate Research Fund of the University of Texas at Dallas School of Natural Sciences and Mathematics for the support of undergraduate students.

Conflicts of Interest: The authors declare no conflict of interest.

References

1. De Volder, M.F.L.; Tawfick, S.H.; Baughman, R.H.; Hart, A.J. Carbon Nanotubes: Present and Future Commercial Applications. *Science* **2013**, *339*, 535–539. [CrossRef] [PubMed]
2. Serpell, C.J.; Kostarelos, K.; Davis, B.G. Can Carbon Nanotubes Deliver on Their Promise in Biology? Harnessing Unique Properties for Unparalleled Applications. *ACS Cent. Sci.* **2016**, *2*, 190–200. [CrossRef]
3. Rao, R.; Pint, C.L.; Islam, A.E.; Weatherup, R.S.; Hofmann, S.; Meshot, E.R.; Wu, F.; Zhou, C.; Dee, N.; Amama, P.B.; et al. Carbon Nanotubes and Related Nanomaterials: Critical Advances and Challenges for Synthesis toward Mainstream Commercial Applications. *ACS Nano* **2018**, *12*, 11756–11784. [CrossRef] [PubMed]
4. Pauluhn, J. Subchronic 13-Week Inhalation Exposure of Rats to Multiwalled Carbon Nanotubes: Toxic Effects Are Determined by Density of Agglomerate Structures, Not Fibrillar Structures. *Toxicol. Sci.* **2009**, *113*, 226–242. [CrossRef] [PubMed]
5. Pothmann, D.; Simar, S.; Schuler, D.; Dony, E.; Gaering, S.; Le Net, J.-L.; Okazaki, Y.; Chabagno, J.M.; Bessibes, C.; Beausoleil, J.; et al. Lung inflammation and lack of genotoxicity in the comet and micronucleus assays of industrial multiwalled carbon nanotubes Graphistrength© C100 after a 90-day nose-only inhalation exposure of rats. *Part. Fibre Toxicol.* **2015**, *12*, 21. [CrossRef]
6. Poland, C.A.; Duffin, R.; Kinloch, I.; Maynard, A.; Wallace, W.A.; Seaton, A.; Stone, V.; Brown, S.; Macnee, W.; Donaldson, K. Carbon nanotubes introduced into the abdominal cavity of mice show asbestos-like pathogenicity in a pilot study. *Nat. Nanotechnol.* **2008**, *3*, 423–428. [CrossRef]
7. Kato, T.; Totsuka, Y.; Ishino, K.; Matsumoto, Y.; Tada, Y.; Nakae, D.; Goto, S.; Masuda, S.; Ogo, S.; Kawanishi, M.; et al. Genotoxicity of multi-walled carbon nanotubes in both in vitro and in vivo assay systems. *Nanotoxicology* **2013**, *7*, 452–461. [CrossRef]
8. Suzui, M.; Futakuchi, M.; Fukamachi, K.; Numano, T.; Abdelgied, M.; Takahashi, S.; Ohnishi, M.; Omori, T.; Tsuruoka, S.; Hirose, A.; et al. Multiwalled carbon nanotubes intratracheally instilled into the rat lung induce development of pleural malignant mesothelioma and lung tumors. *Cancer Sci.* **2016**, *107*, 924–935. [CrossRef]
9. Ravi Kiran, A.V.V.V.; Kusuma Kumari, G.; Krishnamurthy, P.T. Carbon nanotubes in drug delivery: Focus on anticancer therapies. *J. Drug Deliv. Sci. Technol.* **2020**, *59*, 101892. [CrossRef]
10. Zhang, Y.-N.; Poon, W.; Tavares, A.J.; McGilvray, I.D.; Chan, W.C.W. Nanoparticle–liver interactions: Cellular uptake and hepatobiliary elimination. *J. Control. Release* **2016**, *240*, 332–348. [CrossRef]

11. Wang, R.; Lee, M.; Kinghorn, K.; Hughes, T.; Chuckaree, I.; Lohray, R.; Chow, E.; Pantano, P.; Draper, R. Quantitation of cell-associated carbon nanotubes: Selective binding and accumulation of carboxylated carbon nanotubes by macrophages. *Nanotoxicology* **2018**, *12*, 677–690. [CrossRef] [PubMed]
12. Kelley, J.L.; Ozment, T.R.; Li, C.; Schweitzer, J.B.; Williams, D.L. Scavenger receptor-A (CD204): A two-edged sword in health and disease. *Crit. Rev. Immunol.* **2014**, *34*, 241–261. [CrossRef] [PubMed]
13. Zani, I.; Stephen, S.; Mughal, N.; Russell, D.; Homer-Vanniasinkam, S.; Wheatcroft, S.; Ponnambalam, S. Scavenger receptor structure and function in health and disease. *Cells* **2015**, *4*, 178. [CrossRef] [PubMed]
14. PrabhuDas, M.R.; Baldwin, C.L.; Bollyky, P.L.; Bowdish, D.M.E.; Drickamer, K.; Febbraio, M.; Herz, J.; Kobzik, L.; Krieger, M.; Loike, J.; et al. A Consensus Definitive Classification of Scavenger Receptors and Their Roles in Health and Disease. *J. Immunol.* **2017**, *198*, 3775–3789. [CrossRef]
15. Maler, M.D.; Nielsen, P.J.; Stichling, N.; Cohen, I.; Ruzsics, Z.; Wood, C.; Engelhard, P.; Suomalainen, M.; Gyory, I.; Huber, M.; et al. Key Role of the Scavenger Receptor MARCO in Mediating Adenovirus Infection and Subsequent Innate Responses of Macrophages. *mBio* **2017**, *8*, e00670-17. [CrossRef] [PubMed]
16. Rausch, J.; Zhuang, R.-C.; Mäder, E. Surfactant assisted dispersion of functionalized multi-walled carbon nanotubes in aqueous media. *Compos. Part A Appl. Sci. Manuf.* **2010**, *41*, 1038–1046. [CrossRef]
17. White, C.M.; Banks, R.; Hamerton, I.; Watts, J.F. Characterisation of commercially CVD grown multi-walled carbon nanotubes for paint applications. *Prog. Org. Coat.* **2016**, *90*, 44–53. [CrossRef]
18. Wang, R.; Hughes, T.; Beck, S.; Vakil, S.; Li, S.; Pantano, P.; Draper, R.K. Generation of toxic degradation products by sonication of Pluronic^{R} dispersants: Implications for nanotoxicity testing. *Nanotoxicology* **2013**, *7*, 1272–1281. [CrossRef] [PubMed]
19. Wang, R.; Meredith, N.A.; Lee, M., Jr.; Deutsch, D.; Miadzvedskaya, L.; Braun, E.; Pantano, P.; Harper, S.; Draper, R. Toxicity assessment and bioaccumulation in zebrafish embryos exposed to carbon nanotubes suspended in Pluronic(R) F-108. *Nanotoxicology* **2016**, *10*, 689–698. [CrossRef]
20. Nakata, T. Destruction of challenged endotoxin in a dry heat oven. *PDA J. Pharm. Sci. Technol.* **1994**, *48*, 59–63.
21. Wang, R.; Murali, V.S.; Draper, R. Detecting Sonolysis of Polyethylene Glycol upon Functionalizing Carbon Nanotubes. In *Cancer Nanotechnology: Methods and Protocols*; Zeineldin, R., Ed.; Springer: New York, NY, USA, 2017; pp. 147–164. [CrossRef]
22. Zhou, H.; Imrich, A.; Kobzik, L. Characterization of immortalized MARCO and SR-AI/II-deficient murine alveolar macrophage cell lines. *Part. Fibre Toxicol.* **2008**, *5*, 7. [CrossRef] [PubMed]
23. Ashkenas, J. Structures and high and low affinity ligand binding properties of murine type I and type II macrophage scavenger receptors. *J. Lipid Res.* **1993**, *34*, 983–1000. [PubMed]
24. Wang, R.; Mikoryak, C.; Li, S.; Bushdiecker II, D.; Musselman, I.H.; Pantano, P.; Draper, R.K. Cytotoxicity screening of single-walled carbon nanotubes: Detection and removal of cytotoxic contaminants from carboxylated carbon nanotubes. *Mol. Pharm.* **2011**, *8*, 1351–1361. [CrossRef] [PubMed]
25. Franken, N.A.P.; Rodermond, H.M.; Stap, J.; Haveman, J.; van Bree, C. Clonogenic assay of cells in vitro. *Nat. Protoc.* **2006**, *1*, 2315–2319. [CrossRef]
26. Sahlin, S.; Hed, J.; Runfquist, I. Differentiation between attached and ingested immune complexes by a fluorescence quenching cytofluorometric assay. *J. Immunol. Methods* **1983**, *60*, 115–124. [CrossRef]
27. Busetto, S.; Trevisan, E.; Patriarca, P.; Menegazzi, R. A single-step, sensitive flow cytofluorometric assay for the simultaneous assessment of membrane-bound and ingested Candida albicans in phagocytosing neutrophils. *Cytom. Part A* **2004**, *58A*, 201–206. [CrossRef]
28. Herzog, E.; Casey, A.; Lyng, F.M.; Chambers, G.; Byrne, H.J.; Davoren, M. A new approach to the toxicity testing of carbon-based nanomaterials—The clonogenic assay. *Toxicol. Lett.* **2007**, *174*, 49–60. [CrossRef]
29. Gellein, K.; Hoel, S.; Gellein, K.; Hoel, S.; Evje, L.; Syversen, T. The colony formation assay as an indicator of carbon nanotube toxicity examined in three cell lines. *Nanotoxicology* **2009**, *3*, 215–221. [CrossRef]
30. Morris, E.J.; Geller, H.M. Induction of neuronal apoptosis by camptothecin, an inhibitor of DNA topoisomerase-I: Evidence for cell cycle-independent toxicity. *J. Cell Biol.* **1996**, *134*, 757–770. [CrossRef]
31. Dunne, D.W.; Resnick, D.; Greenberg, J.; Krieger, M.; Joiner, K.A. The type I macrophage scavenger receptor binds to gram-positive bacteria and recognizes lipoteichoic acid. *Proc. Natl. Acad. Sci. USA* **1994**, *91*, 1863–1867. [CrossRef]
32. Steinberg, D. Low Density Lipoprotein Oxidation and Its Pathobiological Significance. *J. Biol. Chem.* **1997**, *272*, 20963–20966. [CrossRef] [PubMed]

33. Nagao, G.; Ishii, K.; Hirota, K.; Makino, K.; Terada, H. Role of Lipid Rafts in Phagocytic Uptake of Polystyrene Latex Microspheres by Macrophages. *Anticancer Res.* **2010**, *30*, 3167–3176. [PubMed]
34. Ordija, C.M.; Chiou, T.T.; Yang, Z.; Deloid, G.M.; de Oliveira Valdo, M.; Wang, Z.; Bedugnis, A.; Noah, T.L.; Jones, S.; Koziel, H.; et al. Free actin impairs macrophage bacterial defenses via scavenger receptor MARCO interaction with reversal by plasma gelsolin. *Am. J. Physiol. Lung Cell. Mol. Physiol.* **2017**, *312*, L1018–L1028. [CrossRef] [PubMed]
35. Hampton, R.Y.; Golenbock, D.T.; Penman, M.; Krieger, M.; Raetz, C.R.H. Recognition and plasma clearance of endotoxin by scavenger receptors. *Nature* **1991**, *352*, 342–344. [CrossRef] [PubMed]
36. Moore, K.J.; Tabas, I. Macrophages in the Pathogenesis of Atherosclerosis. *Cell* **2011**, *145*, 341–355. [CrossRef] [PubMed]
37. Nagy, L.; Tontonoz, P.; Alvarez, J.G.A.; Chen, H.; Evans, R.M. Oxidized LDL Regulates Macrophage Gene Expression through Ligand Activation of PPARγ. *Cell* **1998**, *93*, 229–240. [CrossRef]
38. Trpkovic, A.; Resanovic, I.; Stanimirovic, J.; Radak, D.; Mousa, S.A.; Cenic-Milosevic, D.; Jevremovic, D.; Isenovic, E.R. Oxidized low-density lipoprotein as a biomarker of cardiovascular diseases. *Crit. Rev. Clin. Lab. Sci.* **2015**, *52*, 70–85. [CrossRef]
39. Ramírez-Zacarías, J.L.; Castro-Muñozledo, F.; Kuri-Harcuch, W. Quantitation of adipose conversion and triglycerides by staining intracytoplasmic lipids with oil red O. *Histochemistry* **1992**, *97*, 493–497. [CrossRef]
40. Xu, S.; Huang, Y.; Xie, Y.; Lan, T.; Le, K.; Chen, J.; Chen, S.; Gao, S.; Xu, X.; Shen, X.; et al. Evaluation of foam cell formation in cultured macrophages: An improved method with Oil Red O staining and DiI-oxLDL uptake. *Cytotechnology* **2010**, *62*, 473–481. [CrossRef]
41. Kraus, N.A.; Ehebauer, F.; Zapp, B.; Rudolphi, B.; Kraus, B.J.; Kraus, D. Quantitative assessment of adipocyte differentiation in cell culture. *Adipocyte* **2016**, *5*, 351–358. [CrossRef]
42. Dutta, D.; Sundaram, S.K.; Teeguarden, J.G.; Riley, B.J.; Fifield, L.S.; Jacobs, J.M.; Addleman, S.R.; Kaysen, G.A.; Moudgil, B.M.; Weber, T.J. Adsorbed proteins influence the biological activity and molecular targeting of nanomaterials. *Toxicol. Sci.* **2007**, *100*, 303–315. [CrossRef]
43. Gao, N.; Zhang, Q.; Mu, Q.; Bai, Y.; Li, L.; Zhou, H.; Butch, E.R.; Powell, T.B.; Snyder, S.E.; Jiang, G.; et al. Steering carbon nanotubes to scavenger receptor recognition by nanotube surface chemistry modification partially alleviates NFκB activation and reduces its immunotoxicity. *ACS Nano* **2011**, *5*, 4581–4591. [CrossRef] [PubMed]
44. Wang, X.; Guo, J.; Chen, T.; Nie, H.; Wang, H.; Zang, J.; Cui, X.; Jia, G. Multi-walled carbon nanotubes induce apoptosis via mitochondrial pathway and scavenger receptor. *Toxicol. Vitr.* **2012**, *26*, 799–806. [CrossRef] [PubMed]
45. Singh, R.P.; Das, M.; Thakare, V.; Jain, S. Functionalization density dependent toxicity of oxidized multiwalled carbon nanotubes in a murine macrophage cell line. *Chem. Res. Toxicol.* **2012**, *25*, 2127–2137. [CrossRef] [PubMed]
46. Hirano, S.; Fujitani, Y.; Furuyama, A.; Kanno, S. Macrophage receptor with collagenous structure (MARCO) is a dynamic adhesive molecule that enhances uptake of carbon nanotubes by CHO-K1 Cells. *Toxicol. Appl. Pharmacol.* **2012**, *259*, 96–103. [CrossRef] [PubMed]
47. Fleischer, C.C.; Payne, C.K. Nanoparticle–Cell Interactions: Molecular Structure of the Protein Corona and Cellular Outcomes. *Acc. Chem. Res.* **2014**, *47*, 2651–2659. [CrossRef] [PubMed]
48. Feiner-Gracia, N.; Beck, M.; Pujals, S.; Tosi, S.; Mandal, T.; Buske, C.; Linden, M.; Albertazzi, L. Super-Resolution Microscopy Unveils Dynamic Heterogeneities in Nanoparticle Protein Corona. *Small* **2017**, *13*, 1701631. [CrossRef]
49. Liu, N.; Tang, M.; Ding, J. The interaction between nanoparticles-protein corona complex and cells and its toxic effect on cells. *Chemosphere* **2020**, *245*, 125624. [CrossRef]
50. You, D.J.; Lee, H.Y.; Bonner, J.C. Macrophages: First Innate Immune Responders to Nanomaterials. In *Interaction of Nanomaterials with the Immune System*; Bonner, J.C., Brown, J.M., Eds.; Springer International Publishing: Berlin/Heidelberg, Germany, 2020; pp. 15–34. [CrossRef]

nanomaterials

MDPI

Article

Rifabutin-Loaded Nanostructured Lipid Carriers as a Tool in Oral Anti-Mycobacterial Treatment of Crohn's Disease

Helena Rouco [1], Patricia Diaz-Rodriguez [2], Diana P. Gaspar [3], Lídia M. D. Gonçalves [3], Miguel Cuerva [4], Carmen Remuñán-López [5], António J. Almeida [3] and Mariana Landin [1,*]

1 R+D Pharma Group (GI-1645), Strategic Grouping in Materials (AEMAT), Department of Pharmacology, Pharmacy and Pharmaceutical Technology, Faculty of Pharmacy, Universidade de Santiago de Compostela-Campus Vida, 15782 Santiago de Compostela, Spain; helena.rouco@rai.usc.es
2 Drug Delivery Systems Group, Department of Chemical Engineering and Pharmaceutical Technology, School of Sciences, Universidad de La Laguna (ULL), Campus de Anchieta, 38200 La Laguna (Tenerife), Spain; pdiarodr@ull.edu.es
3 Research Institute for Medicines (iMed.ULisboa), Faculty of Pharmacy, Universidade de Lisboa, 1649-003 Lisbon, Portugal; diana.gaspar89@gmail.com (D.P.G.); lgoncalves@ff.ulisboa.pt (L.M.D.G.); aalmeida@ff.ulisboa.pt (A.J.A.)
4 Department of Physical Chemistry, Nanomag laboratory, Universidade de Santiago de Compostela-Campus Vida, 15782 Santiago de Compostela, Spain; miguelcvidales@gmail.com
5 Nanobiofar Group (GI-1643), Department of Pharmacology, Pharmacy and Pharmaceutical Technology, Faculty of Pharmacy, Universidade de Santiago de Compostela-Campus Vida, 15782 Santiago de Compostela, Spain; mdelcarmen.remunan@usc.es
* Correspondence: m.landin@usc.es

Received: 29 September 2020; Accepted: 26 October 2020; Published: 27 October 2020

Abstract: Oral anti-mycobacterial treatment of Crohn's disease (CD) is limited by the low aqueous solubility of drugs, along with the altered gut conditions of patients, making uncommon their clinical use. Hence, the aim of the present work is focused on the in vitro evaluation of rifabutin (RFB)-loaded Nanostructured lipid carriers (NLC), in order to solve limitations associated to this therapeutic approach. RFB-loaded NLC were prepared by hot homogenization and characterized in terms of size, polydispersity, surface charge, morphology, thermal stability, and drug payload and release. Permeability across Caco-2 cell monolayers and cytotoxicity and uptake in human macrophages was also determined. NLC obtained were nano-sized, monodisperse, negatively charged, and spheroidal-shaped, showing a suitable drug payload and thermal stability. Furthermore, the permeability profile, macrophage uptake and selective intracellular release of RFB-loaded NLC, guarantee an effective drug dose administration to cells. Outcomes suggest that rifabutin-loaded NLC constitute a promising strategy to improve oral anti-mycobacterial therapy in Crohn's disease.

Keywords: rifabutin; nanostructured lipid carriers; cell uptake; Caco-2 cells; oral administration; Crohn's disease

1. Introduction

Crohn's disease (CD) is a chronic inflammatory bowel condition with a higher predominance in industrialized countries, principally in Western Europe and North America [1]. The disease is characterized by the presence of outbreaks followed by remission periods [1,2], and although symptomatology is variable, diarrhea, abdominal pain, nausea, vomiting, and weight loss are usually involved [1]. The inflammatory process is usually transmural, involving any region of the digestive tract, affecting distal ileum and colon mainly [1,2].

CD aetiology has been a controversial topic recently [3]. Disease development is currently associated with genetic susceptibility and environmental factors, such as alterations in gut microbiome and treatment with antibiotics or non-steroidal anti-inflammatories [1,2]. Nevertheless, it is necessary to highlight the recent increment in scientific literature showing the contribution of the mycobacterial pathogen *Mycobacterium avium paratuberculosis* (MAP) in CD instauration [3,4]. Moreover, inflamed mucosal and submucosal layers in CD are infiltrated by immune cells such as macrophages [5]. These cells constitute an interesting target for anti-mycobacterial therapy, since MAP is a facultative intracellular organism that resides in host macrophages, establishing a persistent infection [6].

Despite this information, CD's current treatment is still focused on the pharmacological control of the inflammatory process (using immunosuppressants, corticosteroids, anti-TNF or anti-interleukin drugs and adhesion molecule inhibitors) with the main objective of maintaining the disease remission stage without the need for surgery [1]. However, although these treatments improve patients' quality of life, their ability to modify the long-term evolution of the disease has not been demonstrated yet [2].

Regarding the antibiotic use in CD, they are nowadays relegated to the treatment of perianal fistulas or disease suppurative complications [1]. Still, some case reports describe long-term CD remissions after antibiotic therapy [4]. Moreover, an open label extension phase III study sponsored by RedHill Biopharma is currently actively testing orally administered capsules containing a combination of rifabutin, clofazimine and clarithromycin at fixed doses in CD patients [7]. This study includes the introduction of a MAP PCR test at the baseline and the evaluation of changes of this blood status during the study [7], which would give insight into in vivo effectivity of this antibiotic combination [8] and into the clinical benefit derived from MAP eradication [9].

Although orally administered antimycobacterial drugs constitute a promising strategy in CD treatment, two aspects limit this approach. First, gut physiological parameters are altered in CD patients, which can reduce the possibilities to exploit pH, transit time or microbiome as targeting strategies for drug delivery [5]. On the other hand, antimycobacterial drugs show high lipophilicity and low oral bioavailability [10–12].

In this context, particulate systems constitute an interesting approach, as they can accumulate in inflamed bowel sites [5]. Additionally, nanoparticulated systems can be designed to load lipophilic drugs, improving their oral bioavailability [13,14]. Moreover, the drug particle reduction to nano size can lead to an enhanced water solubility and dissolution rate [15].

Among nanoparticulate systems, Nanostructured Lipid Carriers (NLC), the second generation of lipid nanoparticles (LN) [16], can be good candidates to formulate useful antimycobacterial systems. NLC are solid matrices at both room and body temperatures [17]. They are composed by a solid lipid and a liquid lipid [16] and present several advantages over the first generation of LN (known as Solid Lipid Nanoparticles or SLN), such as improved stability, higher suppleness in drug release modulation, and increased drug loading capacity [17]. NLC "in vitro" tolerability seems to be higher in comparison with other colloidal carriers, such as polymeric nanoparticles [18], making them an interesting option for oral drug administration.

Therefore, the aim of this work is to investigate the performance of rifabutin (RFB)-loaded NLC (whose formulation procedure and composition were previously optimized by Artificial Intelligence tools), to demonstrate their safety and suitability to achieve an appropriate intestinal permeability and an efficient macrophages uptake. Our goal is to improve the current Crohn's disease treatments intended to eradicate MAP housed within intestinal macrophages, an area in which, to the best of our knowledge, nanotechnology has never been applied. In this way, an extensive characterization of the nanosystems in terms of particle size, polydispersity, surface charge, and drug payload, was performed. Thermal resistance, morphology, and drug release from NLC in different simulated media were also evaluated. Furthermore, an analysis of the in vitro performance of NLC in cell cultures including a permeability evaluation through Caco-2 monolayers, along with the assessment of cytotoxicity and uptake in human macrophages, was carried out in order to evaluate the targeting potential of the developed nanocarriers.

2. Materials and Methods

2.1. Materials

Rifabutin (RFB) (98% purity) was purchased from Acros Organics™ (Fair Lawn, NJ, USA). Polysorbate 80 (Tween® 80), Coumarin 6, dialysis membrane (Spectrum™ Labs Spectra/Por, MWCO 3.5 KDa), and phorbol 12-myristate 13-acetate (PMA) were acquired from Sigma Aldrich (St Louis, MO, USA). Oleic acid was obtained from Merck (Darmstadt, Germany). Precirol® ATO 5 (glyceryl distearate) and Epikuron® 145 V (deoiled phosphatidyl choline-enriched lecithin) were kind gifts from Gattefossé (Saint-Priest, France) and Cargill (Wayzata, MN, USA) respectively. THP-1, Caco-2 human colon carcinoma and RAW 264.7 cell lines were obtained from ATCC (Manassas, VA, USA). Alexa Fluor™ 647 phalloidin, ProLong® Gold Antifade reagent with DAPI, Gibco™ antibiotic-antimycotic (amphotericin B, penicillin, streptomycin), trypsin-EDTA, foetal bovine serum (FBS), Roswell Park Memorial Institute 1640 Medium (RPMI 1640), Minimum Essential Media (α-MEM), and phosphate buffered saline (PBS) were obtained from Thermo Fisher Scientific (Waltham, MA, USA). Dulbeco's Modified Eagle Medium (DMEM) was purchased from Corning (Corning, NY, USA). Antibiotic solution (10.000 units/mL penicillin, 10.000 µg/mL streptomycin) was acquired from GE Healthcare Life Sciences (Chicago, IL, USA). Cell proliferation kit (WST-1) was purchased from Roche (Basel, Switzerland). Ultrapure water (MilliQ plus, Millipore Ibérica, Madrid, Spain) was used throughout and the remaining solvents and reagents were analytical or HPLC grade.

2.2. NLC Formulation

Several batches of NLC loaded with RFB were developed utilizing the composition and operating conditions of a previously optimized NLC system using Artificial Intelligence tools [19]. Briefly, the components of the formulation were Precirol® ATO 5 and oleic acid as the lipid components (25:75 ratio), and Tween® 80 and Epikuron® 145 V as surfactants. The drug (15 mg) was dissolved in the molten lipid phase at 80 °C (300 mg). The aqueous phase (10 mL), a dispersion of Epikuron® 145 V (0.5% *w/w* regarding the lipid phase weight) and Tween® 80 (1.9% *w/v* regarding aqueous phase) in Milli-Q® water, was heated at the same temperature, added to the lipid phase and hot shear homogenized (80 °C) using an Ultra-Turrax T25 (IKA Labortechnik, Staufen, Germany) at 14,800 rpm for 10 min, in a water bath. NLC dispersions were rapidly cooled by transferring them to an ice bath, with gentle stirring, for 2 min. Formulations were carried out in quintuplicate and subsequently dialyzed overnight (MWCO 3.5 KDa), in order to remove the non-incorporated components and obtain the purified NLC.

2.3. NLC Characterization

2.3.1. Particle Size, Surface Charge and Physical Stability

Particle size, polydispersity index and surface charge of NLC were determined using a Zetasizer Nano ZS (Malvern Instruments, Malvern, UK). For size and polydispersity index determinations, samples were placed in polystyrene cuvettes and diluted with Milli-Q® water (1:10). Surface charge was determined as zeta potential through particle mobility in an electric field. To carry out this determination, samples were also diluted with Milli-Q® water (1:10) and placed in a specific cuvette where a potential of ±150 mV was established. All the measurements were performed at 25 ± 1 °C by quadruplicate.

2.3.2. Transmission Electron Microscopy (TEM)

Transmission electron microscopy was employed to evaluate morphology of blank (control NLC without drug) and RFB-loaded NLC and to confirm particle sizes previously obtained by DLS. Thus, NLC suspensions were placed on formvar/carbon-coated grids (400 mesh) and stained with 2% (*w/v*) uranyl acetate. Finally, samples were analysed using a JEOL microscope (JEM 1010, Tokyo, Japan).

Images were then obtained by using a CCD Orius-Digital Montage Plug-in camera (Gatan, Inc., Pleasanton, CA, USA) and analysed by means of a Gatan Digital Micrograph software (Gatan, Inc., USA). The number of particles considered for size determinations were 44 and 12 for blank and loaded NLC, respectively.

2.3.3. Atomic Force Microscopy (AFM)

NLC morphology, particle size and size distribution were also analysed by atomic force microscopy (AFM). This technique is based on the electrostatic interaction between the sample and the AFM tip, which allows for the determination of a sample topography. Measurements were conducted under normal ambient conditions using an XE-100 instrument (Park Systems, Suwon, South Korea) in non-contact mode with the high-resonance non-contact AFM cantilever (ACTA probe, n = 330 kHz). For AFM imaging, 20 µL of the sample were dropped onto freshly exfoliated mica sheet (SPI Supplies, grade V-1 Muscovite) and after 5 min the mica was washed with Milli-Q water and dried under nitrogen flow. All experiments were performed at room temperature. XEI® data processing tool (Park Systems, South Korea) were used for the analysis of the obtained data, which were adjusted to a gaussian distribution.

2.3.4. Encapsulation Efficiency and Drug Loading

Encapsulation efficiency and drug loading determinations were performed as previously described [19]. Purified NLC and non-purified NLC (200 µL) were dissolved with acetonitrile (1.5 mL) and centrifuged at 16,099× *g* and 4 °C for 30 min. Centrifugation produces the precipitation of the lipid phase, while the drug remains in the supernatant. RFB quantification was performed by High Performance Liquid Chromatography (HPLC) as described in Section 2.4. The amount of drug quantified in the supernatant of non-purified nanoparticles was used as total drug content.

Encapsulation efficiency (EE) and drug loading (DL) of NLC were calculated using the following equations:

$$EE\ (\%) = [(W_{loaded\ drug})/W_{total\ drug}] \times 100, \quad (1)$$

$$DL\ (\%) = [(W_{loaded\ drug})/W_{lipid}] \times 100, \quad (2)$$

where $W_{loaded\ drug}$ is the amount of drug successfully incorporated in the formulation (remaining in the supernatant following acetonitrile addition), $W_{total\ drug}$ is the total amount of drug, and W_{lipid} is the weight of the lipid vehicle.

2.3.5. Thermal Analysis Using Dynamic Light Scattering (DLS)

The influence of temperature on both blank and RFB-loaded NLC suspensions stability was analysed by DLS in a Zetasizer Nano ZS. Three batches of each type of NLC (blank and loaded with RFB) were diluted as described above, and particle size measurements were made during heating and cooling cycles (25 °C-90 °C-25 °C) at 0.5 °C/min in quartz cells. Particle size determinations were recorded every 0.5 °C. Each batch was analysed in duplicate.

2.3.6. In Vitro Release Studies

RFB release from loaded NLC was investigated in simulated intestinal fluid (SIF) and macrophage's lysate, in order to compare NLC behaviour in different environments, the intestinal tract and inside macrophages. SIF with pancreatin was prepared according to United States Pharmacopeia (USP).

In order to obtain macrophages cell lysate, Raw 264.7 cells (a murine macrophage cell line) were cultured in DMEM supplemented with 10% foetal bovine serum (FBS) and 1% penicillin/streptomycin and incubated at 37 °C and 5% CO_2. Cells were split when reaching 80% confluence by trypsinization and expanded until achieving enough number of cells. Cells were then trypsinized using standard conditions, washed with PBS, centrifuged, and resuspended in Milli-Q® water in order to achieve a concentration of 3.125 million cells/mL. Cell lysis was performed by subjecting the cell suspension to three freeze-thaw cycles.

Drug release studies were performed by quadruplicate at 37 °C in horizontal Franz diffusion cells, where a 1:3 dilution of the nanoparticle suspension in release medium was put in the donor chamber. A dialysis membrane (MWCO 3.5 KDa) was placed between the two chambers in order to avoid the presence of NLC in the receptor chamber. At pre-set times, samples were taken from the receptor chamber and replaced with fresh medium. Drug quantification was performed by HPLC.

2.4. *High Performance Liquid Chromatography Method*

RFB was quantified following a validated method previously described [20], using an Agilent 1100 HPLC system (Agilent Technologies, Santa Clara, CA, USA) equipped with a C18 column (Waters symmetry 5 μm, 3.9 × 150 mm). Throughout HPLC analysis, 20 μL of each sample were injected and eluted with a mobile phase composed by a mixture of sodium acetate 0.05 M/potassium dihydrogen phosphate 0.05 M (pH adjusted to 4.0 with acetic acid) and acetonitrile (Scharlau, Barcelona, Spain) in a 53:47 (*v*/*v*) proportion. Drug quantification was performed at 275 nm, with a 1 mL/min flow rate in an isocratic mode.

2.5. *In Vitro Cell Studies*

2.5.1. Cell Viability Studies

Cytotoxicity of NLC formulations was analysed using WST-1 (2-(4-iodophenyl)-3-(4-nitrophenyl)-5-(2,4-disulfophenyl)-2*H* tetrazolium, monosodium salt; Roche, Indianapolis, IN, USA), which produces a water-soluble formazan dye upon cellular reduction by the mitochondrial succinate-tetrazolium reductase [21,22]. Human monocytes (THP-1) were cultured in RPMI 1640 supplemented with 10% heat-inactivated foetal bovine serum (FBS), 1% penicillin/streptomycin and 2-mercaptoethanol 0.05 mM at 37 °C and 5% CO_2. Five days before the experiment, cells were differentiated to macrophages by stimulation with 200 nM of PMA (Phorbol 12-myristate 13-acetate) for 3 days at a cell density of 2×10^5 cells/mL. Then, PMA-containing medium was replaced by fresh medium and cells were incubated for another 2 days with normal media. The day before the experiment, cells were seeded at a density of 2.5×10^4 cells/well in 96-well plates. Purified NLC samples were diluted to achieve a final concentration of 0.3, 0.12, 0.06, and 0.03 mg/mL of nanoparticles solid mass per volume. To evaluate cell viability, macrophages were incubated with blank and RFB-loaded NLC formulations, as well as with RFB solutions (concentration equivalent to those present in the previous NLC dilutions), for 24 h (37 °C, 5% CO_2). After the incubation period, samples were removed and 10 μL of WST-1 reagent along with 100 μL of culture medium were added to each well. After 2 h of incubation with WST-1 reagent, absorbance was read at 450 nm in a microplate reader (Model 680, Bio-Rad, Hercules, CA, USA). Cell viability relative to negative control (Milli-Q® water or DMSO, as appropriate) was calculated according to the following equation:

$$\text{Cell viability (\%)} = (\text{Sample Absorbance}/\text{Control Absorbance}) \times 100, \quad (3)$$

2.5.2. Confocal Microscopy

Qualitative analysis of NLC internalization by THP-1 derived macrophages was performed by confocal microscopy. For this purpose, nanoparticles were fluorescently labelled with coumarin 6 by incorporating the fluorophore into the oil phase during the formulation process. Cells were seeded at a concentration of 5.3×10^4 cells/cm^2 in chambered cell culture slides (Nunc™ Lab-Tek II Chamber Slide™, Thermo Fisher Scientific, Waltham, MA, USA) the day before the experiment. Then, cells were incubated at 37 °C and 5% CO_2 for 5 h with the samples (blank and RFB-loaded NLC), which were added in a final concentration of 0.12 mg/mL. After this incubation period, culture medium was removed, and cells were washed twice with pre-warmed phosphate buffered saline (PBS). Cell fixation was performed using a 3.7% formaldehyde solution in PBS for 10 min at room temperature, followed by two washing steps with PBS. Then, a 0.1% Triton X-100 solution was added to permeabilize the cell membrane. Finally, cells were incubated with a 1:40 dilution of Alexa Fluor™ 647 phalloidin in PBS for 20 min in order to label the macrophages cytoskeleton, and after two extra washing steps, macrophages nucleus were stained with ProLong® Gold Antifade reagent with DAPI. Images were obtained using a confocal laser microscopy Leica SP5 (Leica Microsystems, Wetzlar, Germany).

2.5.3. Macrophage Uptake Quantification

To quantify NLC uptake by THP-1 derived macrophages, NLC were fluorescently labelled with coumarin 6 as previously described. Dialysis of the samples was also accomplished prior to performing the experiment. Macrophage uptake quantification was carried out according to a method previously described [23] with slight modifications. First, macrophages were seeded in 96-well plates at a cell density of 2.5×10^5 cells/mL and 100 µL per well; nanoparticle suspensions were added to them at a final concentration of 0.12 mg/mL, and fluorescence was determined in a microplate reader (Fluostar Optima, BMG Labtech, Offenburg, Germany) at an excitation and emission wavelength of 485 and 520 nm, respectively (Initial fluorescence). Cells were then incubated during 2 h at 37 °C and 5% CO_2. Samples were removed, and cells were subjected to three washing steps with 250 µL of a 20 mM glycine solution in PBS pH 7.4, in order to remove non-internalized nanoparticles and to quench their fluorescent signals. Finally, 100 µL of Triton X-100 1% were added to disrupt cellular membrane, and fluorescence was again measured (Fluorescence post-lysis). Macrophage uptake was calculated according to the following equation:

$$\text{Macrophage uptake (\%)} = (\text{Fluorescence post-lysis/Initial fluorescence}) \times 100, \quad (4)$$

2.5.4. Nanoparticle Permeation across Caco-2 Cells Monolayers

Permeation studies were performed in human colon carcinoma Caco-2 cell line according to a previously described protocol [24], with modifications. Cells were seeded at a concentration of 6.25×10^3 cells/cm^2 in Corning® Transwell® polycarbonate membrane cell culture inserts (Corning, Corning, NY, USA) and cultured in α-MEM supplemented with 20% FBS, 1% penicillin/streptomycin and 1% antibiotic/antimycotic. Culture medium was replaced every 3–4 days and cells were incubated at 37 °C and 5% CO_2 for 28 days, approximately, until the monolayer reached a suitable transepithelial electrical resistance (TEER). At the beginning of the experiment, TEER was higher than 400 Ω cm^2, which indicates the formation of an intact monolayer [24].

RFB-loaded NLC fluorescently labelled with coumarin 6 at a final concentration of 0.12 mg/mL or pure Milli-Q® water (control), were added in the donor compartment. After 2, 4, 6, 24, and 48 h, samples were taken from the receptor compartment and replaced by fresh medium. Fluorescence was measured in a microplate reader (Fluostar Optima, BMG Labtech, Germany), as previously described, in order to evaluate NLC passage across the cell monolayer. Moreover, in order to correlate the amount of NLC present in the receptor compartment with the fluorescent signal obtained, a calibration curve was prepared in triplicate by measuring the fluorescence of known amounts of coumarin 6-labelled RFB-loaded NLC. Finally, permeability of NLC across Caco-2 cells was expressed either as the concentration of permeated RFB (µg/mL) regarding time elapsed or as a function of the apparent permeability coefficient (P_{app}), which is employed to investigate the transport rate. P_{app} was determined according to the following equation:

$$\text{Papp (cm/s)} = dQ/dt \times 1/(A \times C_0), \quad (5)$$

where C_0 is the initial RFB concentration in the upper compartment (6 µg/mL), A is the growth area (0.33 cm^2) and dQ/dt is the appearance rate of the particles on the lower chamber based on its cumulative transport for 48 h. This linear appearance rate was calculated as the slope resulting from the representation of the RFB amount present in the receptor compartment versus time.

2.6. Statistical Analysis

All experiments were performed at least in triplicate. The data were expressed by mean ± SD and treated with IBM SPSS 24 software. The confidence interval was 95% ($p \leq 0.05$). The groups were compared by performing one-way or two-way analysis of variance (ANOVA), as appropriate, followed by post hoc Tukey's Multiple Comparison Test, and the significant differences between groups were determined.

3. Results and Discussion

3.1. NLC Characterization

NLC formulation procedure and composition were beforehand optimized by Artificial Intelligence (AI) tools in order to achieve optimal physicochemical properties along with a suitable drug payload [19]. Stability of the developed nanocarriers has proven to be adequate after 1 month of storage at 5 ± 1 °C, in terms of particle size, polydispersity index and drug payload. Minor changes without impact over colloidal stability were found for zeta potential [19]. Besides, an estimation of the characteristics of RFB-loaded NLC, prepared with these optimized parameters, was also provided [19]. In this way, to verify the robustness of this optimizations process, RFB-loaded NLC were prepared, and particle size, PDI, ZP, and drug payload were again determined. Furthermore, this work includes further characterization of these nanocarriers in terms of morphology, thermal behaviour, release profile, and in vitro performance in cell cultures.

3.1.1. Particle Size, Surface Charge, Physical Stability, and Drug Payload

Blank and RFB-loaded NLC were prepared using hot high shear homogenization. Formulations were carried out in quintuplicate, dialyzed overnight and fully characterized in terms of particle size, size distribution, surface charge, and drug load (Table 1).

Table 1. Blank and RFB-loaded NLC characterization in terms of particle size, PDI, ZP, EE, and DL (n = 3 ± SD).

NLC	Size (nm)	PDI	ZP (mV)	EE (%)	DL (%)
Blank	111 ± 3	0.23 ± 0	−26 ± 2	-	-
RFB-loaded	151 ± 34	0.22 ± 0.02	−24 ± 2	92.83 ± 3.75	4.62 ± 0.33

Particle size and size distribution are known to affect NLC characteristics such as stability, release rate and biologic performance [17], and because of that, they should be carefully characterized. NLC formulations showed particle sizes within the nano range, with values of 111 ± 3 nm and 151 ± 34 nm, for blank and RFB-loaded nanocarriers, respectively. Differences in size observed between blank and loaded formulations could be associated with the required accommodation space for the drug [25]. Regarding particle size distribution, blank NLC showed a polydispersity index (PDI) value of 0.23 ± 0.00, whereas the loaded ones displayed an almost identical value of 0.22 ± 0.02. Therefore, the obtained PDI values were below 0.3 in both cases, which is an acceptable value for lipid nanocarriers and indicative of homogeneous particle size distribution [26]. Remarkably, both size and PDI values obtained for RFB-loaded NLC are in close agreement with those previously predicted by Artificial Intelligence tools, which have been reported to be 152 nm and 0.23, for size and PDI, respectively [19].

Moreover, both blank and loaded nanocarriers showed zeta potential values close to −25 mV (−26 ± 2 and −24 ± 2 mV, for blank and RFB-loaded NLC, respectively), which guarantees a good colloidal stability if emulsifiers are included among formulation components [17,27]. These results differ slightly from those predicted by Artificial Intelligence tools, which showed slightly less negative values (−19 mV) [19]. However, these differences in ZP could be easily associated with the dialysis step performed in this work after NLC formulation, which can favour the removal of NLC superficial components, such as Tween® 80, a non-ionic emulsifier. Since this type of emulsifier has been reported to localize close to the nanoparticle interface, counteracting the negative charge of the lipid matrix [28], its partial removal is expected to lead to a more negative zeta potential. Furthermore, these small differences could only have a slight impact on colloidal stability and are not likely to influence the in vivo fate of the nano-formulations.

Concerning drug payload, RFB was incorporated to NLC at 5% (*w/w*) regarding lipid matrix weight showing a suitable drug payload, with an encapsulation efficiency (EE) of 92.83 ± 3.75% and a drug loading (DL) of 4.62 ± 0.33%. These values suggest that almost all the added drug was successfully incorporated into the nanoparticle matrix. In the same way as in the case of particle size and PDI, EE and DL values obtained are almost identical to those predicted by Artificial intelligence tools, which have been reported to exhibit values of 100% and 5%, for EE and DL, respectively [19].

Hence, the NLC physicochemical characterization data show that they have a particle size within the nano-range, a monodisperse particle size distribution and a suitable drug payload. Besides, the highly negative zeta potential exhibited by the formulations is expected to promote a good colloidal stability. Finally, the results of RFB-loaded NLC characterization closely agree with those predicted by Artificial Intelligence, demonstrating the suitability of these tools to successfully optimize the design of nanoparticle-based drug delivery systems and develop robust and reproducible protocols of NLC preparation.

3.1.2. Thermal Analysis Using Dynamic Light Scattering (DLS)

To assess NLC thermal stability, blank and RFB-loaded formulations were subjected to a heating stage from 25 °C to 90 °C, followed by a cooling step to the initial temperature. This approach was previously described to investigate the ability of lipid nanoparticle formulations to maintain their initial properties during high temperature-related procedures [23,29].

In the case of blank NLC (Figure 1A), particle size remains almost unchanged during the whole thermal analysis. A similar behavior was observed for RFB-loaded NLC (Figure 1B) but showing a slight reduction in nanoparticle size. Particle size maintenance along with the negligible size variations exhibited by both formulations throughout the assay indicate a good thermal stability. Therefore, results obtained suggest the developed NLC formulations are suitable for further temperature-requiring processes, as is the case of spray-drying [23], that could simplify the oral administration of NLC obtaining dried powders, which can be easily administered in capsules or tablets [30].

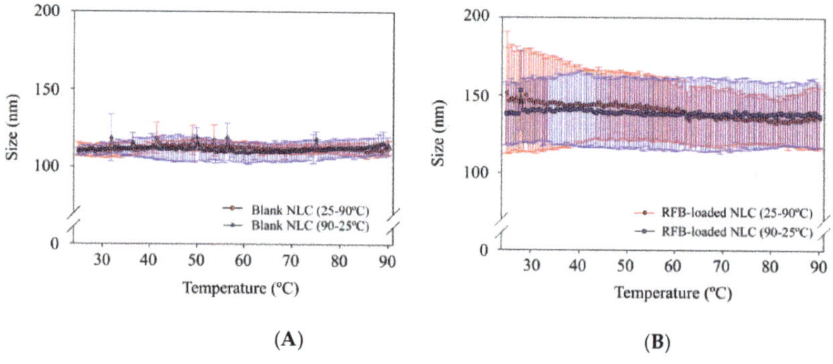

Figure 1. Dynamic light scattering thermograms of (**A**) Blank NLC formulations and (**B**) RFB-loaded NLC formulations.

3.1.3. Transmission Electron Microscopy (TEM)

TEM technique was employed to evaluate both blank and RFB-loaded NLC morphology as well as to verify nanocarriers size, as recommended elsewhere [27]. As shown in Figure 2, NLC exhibit a spheroidal morphology. Furthermore, in some images (such as Figure 2B), a structure with concentric layers could be noticed, which is also disturbed towards the center of the nanoparticle, exhibiting a high electron density. This lipid nanoparticle structure has been previously described and is associated with the polymorphic α-form of lipids [31]. Moreover, a size of 119 ± 41 nm in the case of blank NLC and slightly higher (173 ± 85 nm) in the case of RFB-loaded ones was observed, confirming the results obtained by DLS.

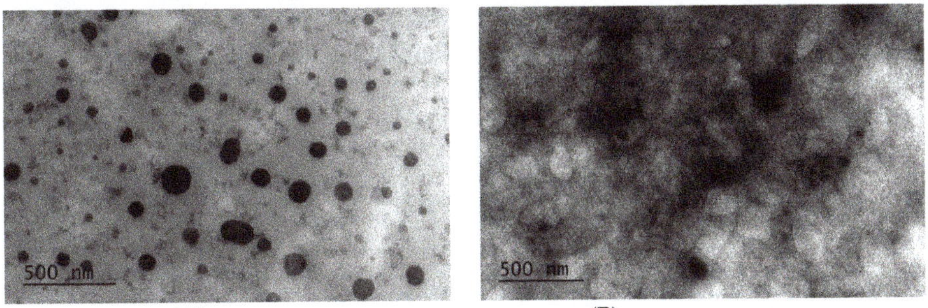

(A) **(B)**

Figure 2. Transmission electron micrographs of (**A**) Blank and (**B**) RFB-loaded NLC.

3.1.4. Atomic Force Microscopy (AFM)

Blank and RFB-loaded NLC morphology, particle size and distribution were also assessed by Atomic force microscopy, a technique which gives insight into the sample z-dimension from the deflection of a fine leaf spring (known as the AFM cantilever) [32]. Therefore, AFM is a useful tool to complete the information obtained by DLS and by the two-dimensional images provided by TEM.

In this way, the AFM images of blank and RFB-loaded nanoparticles depicted in Figure 3 confirm the spheroidal shape previously shown by TEM. Moreover, results derived from AFM analysis were expressed as the frequency (%) of nanoparticles exhibiting a specific height. Thus, blank and RFB-loaded nanoparticles exhibited a similar size, as values of 43 ± 3 nm and 33 ± 1 nm, respectively, were obtained (Figure 4). The smaller nanoparticle height reported by AFM in comparison with the diameters obtained by DLS and TEM corroborates the existence of a spheroidal structure, closer to a disk than to a sphere. This structure further confirms the prevalence of the polymorphic α-form of lipids [27,31], as previously mentioned, which has been associated with a high loading capacity and a low tendency to expulse the encapsulated drug from the lipid matrix [27].

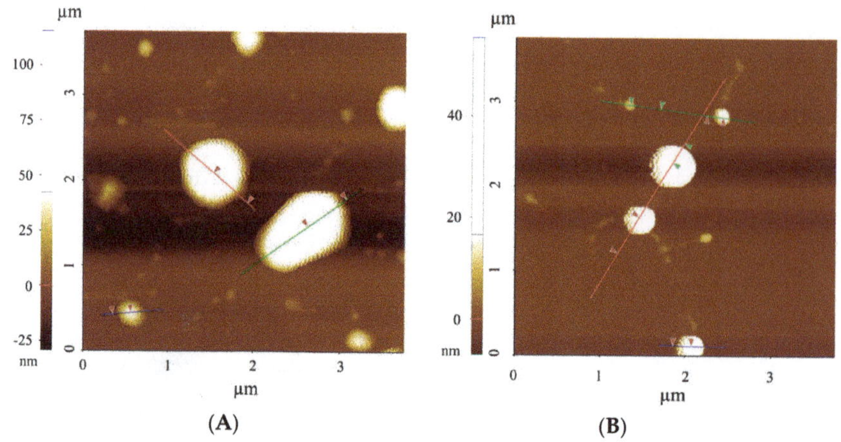

Figure 3. Atomic force microscopy images of (**A**) Blank and (**B**) RFB-loaded NLC.

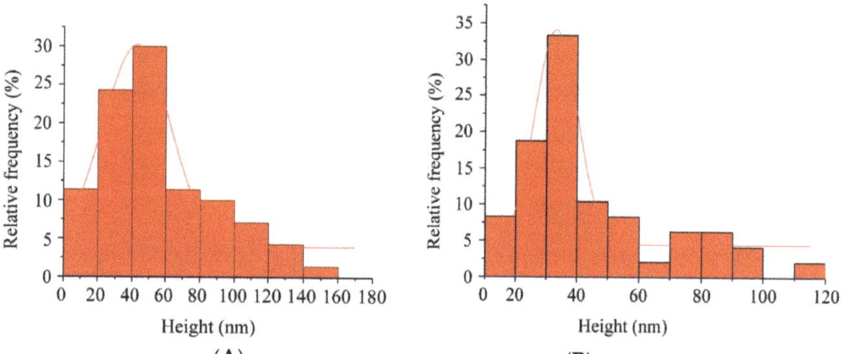

Figure 4. Particle size and size distribution according to AFM analysis of (**A**) Blank and (**B**) RFB-loaded NLC. Results were adjusted to a gaussian distribution.

3.1.5. In Vitro Release Studies

Release studies were performed to investigate the ability of NLC to act as RFB reservoirs. This compound is an antimicrobial agent active against widely known *Mycobacterium* species, including *M. leprae*, *M. tuberculosis*, or MAP [8], an infectious agent increasingly related with CD development [3]. Furthermore, RFB has been included in the triple oral anti-mycobacterial regimen currently under evaluation intended to eradicate MAP infection from CD patients [8]. In this way, release from nanoparticles was performed in both simulated intestinal fluid (SIF) and macrophage's lysate, with the aim of analyzing the expected drug release profile in the gut and intracellular environment, respectively. In the drug release study in SIF, the experimental results indicated that the RFB release from NLC in intestinal environment is negligible, since the amount of drug released during the whole assay was not detected by HPLC. Regarding RFB release assay in murine macrophage's lysate, the released drug started to be detectable at 1 h, and increased progressively until 16 h, when the amount of RFB in release medium was found to be quantifiable by HPLC. After 16 h, 1.46 ± 0.47 μg of drug were detected in the receptor chamber of Franz diffusion cells, resulting in a release percentage of 0.1 ± 0.03% at the end of the experiment.

In physiological conditions, drug release from lipid nanocarriers has been reported to occur, simultaneously, through erosion and diffusion mechanisms [33]. Poor RFB release from NLC obtained in the assays is likely to be related with the high lipophilicity of the drug (log P = 4.218) [34], as well as with the favorable conditions within the nanoparticle due to the high RFB solubility in the lipid matrix, which significantly reduces drug diffusion towards the aqueous release medium [35]. Several authors employed different strategies to overcome these issues associated with the poor in vitro release profile of lipophilic drugs, such as the addition of ethanol [36] or surfactants [37] in the release medium. However, in most cases, these approaches are not representative of the in vivo environment.

Regarding drug release through lipid matrix degradation, it is necessary to consider that it occurs primarily by enzymes, and also through hydrolytic processes, although to a lesser extent [33]. Because of that, analysis of NLC matrix degradation by enzymes present in both intestine and macrophage intracellular environment constitutes an interesting approach. According to the results obtained, NLC matrix can efficiently endure pancreatin activity of SIF, however, it is more affected by enzymes present in macrophage intracellular environment. Despite the higher effectivity of these macrophage enzymes, the amount of drug released from nanoparticles is still low. This slight drug release can be associated with the low enzymatic concentration in macrophage lysate achieved after dilution of cell suspension with Milli-Q® water. Therefore, as this concentration would obviously be higher inside macrophages in physiological conditions, a greater drug release would also be expected in this case.

Hence, outcomes obtained constitute an interesting proof of concept of the controlled and selective drug release provided by NLC inside macrophages, where MAP has been reported to establish a persisting infection [6].

3.2. *In Vitro Cellular Studies*

3.2.1. Cell Viability Studies

SLN and NLC are composed of biodegradable lipids with generally recognised as safe (GRAS) status [38]. However, despite these promising features, further studies are required to support their therapeutic use [18]. For this purpose, cell viability of THP-1 derived macrophages was analysed after NLC treatment.

Figure 5a shows cell viability after treatment with blank and RFB-loaded formulations at several concentrations (0.3, 0.12, 0.06 and 0.03 mg/mL). Besides, cells treated with equivalent RFB concentrations were used as control (Figure 5b). In general, formulations exhibited a good biocompatibility, leading to cell viabilities ≥70% for concentrations lower than 0.3 mg/mL. Two-way ANOVA ($p < 0.05$) points out a statistically significant effect of treatment (blank NLC or RFB-loaded NLC), NLC concentration, and their interaction on cell viability.

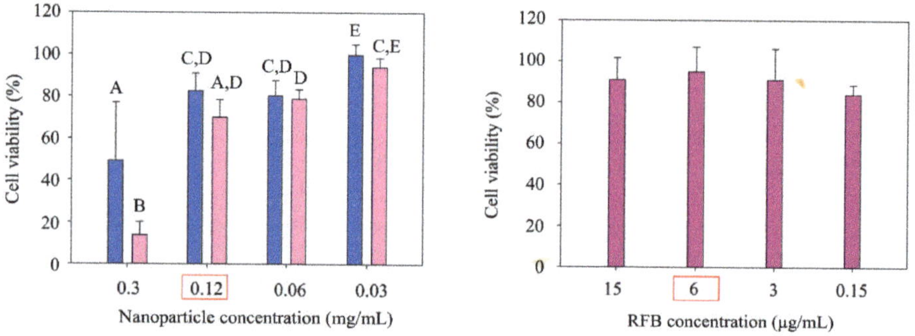

(**a**) (**b**)

Figure 5. Cell viability (%) relative to control with Milli-Q® water of (**a**) blank NLC formulations (dark blue colour) and RFB-loaded formulations (pink colour), using several nanoparticle concentrations (0.3, 0.12, 0.06 and 0.03 mg/mL). (**b**) Cell viability (%) relative to control with DMSO, of RFB solutions in DMSO prepared employing the same drug concentration as present in NLC formulations (purple colour). (A–E characters denote the homogeneous subsets pointed out by the post hoc Tukey's Multiple Comparison Test ($p < 0.05$).

Post hoc Tukey's Multiple Comparison Test ($p < 0.05$) points out a NLC concentration-dependent cytotoxic effect. However, it shows no statistical differences in cell viability for the experiments carried out with RFB-loaded NLC at 0.12 mg/mL and 0.06 mg/mL, therefore, the concentration 0.12 mg/mL was selected for further assays.

On the other hand, no significant modifications in cell viability were observed for RFB solutions (Figure 5b) containing equivalent amounts of drug, which implies that the reduction in viability must be mainly attributed to the toxicity of NLC components (oleic acid or emulsifiers), as suggested by several authors [39,40], and not to cytotoxic effects derived from RFB inclusion in the nanocarriers.

To allow the comparison of the cytotoxicity results obtained for RFB-loaded NLC with available data in literature, determination of IC_{50} was accomplished (Figure 6). The estimation of this value was performed from dose-response curves, where IC_{50} was defined as the concentration required to induce a 50% reduction in cell viability, resulting in a value of approximately 0.18 mg/mL. This finding is in line with previously published studies on lipid nanoparticle cytotoxicity, where IC_{50} was reported to be found mainly in the range of 0.1–1 mg/mL nanoparticles [18].

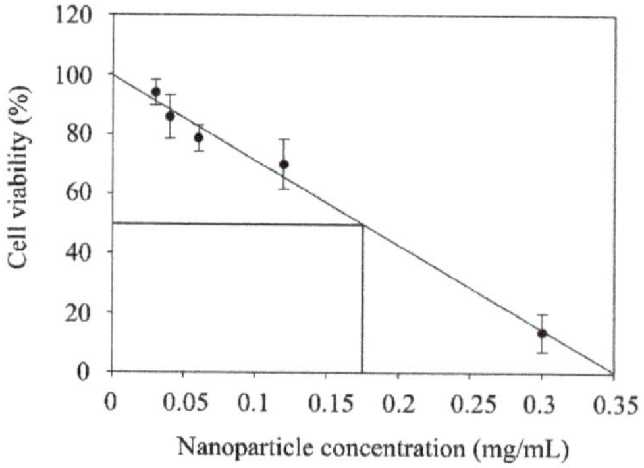

Figure 6. Dose response curve ($R^2 = 0.9881$) obtained from cell viability data at several RFB-loaded NLC concentrations. IC_{50} was calculated as the concentration of nanoparticles producing a 50% reduction in cell viability.

From the results obtained, NLC formulations present a suitable safety profile, similar to previously published works with lipid nanoparticles. Moreover, the highest NLC concentration of all the tested ones, showing an adequate biocompatibility in THP-1 derived macrophages, has been found to be 0.12 mg/mL. A cell viability ≥ 70% has been reported to be the threshold, according to ISO 10993-5 [41], below which a cytotoxic effect is considered to take place.

3.2.2. Confocal Microscopy

Qualitative study of both blank and RFB-loaded NLC internalization by THP-1 derived macrophages was analysed employing a nanoparticle concentration of 0.12 mg/mL, in accordance with the results obtained in the cell viability experiment. Moreover, the selection of this value was based not only on the results obtained in the biocompatibility assay, but also on the drug concentration required to efficiently eradicate the mycobacterial infection.

Regarding this last point, a minimum inhibitory concentration (MIC) ranging from 0.5 to 4 µg/mL has been obtained in vitro for RFB in both human and animal isolated MAP strains. Interestingly, five of six MAP human isolates show a MIC of only 1 µg/mL for this drug [42]. Furthermore, RFB has been reported to slow the multiplication of three virulent strains of Mycobacterium avium complex [43], a group of which MAP is an important member [44], in a model of intracellular infection in human macrophages when a dose of 0.5 µg/mL is employed [43]. Considering that RFB payload in NLC has been proven to reach almost 5% of the solid content of the formulations, a dose of approximately 6 µg/mL of drug was administered to macrophages. This drug concentration is clearly superior to the value required for RFB MIC, guaranteeing the administration of an effective dose to cells.

As observed in Figure 7, both blank (Figure 7A) and RFB-loaded NLC (Figure 7B) have been efficiently taken up by macrophages, which constitutes a promising start point for the treatment of infections produced by intracellular pathogens such as MAP. Images of separate channels of blank and loaded formulations are shown in Figures S1 and S2, respectively. Furthermore, images of NLC uptake by a macrophages group can be found in Figure S3.

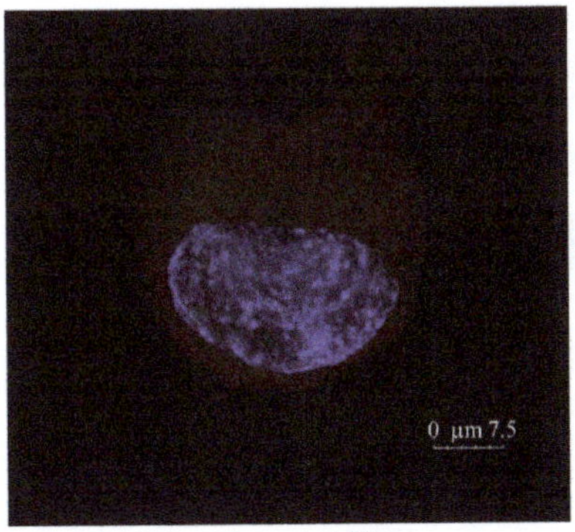

(A)

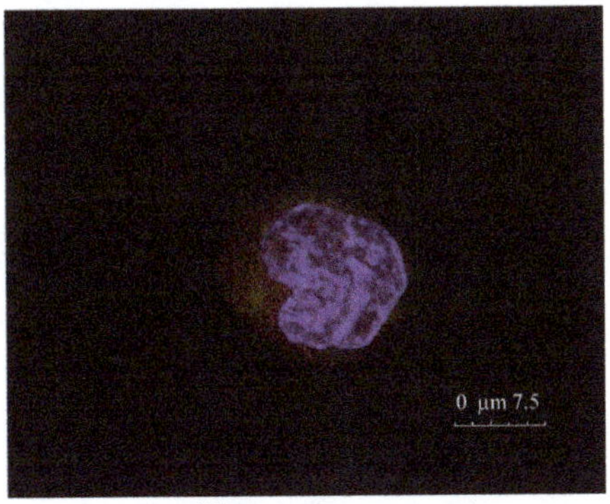

(B)

Figure 7. Confocal microscopy images of (**A**) Blank and (**B**) RFB-loaded NLC macrophages uptake. Red, blue, and green colours represent cell cytoplasm (Alexa Fluor™ 647 phalloidin), cell nuclei (DAPI) and NLC formulations (Coumarin 6), respectively.

3.2.3. Macrophage Uptake Quantification

Nanoparticle internalization by macrophages was also investigated using a quantitative approach and NLC formulations at 0.12 mg/mL. In this method, blank formulations showed an internalization percentage of 8.33 ± 1.15% after 2 h of exposure. Moreover, a higher internalization percentage, 13.39 ± 1.44%, was obtained for RFB-loaded NLC. Statistical analysis (one-way ANOVA, $p < 0.05$) revealed significant differences between the uptake of blank and loaded formulations. This higher macrophages uptake reported for loaded formulations might be related to their size (151 ± 34 nm), larger than the blank ones (111 ± 3 nm), since the uptake of particulate systems by macrophages rises progressively with the particle size increase [45].

In addition, the uptake percentage obtained for RFB-loaded NLC reveals that 13% of the administered dose (6 μg/mL or 0.6 μg each well) was efficiently taken up by macrophages, which constitutes a total RFB amount of 0.078 μg per well. Since each well contains 25.000 cells and human macrophages have a cell volume of approximately 4990 μm^3 [46], a total cell volume of 1.2475×10^{-4} mL is expected. Taking together the volumes of internalized drug and the total cell volume estimated, it is reasonable to think that an internalized concentration of 625 μg/mL could be achieved, which exceeds the range of the intracellular MIC previously reported. It is also important to note that colocalization phenomena amongst nanoparticles and mycobacteria have been suggested to occur by means of phagolysosomes fusion [47]. In this way, RFB would not be free in the cytoplasm and hence, it would probably not be the substrate of efflux pumps, which could modify the intracellular drug concentration indicated in this work.

3.2.4. Nanoparticle Permeation across Caco-2 Cells Monolayers

Nanoparticle permeation across the intestinal barrier is required to reach intestinal macrophages. Despite some of them being able to extend dendrites into the intestinal lumen, the majority of the macrophages are located below the epithelial monolayer, in the lamina propria [48]. The analysis of nanoparticles permeability across human colon carcinoma cell monolayers (Caco-2) has been reported to establish a good correlation with human in vivo absorption and has been broadly employed to predict drug permeability [24]. The drug concentration in the receptor compartment was estimated from the NLC concentration in this compartment at different times. Results are shown in Figure 8. No NLC permeation across the Caco-2 monolayer occurred during the first 2 h. After, RFB concentration in the receptor compartment increased linearly over time, achieving RFB concentrations of 3.29×10^{-4} 0.06 ± 0.05, 0.43 ± 0.01 and 0.9 ± 0.1 μg/mL at 4, 6, 24, and 48 h, respectively. In addition, a Papp value of 2.02×10^{-6} cm/s was obtained for RFB-NLC formulations. A Papp value of 2×10^{-6} cm/s has been reported as the threshold to achieve complete drug absorption in humans [49], therefore, the obtained value for RFB-NLC suggests that they exhibit good permeability across Caco-2 monolayers.

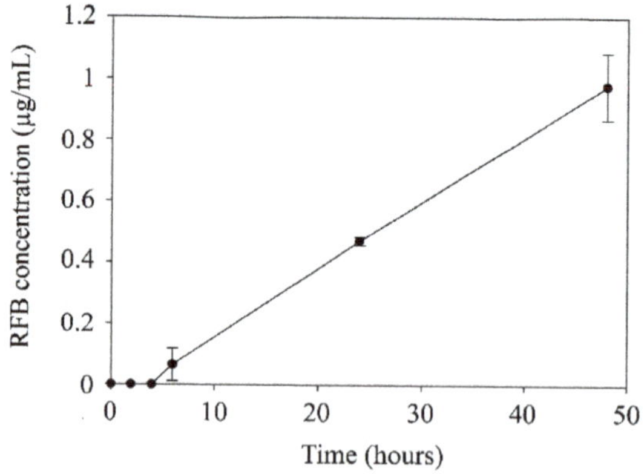

Figure 8. Permeation profile of rifabutin (RFB) loaded in NLC across Caco-2 cell monolayers expressed as a function of drug concentration in the lower compartment in a 48-h time interval.

Besides, the achieved permeability allowed to obtain a drug concentration virtually in range with the previously mentioned MIC reported for RFB just after 24 h of incubation with the nanocarriers, which is the accurate colonic transit time described for patients with CD [5]. Moreover, the in vivo permeability exhibited by NLC across the intestinal membrane of CD patients is expected to be even higher than reflected by this assay. The disruption of the epithelial barrier shown by inflammatory bowel disease patients increases gut permeability and favors nanoparticle passage [5]. In this way, nanoparticles are expected to accumulate preferentially in the intestinal inflamed sites, which are densely infiltrated with macrophages [5], ensuring the administration of an effective drug dose to the infected cells.

4. Conclusions

NLC showing a particle size within the nano-range (111 ± 3–151 ± 34 nm); a monodisperse size distribution (0.22 ± 0.02–0.23 ± 0), a negative zeta potential (−24 ± 2–−26 ± 2 mV), and a suitable rifabutin payload (4.62 ± 0.33%) were successfully prepared using a formulation process previously optimized by Artificial Intelligence tools. Formulations exhibited a spheroidal appearance, a good ability to withstand high temperature-related processes and a good safety profile in cellular studies. Moreover, the efficient macrophage uptake of the developed NLC has been demonstrated allowing the obtention of a therapeutic rifabutin concentration after only 2 h of incubation. This fact, along with the permeation exhibited by NLC across Caco-2 cell monolayers and their tendency to release the drug in the intracellular environment, guarantee the achievement of an effective rifabutin dose inside the phagocytic cells, where mycobacterium avium paratuberculosis is known to reside. Therefore, rifabutin-loaded NLC constitute a promising tool to improve anti-mycobacterial therapy in Crohn's disease.

Supplementary Materials: The following are available online at http://www.mdpi.com/2079-4991/10/11/2138/s1, Figure S1: Confocal imaging of blank NLC macrophages uptake, Figure S2: Confocal imaging of RFB-loaded NLC macrophages uptake, Figure S3: Confocal imaging of blank NLC uptake by a group of macrophages.

Author Contributions: Conceptualization, H.R., P.D.-R., A.J.A. and M.L.; methodology, H.R., P.D.-R., D.P.G., L.M.D.G. and M.C.; validation, H.R.; formal analysis, H.R. and P.D.-R.; investigation, H.R., P.D.-R., D.P.G., L.M.D.G. and M.C.; resources, C.R.-L., A.J.A. and M.L.; writing—original draft preparation, H.R.; writing—review and editing, P.D.-R., C.R.-L., A.J.A. and M.L.; visualization, H.R.; supervision, C.R.-L., A.J.A. and M.L.; project administration, M.L.; funding acquisition, M.L. All authors have read and agreed to the published version of the manuscript.

Funding: This research was funded by V-A POCTEP Program (0245_IBEROS_1_E) of EU (FEDER), Xunta de Galicia (Competitive Reference Groups, ED431C 2016/008 and ED431C2017/09-FEDER), as well as by Fundação para a Ciência e Tecnologia, Portugal (under iMED.ULisboa project Pest-UID/DTP/04138/2019).

Conflicts of Interest: The authors declare no conflict of interest. The funders had no role in the design of the study; in the collection, analyses, or interpretation of data; in the writing of the manuscript, or in the decision to publish the results.

Abbreviations

CD	Crohn's disease
LN	Lipid nanoparticles
RFB	Rifabutin
NLC	Nanostructured lipid carriers
SLN	Solid lipid nanoparticles
AI	Artificial intelligence
HPLC	High performance liquid chromatography
EE	Encapsulation efficiency
DL	Drug loading
DLS	Dynamic light scattering
SIF	Simulated intestinal fluid
TEM	Transmission electron microscopy
MAP	Mycobacterium avium paratuberculosis
TNF	Tumor necrosis factor
PDI	Polydispersity index
ZP	Zeta potential
TEER	Transepithelial electric resistance
GRAS	Generally regarded as safe
MIC	Minimum inhibitory concentration
IC50	inhibitory concentration 50
Papp	Apparent permeability coefficient

References

1. Feuerstein, J.D.; Cheifetz, A.S. Crohn Disease: Epidemiology, Diagnosis, and Management. *Mayo Clin. Proc.* **2017**, *92*, 1088–1103. [CrossRef] [PubMed]
2. Cosnes, J.; Gower-Rousseau, C.; Seksik, P.; Cortot, A. Epidemiology and natural history of inflammatory bowel diseases. *Gastroenterology* **2011**, *140*, 1785–1794. [CrossRef] [PubMed]
3. Davis, W.C. On deaf ears, *Mycobacterium avium paratuberculosis* in pathogenesis Crohn's and other diseases. *World J. Gastroenterol.* **2015**, *21*, 13411–13417. [CrossRef] [PubMed]
4. Kuenstner, J.T.; Naser, S.; Chamberlin, W.; Borody, T.; Graham, D.Y.; McNees, A.; Hermon-Taylor, J.; Hermon-Taylor, A.; Dow, C.T.; Thayer, W.; et al. The Consensus from the *Mycobacterium avium* ssp. *paratuberculosis* (MAP) Conference 2017. *Front. Public Health* **2017**, *5*, 208. [CrossRef] [PubMed]
5. Mohan, L.J.; Daly, J.S.; Ryan, B.M.; Ramtoola, Z. The future of nanomedicine in optimising the treatment of inflammatory bowel disease. *Scand. J. Gastroenterol.* **2019**, *54*, 18–26. [CrossRef]
6. Murphy, J.T.; Sommer, S.; Kabara, E.A.; Verman, N.; Kuelbs, M.A.; Saama, P.; Halgren, R.; Coussens, P.M. Gene expression profiling of monocyte-derived macrophages following infection with *Mycobacterium avium* subspecies *avium* and *Mycobacterium avium* subspecies *paratuberculosis*. *Physiol. Genom.* **2006**, *28*, 67–75. [CrossRef] [PubMed]
7. NIH. Open Label Efficacy and Safety of Anti-MAP (*Mycobacterium avium* ssp. *paratuberculosis*) Therapy in Adult Crohn's Disease (MAPUS2). Available online: https://clinicaltrials.gov/ct2/show/record/NCT03009396?view=record (accessed on 14 July 2020).
8. Savarino, E.; Bertani, L.; Ceccarelli, L.; Bodini, G.; Zingone, F.; Buda, A.; Facchin, S.; Lorenzon, G.; Marchi, S.; Marabotto, E.; et al. Antimicrobial treatment with the fixed-dose antibiotic combination RHB-104 for *Mycobacterium avium* subspecies *paratuberculosis* in Crohn's disease: Pharmacological and clinical implications. *Expert Opin. Biol.* **2019**, *19*, 79–88. [CrossRef] [PubMed]
9. Honap, S.; Johnston, E.; Agrawal, G.; Al-Hakim, B.; Hermon-Taylor, J.; Sanderson, J. Anti-*Mycobacterium paratuberculosis* (MAP) therapy for Crohn's disease: An overview and update. *Frontline Gastroenterol.* **2020**. [CrossRef]
10. Blaschke, T.F.; Skinner, M.H. The clinical pharmacokinetics of rifabutin. *Clin. Infect. Dis.* **1996**, *22*, S15–S22. [CrossRef]

11. Zhang, Y.; Feng, J.; McManus, S.A.; Lu, H.D.; Ristroph, K.D.; Cho, E.J.; Dobrijevic, E.L.; Chan, H.K.; Prud'homme, R.K. Design and Solidification of Fast-Releasing Clofazimine Nanoparticles for Treatment of Cryptosporidiosis. *Mol. Pharm.* **2017**, *14*, 3480–3488. [CrossRef]
12. Inoue, Y.; Yoshimura, S.; Tozuka, Y.; Moribe, K.; Kumamoto, T.; Ishikawa, T.; Yamamoto, K. Application of ascorbic acid 2-glucoside as a solubilizing agent for clarithromycin: Solubilization and nanoparticle formation. *Int. J. Pharm.* **2007**, *331*, 38–45. [CrossRef] [PubMed]
13. Ceci, C.; Graziani, G.; Faraoni, I.; Cacciotti, I. Strategies to Improve Ellagic Acid Bioavailability: From Natural or Semisynthetic Derivatives to Nanotechnological Approaches Based on Innovative Carriers. *Nanotechnology* **2020**, *31*, 382001. [CrossRef] [PubMed]
14. Cacciotti, I.; Chronopoulou, L.; Palocci, C.; Amalfitano, A.; Cantiani, M.; Cordaro, M.; Lajolo, C.; Callà, C.; Boninsegna, A.; Lucchetti, D. Controlled release of 18-β-glycyrrhetic acid by nanodelivery systems increases cytotoxicity on oral carcinoma cell line. *Nanotechnology* **2018**, *29*, 285101. [CrossRef] [PubMed]
15. Wais, U.; Jackson, A.W.; He, T.; Zhang, H. Nanoformulation and encapsulation approaches for poorly water-soluble drug nanoparticles. *Nanoscale* **2016**, *8*, 1746–1769. [CrossRef] [PubMed]
16. Müller, R.H.; Petersen, R.D.; Hommoss, A.; Pardeike, J. Nanostructured lipid carriers (NLC) in cosmetic dermal products. *Adv. Drug Deliv. Rev.* **2007**, *59*, 522–530. [CrossRef] [PubMed]
17. Khosa, A.; Reddi, S.; Saha, R.N. Nanostructured lipid carriers for site-specific drug delivery. *Biomed. Pharm.* **2018**, *103*, 598–613. [CrossRef]
18. Doktorovova, S.; Souto, E.B.; Silva, A.M. Nanotoxicology applied to solid lipid nanoparticles and nanostructured lipid carriers-A systematic review of in vitro data. *Eur. J. Pharm. Biopharm.* **2014**, *87*, 1–18. [CrossRef]
19. Rouco, H.; Diaz-Rodriguez, P.; Rama-Molinos, S.; Remunan-Lopez, C.; Landin, M. Delimiting the knowledge space and the design space of nanostructured lipid carriers through Artificial Intelligence tools. *Int. J. Pharm.* **2018**, *553*, 522–530. [CrossRef]
20. Gaspar, M.M.; Cruz, A.; Penha, A.F.; Reymao, J.; Sousa, A.C.; Eleuterio, C.V.; Domingues, S.A.; Fraga, A.G.; Filho, A.L.; Cruz, M.E.; et al. Rifabutin encapsulated in liposomes exhibits increased therapeutic activity in a model of disseminated tuberculosis. *Int. J. Antimicrob. Agents* **2008**, *31*, 37–45. [CrossRef]
21. Tominaga, H.; Ishiyama, M.; Ohseto, F.; Sasamoto, K.; Hamamoto, T.; Suzuki, K.; Watanabe, M. A water-soluble tetrazolium salt useful for colorimetric cell viability assay. *Anal. Commun.* **1999**, *36*, 47–50. [CrossRef]
22. Ngamwongsatit, P.; Banada, P.P.; Panbangred, W.; Bhunia, A.K. WST-1-based cell cytotoxicity assay as a substitute for MTT-based assay for rapid detection of toxigenic *Bacillus* species using CHO cell line. *J. Microbiol. Methods* **2008**, *73*, 211–215. [CrossRef]
23. Gaspar, D.P.; Faria, V.; Goncalves, L.M.; Taboada, P.; Remunan-Lopez, C.; Almeida, A.J. Rifabutin-loaded solid lipid nanoparticles for inhaled antitubercular therapy: Physicochemical and in vitro studies. *Int. J. Pharm.* **2016**, *497*, 199–209. [CrossRef] [PubMed]
24. Chaves, L.L.; Costa Lima, S.A.; Vieira, A.C.C.; Barreiros, L.; Segundo, M.A.; Ferreira, D.; Sarmento, B.; Reis, S. Nanosystems as modulators of intestinal dapsone and clofazimine delivery. *Biomed. Pharm.* **2018**, *103*, 1392–1396. [CrossRef] [PubMed]
25. Gaba, B.; Fazil, M.; Khan, S.; Ali, A.; Baboota, S.; Ali, J. Nanostructured lipid carrier system for topical delivery of terbinafine hydrochloride. *Bull. Fac. Pharm. Cairo Univ.* **2015**, *53*, 147–159. [CrossRef]
26. Danaei, M.; Dehghankhold, M.; Ataei, S.; Hasanzadeh Davarani, F.; Javanmard, R.; Dokhani, A.; Khorasani, S.; Mozafari, M.R. Impact of Particle Size and Polydispersity Index on the Clinical Applications of Lipidic Nanocarrier Systems. *Pharmaceutics* **2018**, *10*, 57. [CrossRef] [PubMed]
27. Gordillo-Galeano, A.; Mora-Huertas, C.E. Solid lipid nanoparticles and nanostructured lipid carriers: A review emphasizing on particle structure and drug release. *Eur. J. Pharm. Biopharm.* **2018**, *133*, 285–308. [CrossRef]
28. Schubert, M.A.; Muller-Goymann, C.C. Characterisation of surface-modified solid lipid nanoparticles (SLN): Influence of lecithin and nonionic emulsifier. *Eur. J. Pharm. Biopharm.* **2005**, *61*, 77–86. [CrossRef]
29. Mancini, G.; Lopes, R.M.; Clemente, P.; Raposo, S.; Gonçalves, L.M.D.; Bica, A.; Ribeiro, H.M.; Almeida, A.J. Lecithin and parabens play a crucial role in tripalmitin-based lipid nanoparticle stabilization throughout moist heat sterilization and freeze-drying. *Eur. J. Lipid Sci. Technol.* **2015**, *117*, 1947–1959. [CrossRef]
30. Battaglia, L.; Gallarate, M. Lipid nanoparticles: State of the art, new preparation methods and challenges in drug delivery. *Expert Opin. Drug Deliv.* **2012**, *9*, 497–508. [CrossRef]

31. Bunjes, H.; Steiniger, F.; Richter, W. Visualizing the structure of triglyceride nanoparticles in different crystal modifications. *Langmuir Acs J. Surf. Colloids* **2007**, *23*, 4005–4011. [CrossRef]
32. Sitterberg, J.; Ozcetin, A.; Ehrhardt, C.; Bakowsky, U. Utilising atomic force microscopy for the characterisation of nanoscale drug delivery systems. *Eur. J. Pharm. Biopharm.* **2010**, *74*, 2–13. [CrossRef] [PubMed]
33. Pathak, K.; Keshri, L.; Shah, M. Lipid nanocarriers: Influence of lipids on product development and pharmacokinetics. *Crit. Rev. Ther. Drug Carr. Syst.* **2011**, *28*, 357–393. [CrossRef]
34. Global Alliance for TB drug development: Rifabutin. *Tuberculosis* **2008**, *88*, 145–147. [CrossRef]
35. Iqbal, N.; Vitorino, C.; Taylor, K.M. How can lipid nanocarriers improve transdermal delivery of olanzapine? *Pharm. Dev. Technol.* **2017**, *22*, 587–596. [CrossRef]
36. Li, H.; Zhao, X.; Ma, Y.; Zhai, G.; Li, L.; Lou, H. Enhancement of gastrointestinal absorption of quercetin by solid lipid nanoparticles. *J. Control. Release* **2009**, *133*, 238–244. [CrossRef] [PubMed]
37. Das, S.; Ng, W.K.; Kanaujia, P.; Kim, S.; Tan, R.B. Formulation design, preparation and physicochemical characterizations of solid lipid nanoparticles containing a hydrophobic drug: Effects of process variables. *Colloids Surf. B Biointerfaces* **2011**, *88*, 483–489. [CrossRef]
38. Lasa-Saracibar, B.; Estella-Hermoso de Mendoza, A.; Guada, M.; Dios-Vieitez, C.; Blanco-Prieto, M.J. Lipid nanoparticles for cancer therapy: State of the art and future prospects. *Expert Opin. Drug Deliv.* **2012**, *9*, 1245–1261. [CrossRef]
39. Schöler, N.; Olbrich, C.; Tabatt, K.; Müller, R.; Hahn, H.; Liesenfeld, O. Surfactant, but not the size of solid lipid nanoparticles (SLN) influences viability and cytokine production of macrophages. *Int. J. Pharm.* **2001**, *221*, 57–67. [CrossRef]
40. Yin, H.; Too, H.P.; Chow, G.M. The effects of particle size and surface coating on the cytotoxicity of nickel ferrite. *Biomaterials* **2005**, *26*, 5818–5826. [CrossRef]
41. ISO. Biological Evaluation of Medical Devices Part 5: Tests for Cytotoxicity: In vitro Methods. In *EN ISO 10993-5*; ISO: Brussels, Belgium, 2009.
42. Zanetti, S.; Molicotti, P.; Cannas, S.; Ortu, S.; Ahmed, N.; Sechi, L.A. "In vitro" activities of antimycobacterial agents against *Mycobacterium avium* subsp. *paratuberculosis* linked to Crohn's disease and *paratuberculosis*. *Ann. Clin. Microbiol. Antimicrob.* **2006**, *5*, 27. [CrossRef]
43. Perronne, C.; Gikas, A.; Truffot-Pernot, C.; Grosset, J.; Pocidalo, J.; Vilde, J. Activities of clarithromycin, sulfisoxazole, and rifabutin against *Mycobacterium avium* complex multiplication within human macrophages. *Antimicrob. Agents Chemother.* **1990**, *34*, 1508–1511. [CrossRef]
44. Bull, T.J.; Sidi-Boumedine, K.; McMinn, E.J.; Stevenson, K.; Pickup, R.; Hermon-Taylor, J. Mycobacterial interspersed repetitive units (MIRU) differentiate *Mycobacterium avium* subspecies *paratuberculosis* from other species of the *Mycobacterium avium* complex. *Mol. Cell. Probes* **2003**, *17*, 157–164. [CrossRef]
45. Chono, S.; Tanino, T.; Seki, T.; Morimoto, K. Influence of particle size on drug delivery to rat alveolar macrophages following pulmonary administration of ciprofloxacin incorporated into liposomes. *J. Drug Target.* **2006**, *14*, 557–566. [CrossRef] [PubMed]
46. Krombach, F.; Münzing, S.; Allmeling, A.-M.; Gerlach, J.T.; Behr, J.; Dörger, M. Cell size of alveolar macrophages: An interspecies comparison. *Environ. Health Perspect.* **1997**, *105*, 1261–1263.
47. Lemmer, Y.; Kalombo, L.; Pietersen, R.D.; Jones, A.T.; Semete-Makokotlela, B.; Van Wyngaardt, S.; Ramalapa, B.; Stoltz, A.C.; Baker, B.; Verschoor, J.A.; et al. Mycolic acids, a promising mycobacterial ligand for targeting of nanoencapsulated drugs in tuberculosis. *J. Control. Release* **2015**, *211*, 94–104. [CrossRef] [PubMed]

48. Bain, C.C.; Mowat, A.M. Intestinal macrophages–specialised adaptation to a unique environment. *Eur. J. Immunol.* **2011**, *41*, 2494–2498. [CrossRef] [PubMed]
49. Grès, M.-C.; Julian, B.; Bourrié, M.; Meunier, V.; Roques, C.; Berger, M.; Boulenc, X.; Berger, Y.; Fabre, G. Correlation between oral drug absorption in humans, and apparent drug permeability in TC-7 cells, a human epithelial intestinal cell line: Comparison with the parental Caco-2 cell line. *Pharm. Res.* **1998**, *15*, 726–733. [CrossRef]

Publisher's Note: MDPI stays neutral with regard to jurisdictional claims in published maps and institutional affiliations.

nanomaterials

MDPI

Article

Overcoming the Inflammatory Stage of Non-Healing Wounds: In Vitro Mechanism of Action of Negatively Charged Microspheres (NCMs)

Edorta Santos-Vizcaino [1,2,†], Aiala Salvador [1,2,†], Claudia Vairo [1,3,*], Manoli Igartua [1,2], Rosa Maria Hernandez [1,2], Luis Correa [4], Silvia Villullas [3] and Garazi Gainza [3,*]

1 NanoBioCel Group, Laboratory of Pharmaceutics, University of the Basque Country (UPV/EHU), School of Pharmacy, Paseo de la Universidad 7, 01006 Vitoria-Gasteiz, Spain; edorta.santos@ehu.eus (E.S.-V.); aiala.salvador@ehu.eus (A.S.); manoli.igartua@ehu.eus (M.I.); rosa.hernandez@ehu.eus (R.M.H.)

2 Biomedical Research Networking Center in Bioengineering, Biomaterials and Nanomedicine (CIBER-BBN), 01006 Vitoria-Gasteiz, Spain

3 BioKeralty Research Institute AIE, Albert Einstein, 25-E3, 01510 Miñano, Spain; silvia.villullas@keralty.com

4 Praxis Pharmaceutical, San Fernando de Henares Business Park, Avenida de Castilla 2, Dublin Building 2nd floor, San Fernando de Henares, 28830 Madrid, Spain; lcorrea@praxisph.com

* Correspondence: claudia.vairo@keralty.com (C.V.); garazi.gainza@keralty.com (G.G.)

† These authors contributed equally to this work.

Received: 9 May 2020; Accepted: 1 June 2020; Published: 3 June 2020

Abstract: Negatively charged microspheres (NCMs) represent a new therapeutic approach for wound healing since recent clinical trials have shown NCM efficacy in the recovery of hard-to-heal wounds that tend to stay in the inflammatory phase, unlocking the healing process. The aim of this study was to elucidate the NCM mechanism of action. NCMs were extracted from a commercial microsphere formulation (PolyHeal® Micro) and cytotoxicity, attachment, proliferation and viability assays were performed in keratinocytes and dermal fibroblasts, while macrophages were used for the phagocytosis and polarization assays. We demonstrated that cells tend to attach to the microsphere surface, and that NCMs are biocompatible and promote cell proliferation at specific concentrations (50 and 10 NCM/cell) by a minimum of 3 fold compared to the control group. Furthermore, NCM internalization by macrophages seemed to drive these cells to a noninflammatory condition, as demonstrated by the over-expression of CD206 and the under-expression of CD64, M2 and M1 markers, respectively. NCMs are an effective approach for reverting the chronic inflammatory state of stagnant wounds (such as diabetic wounds) and thus for improving wound healing.

Keywords: chronic wound; device; foot ulcer; inflammation; wound healing; macrophage

---

1. Introduction

Hard-to-heal and chronic wounds are those that are not able to adequately continue the healing process, prolonging the situation for longer than 3 months [1,2]. The cost derived from chronic wounds in the US is estimated at more than 25 billion dollars a year, affecting more than 6 million people. Approximately 1% of the population of developed countries will suffer these injuries at some point in their lives [3]. Especially important are those known as diabetic foot ulcers, affecting 15% of diabetic patients, which in the US alone are around 20 million and expected to double by 2030 [4].

In this kind of wound, the healing process is incomplete and interrupted due to multiple factors. Senescent fibroblasts exhibit a decreased migration and synthesis of collagen, accompanied by high protease activity, which inhibits important factors in the healing process (e.g., platelet-derived growth factor (PDGF), transforming growth factor beta (TGF-β) or vascular endothelial growth factor (VEGF)) [5], and keratinocytes become senescent and unable to migrate and close the wound [6].

During the healing process, the macrophage population skews from a predominant pro-inflammatory (M1) to an anti-inflammatory (M2) phenotype, releasing anti-inflammatory mediators and growth factors [7,8]. Moreover, they can generate precursors for fibroblast activation and collagen synthesis [9] which is necessary for suitable wound healing [10]. However, chronic wounds persist in the inflammatory state, with M1 macrophages predominating [11].

An interesting option for the treatment of this type of wound consists of strategies that promote proliferation of the main cells involved in wound healing (keratinocytes and fibroblasts) and allows pro-inflammatory macrophages to skew to an anti-inflammatory phenotype. For that purpose, biomaterials can play an important role. Many alternatives have already been explored in this sense, such as liposomes, nanoparticles, microparticles or scaffolds [12]. Indeed, the type and level of cytokines produced by biomaterial-adherent cells can be modulated in order to regulate the immunologic response, with hydrophilic and anionic surfaces being among the most efficient in preventing inflammatory responses [13].

Negatively charged microspheres (NCMs) are a novel example of microtechnology used in the field of regenerative medicine. These synthetic biocompatible particles present unique biophysical properties, which make NCMs a valuable biomaterial for treating hard-to-heal wounds of different etiologies [14]. Furthermore, NCMs have been recently employed in wound healing for their excellent clinical results, i.e., in nonresponding diabetic foot ulcers [15] and wound dehiscence following breast reduction or mastopexy surgery [16]. Their size (~5 μm) and negative surface charge (zeta potential ~ −40 mV) allow the attachment and migration of cells involved in the healing process, ultimately improving wound healing [17]. Particularly, NCMs have formerly been proposed as a treatment for hard-to-heal and chronic wounds, leading to an improvement of healthy granulation tissue formation and wound area reduction, by 'kick-starting' the healing process [18].

Therefore, the main objective of this work was to demonstrate that specific cell-to-NCM interactions prompt essential steps in the tissue regeneration and wound healing processes. For that, we assessed the biocompatibility of NCMs with the human cell types involved in the wound healing processes, their cell-adhesive properties and ability to induce proliferative responses, as well as their capacity to enhance macrophage switching from pro-inflammatory to anti-inflammatory phenotypes.

2. Materials and Methods

2.1. NCM Samples

All experiments were carried out using NCMs extracted from a commercial formulation (PolyHeal® Micro, Madrid, Spain), consisting of polystyrene microspheres [4.5×10^6 microspheres (MS)/mL] suspended in 22% glycerol and phosphate buffer (KH_2PO_4/Na_2HPO_4) in water for injection. Taking into account that a 22% glycerol concentration is toxic for cells in culture (due to the high osmolarity), the product was washed with $_{dd}H_2O$, centrifuged at 24,000× *g* for 10 min and opportunely resuspended. NCMs were counted by means of a TC20 automated cell counter (Bio-Rad, Madrid, Spain), and diluted as needed. The size of the purified NCMs was measured by means of dynamic light scattering (4.5 ± 0.2 μm) and their zeta-potential was determined through laser doppler micro-electrophoresis (−43 ± 1 mV). To keep the effect of glycerol constant, all assayed doses (NCM/cell) were prepared maintaining a final glycerol concentration of 0.44% (dilution 1:50).

2.2. Cell Culture

HaCaT keratinocytes (ATCC®, Manassas, VA, USA) were cultured in complete medium [Dulbecco's modified Eagle's medium (DMEM) (41965-039, Gibco®, MA, USA) supplemented with 10% (v/v) fetal bovine serum (FBS) and 1% (*v/v*) penicillin-streptomycin (P/S)]. Depending on the assay, other mediums were used such as assay medium (DMEM supplemented with 2% FBS) and starving medium (DMEM supplemented with 0.2% FBS). Cells were assayed between passages 3 and 5.

Primary human dermal fibroblasts isolated from adult skin (HDFa, ATCC®, Manassas, VA, USA) were cultured on complete medium that consisted of fibroblast basal medium (PCS-201-030, ATCC®, Manassas, VA, USA) supplemented with a fibroblast growth kit-low serum (PCS-201-041, ATCC®, Manassas, VA, USA) and 1% P/S. Depending on the assay, other mediums were used such as assay medium (1:5 of complete medium in fibroblast basal medium) and starving medium (fibroblast basal medium). Cells were assayed between passages 3 and 5.

Human macrophages were obtained by primary monocyte isolation and differentiation from blood samples of healthy volunteers according to the ethical guidelines established by the institutional committee of the University of the Basque Country (UPV/EHU) (M30_2019_203). Peripheral blood mononuclear cells (PBMCs) were separated by Ficoll-Paque density gradient centrifugation. Then, monocytes were magnetically isolated using CD14 monoclonal antibody and cultured with complete medium (RPMI-1640, ATCC®, Manassas, VA, USA) supplemented with 10% FBS and 0.1% macrophage colony-stimulating factor (M-CSF) (Sigma-Aldrich, Química SL, Madrid, Spain) for 7 days in order to differentiate to M0 macrophages. Media was replaced every 2 to 3 days. Differentiation of M0 to M1 was induced by cultivating cells with 20 ng/mL of interferon gamma (IFN-γ) (Sigma-Aldrich, Química SL, Madrid, Spain) and 100 ng/mL of lipopolysaccharides (LPS) (Sigma-Aldrich, Química SL, Madrid, Spain) for 48 h. Similarly, differentiation from M0 to M2 was induced with 20 ng/mL interleukin 4 (IL-4). The M0 were maintained with M-CSF 0.1%. Success of the differentiation process was demonstrated by flow cytometry and optical microscope images (Figure S1).

Cells were incubated in a humidified incubator at 37 °C with a 5% CO_2 atmosphere and cell passages were carried out every 2 to 3 days depending on the confluence.

2.3. Cytotoxicity Assay

Cytotoxicity assays were performed following the ISO 10993-5:2009 guidelines for biological evaluation of medical devices.

HaCaT and HDFa (5000 cells/well) and M0 macrophages (20,000 cells/well) were seeded into a 96-well plate on modified culture media supplemented with FBS. All plates were incubated for 1 h in 5% CO_2 at 37 °C to allow complete cell attachment and stretching. Next, different NCM concentrations (0.1–200 NCM/cell) were added and incubated for 48 h. Dimethyl sulfoxide (DMSO, 10%), was used as cytotoxicity control. After 48 h, NCMs were removed from cultures and CCK-8 reagent (Sigma-Aldrich, Saint Louise, MO, USA) added and incubated for 4 h. Absorbance was read with a plate reader (Infinite® 200 PRO series, Tecan Trading AG, Männedorf, Switzerland) at 450 nm and at 650 nm, as the reference wavelength. Based on these results, the NCM/cell ratios were established for further experiments.

2.4. Attachment Assay

NCM attachment on HaCaT and HDFa was evaluated through the fluorescent method described below. Fluoresbrite yellow-green NCMs (FYG-NCMs) (Polysciences, Inc., Warrington, PA, USA) were used. Briefly, 2×10^3 cells/100 µL were seeded per well and cultured with complete medium for 24 h. Then, FYG-NCMs were added to render a final concentration of 50 FYG-NCM/cell. Fluorescence micrographs were taken with an epi-fluorescence microscope Nikon Eclipse TE2000-S (Izasa S.A, Barcelona, Spain) at different incubation times, and images were further analyzed with ImageJ. As cells retain the characteristics of their source tissue—single cells in close proximity (HDFa) or well-differentiated and spatially separated cell clusters (HaCaT)—, analyses were optimized in function of their culture particularities:

(i) For HaCaT, the attachment capacity of FYG-NCMs was semiquantitatively assessed by calculating the ratio between the fluorescence intensity within the area delimited by a cluster of cells and its bordering area ($\approx$ 50 µm width).

(ii) For HDFa, adhesion of FYG-NCMs was semiquantitatively determined by calculating the particle aggregation factor, namely the average number of FYG-NCMs per aggregate. Briefly, fluorescence intensities obtained from areas with a known number of FYG-NCMs were used to calculate the average fluorescence intensity of a single FYG-NCM (at least 8 fields). Based on these data, the fluorescence intensities of at least 7 blindly taken fields were normalized to find the particle aggregation factor. Only fields with evenly distributed cells were included in the analysis.

For both cell types, the cell-adherence of the FYG-NCMs was assessed by comparing the results obtained at 0 h and 24 h (time required to allow completion of the cell adhesion process).

2.5. Proliferation and Viability Assays

HaCaT and HDFa proliferation was assessed by BrdU. Briefly, 2×10^3 HaCaT or 1×10^3 HDFa cells were seeded per well. Prior to treatment, all HaCaT groups were cultured with complete medium for 6 h and then starved overnight. Subsequently, 50 NCM/cell and 10 NCM/cell were added and incubated for 24, 48 and 72 h. For each time point, a control group of 0 NCM/cell was used as reference.

In the case of the HDFa cells, all groups were cultured with complete medium for 24 h and then starved overnight. The starving medium was removed and replaced with assay medium to render a final concentration of 50 NCM/cell and 10 NCM/cell. Finally, plates were incubated for 24, 48 and 72 h. For each time point, a control group of 0 NCM/cell was used as reference.

All cells were cultured in the presence of BrdU (10 µM final concentration) for the last 2 h of each incubation time. All groups were assayed for BrdU uptake employing the cell proliferation Biotrak ELISA system (Amersham, NJ, USA), after complete removal of NCMs and following manufacturer's indications. Absorbances (450 nm) measured for the nonspecific binding control group (technical control, without BrdU) were subtracted from all assayed groups, and the results of the treated cells were normalized against the corresponding control group for each time point.

Viability studies were run in parallel to the cell proliferation assays. Cells were washed twice with PBS and then dyed with the live/dead kit (Invitrogen, Thermofisher, Bilbao, Spain) following manufacturer's instructions. After 30 min, fluorescence micrographs were taken with an epi-fluorescence microscope Nikon Eclipse TE2000-S (Izasa S.A, Barcelona, Spain).

2.6. Macrophage Phagocytosis Determination

The M0, M1 and M2 macrophages were incubated with 5 and 10 NCM/cell for 48 h and observed under the inverted contrast phase microscope Nikon Eclipse TE2000-S (Izasa S.A, Barcelona, Spain). In addition, the M0 macrophages were seeded on a sterile cover slip introduced in each well of a 24-well plate. After 1 h incubation, 5 NCM/cell were added and cells cultured for 48 h at 37 °C and 5% CO_2. Cover slips were then washed with PBS and cells fixed in glutaraldehyde 2% for scanning electron microscopy (SEM) examination with a Hitachi S-4800 (Hitachi High-Technologies Corporation, Tokyo, Japan). For this purpose, samples were dehydrated and sputtered with gold.

2.7. Macrophage Polarization Assay

The ability of the NCMs to induce changes in the surface receptors of macrophages was evaluated by flow cytometry. The ability of the M0 macrophages to develop an anti-inflammatory profile, and the capacity of the M1 polarized macrophages to revert to an anti-inflammatory phenotype was analyzed. Cells were incubated with NCMs at 5 and 10 NCM/cell ratios for 48 h at 37 °C and 5% CO_2. Next, cells were washed with PBS + 2 mM EDTA + 0.5% BSA, detached with TripLe™ and counted. 100,000 M0 or M1 were added to flow cytometry tubes. After Fc receptor blockade, cells were stained with anti CD14, CD64, CD83 and CD206 fluorescent antibodies, washed and analyzed by multicolor flow cytometry (MACSQuant 10, Miltenyi Biotec, Madrid, Spain). Macrophages were gated according to their forward- and side-scatter characteristics and data were analyzed by MACSQuantify software (Miltenyi Biotec, Bergisch Gladbach, Germany).

2.8. Statistical Analysis

Results are expressed as mean ± SD and all the experiments were performed at least in triplicate. Unpaired, two-tailed *t*-tests or Mann-Whitney *U*-tests were used for the attachment assay after testing for normal distribution. For the remaining experiments, differences among the groups at significance levels of 95% were calculated by ANOVA with Bonferroni or Tamhane multiple comparison corrections in function of their equality of variances. Statistical analysis was completed with IBM SPSS Statistics 20 program (SPSS Inc.®, Chicago, IL, USA).

3. Results

3.1. Cytotoxicity Study

NCMs were not cytotoxic in most of the studied concentrations (metabolic activity ≥ 100% as compared to the control). Only high concentrations of NCMs (over 100, 75 and 25 for HaCat, HDFa and macrophages, respectively) gave a viability under 100%. The appropriate NCM/cell ratio for further experiments was determined according to these results and the highest concentration that provided a viability greater or equal to 100% was selected. In addition, a lower concentration was chosen in order to determine the NCM dose-dependent effect. Thus, 50 and 10 NCM/cell ratio were chosen for HaCaT and HDFa, and 10 and 5 NCM/cell in the case of macrophages (Figure S2).

3.2. Attachment Assay

We assessed the cell-adhesive properties of NCMs in both HaCaT and HDFa. To visualize particle adhesion and obtain an accurate quantification, we used fluoresbrite yellow-green NCMs (FYG-NCMs) at 50 FYG-NCM/cell combined with image analysis. Freshly administered FYG-NCMs appeared in the close proximities of HaCaT cell clusters, with few particles within the area occupied by the cells (Figure 1a). After 24 h of incubation, we could observe how fluorescent particles reached the keratinocyte clusters and started to accumulate therein, forming aggregates onto the surface of the cell clusters ($p = 0.001$).

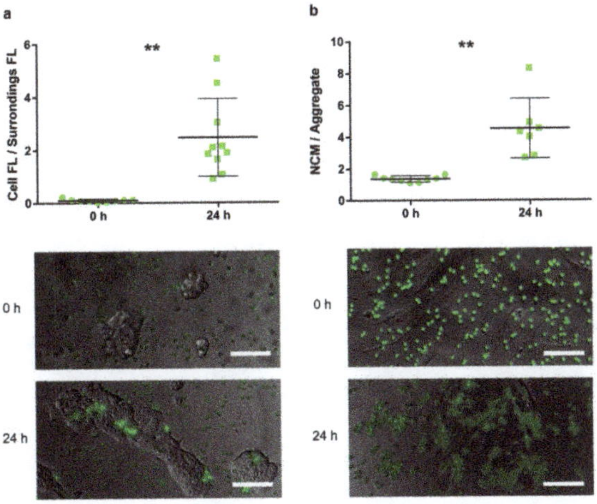

Figure 1. Attachment assay using fluoresbrite yellow-green negatively charged microspheres (FYG-NCMs) in HaCaT and HDFa. (**a**) Ratio between the fluorescence intensity within cell area and immediate surroundings assessed in the HaCaT cell line; FYG-NCMs suspended in $_{dd}H_2O$ and incubated for 0 and 24 h; (**b**) Particle aggregation factor measured in human fibroblasts; FYG-NCMs suspended in $_{dd}H_2O$ and incubated for 0 and 24 h; (**a–b**) Representative epi-fluorescence images of cells assayed with FYG-NCMs (green). **, $p < 0.01$. Scale bars, 100 μm. FL, fluorescence.

On the other hand, FYG-NCMs showed similar behavior when assayed in HDFa. At 0 h, fluorescence micrographs presented single and evenly distributed particles (particle aggregation factor = 1.38), which formed aggregates adapted to the cell shape after 24 h of incubation (Figure 1b). This gave, as a result, a statistically significant increase in the particle aggregation factor ($p = 0.005$). The NCMs remained adsorbed on the cell surface and no particle uptake was observed.

3.3. Proliferation and Viability Assays

We evaluated the capability of the NCMs to promote cell proliferation in HDFa. We assayed the DNA synthesis rate and viability after incubation with 50 MS/cell and 10 MS/cell for increasing exposure times (Figure 2a). A statistically significant increase in the proliferation rate of HDFa was observed after 24 h of treatment with the lowest dose of NCMs ($p = 0.001$), while the highest dose showed nonsignificant results (Figure 2b). From this point onwards, treatments for both 48 and 72 h expressed nonsignificant differences against their corresponding control group (untreated) at any dose (Figure 2d). Fluorescence micrographs with calcein/ethidium dyes, taken in parallel to the proliferation assays, confirmed the compatibility of NCMs during the whole experiment, even at high doses (Figure 2e–g).

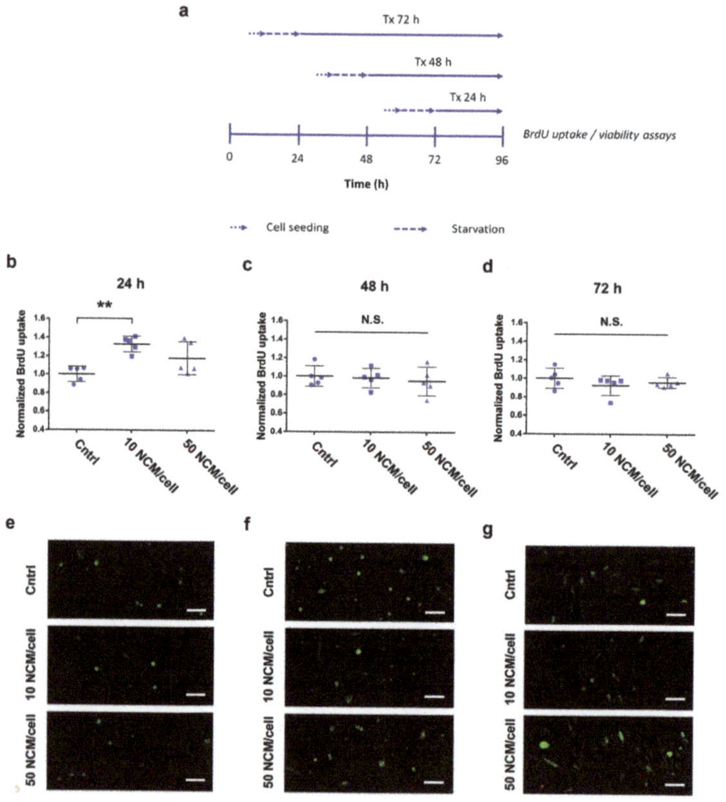

Figure 2. NCM proliferative response in HDFa. (**a**) Experimental design to assess BrdU uptake (**b–d**) and cell viability (**e–g**) after treatment with NCMs at different doses and exposure times. (**b–d**) BrdU uptake in human fibroblasts after 24 h (**b**), 48 h (**c**) and 72 h (**d**) of treatment; (**e–g**) Representative confocal fluorescence images of cells probed with the live/dead viability kit (green, living cells; red, dead cells) 24 h (**e**), 48 h (**f**) and 72 h (**g**) after treatment with NCMs. **, $p < 0.01$; N.S., nonsignificant ($p > 0.05$). Scale bars, 45 µm. Cntrl, control with no NCM exposure.

We also assessed the capacity of NCMs to induce cell proliferation in HaCaT. We exposed keratinocytes to 50 MS/cell and 10 MS/cell doses for increasing incubation times, comparing their DNA synthesis rate and viability at each time point (Figure 3a). Treatments for both 24 and 48 h showed nonsignificant differences against their corresponding control group (untreated) at any dose (Figure 3b,c). Contrarily, we observed a statistically significant increase in cell proliferation for HaCaT cells after 72 h of treatment with both high and low doses of NCMs ($p = 0.027$ and 0.018 respectively) (Figure 3d). Fluorescence micrographs with calcein/ethidium dyes, taken in parallel to the proliferation assays, confirmed the compatibility of NCMs during the whole experiment, even at high doses (Figure 3e–g).

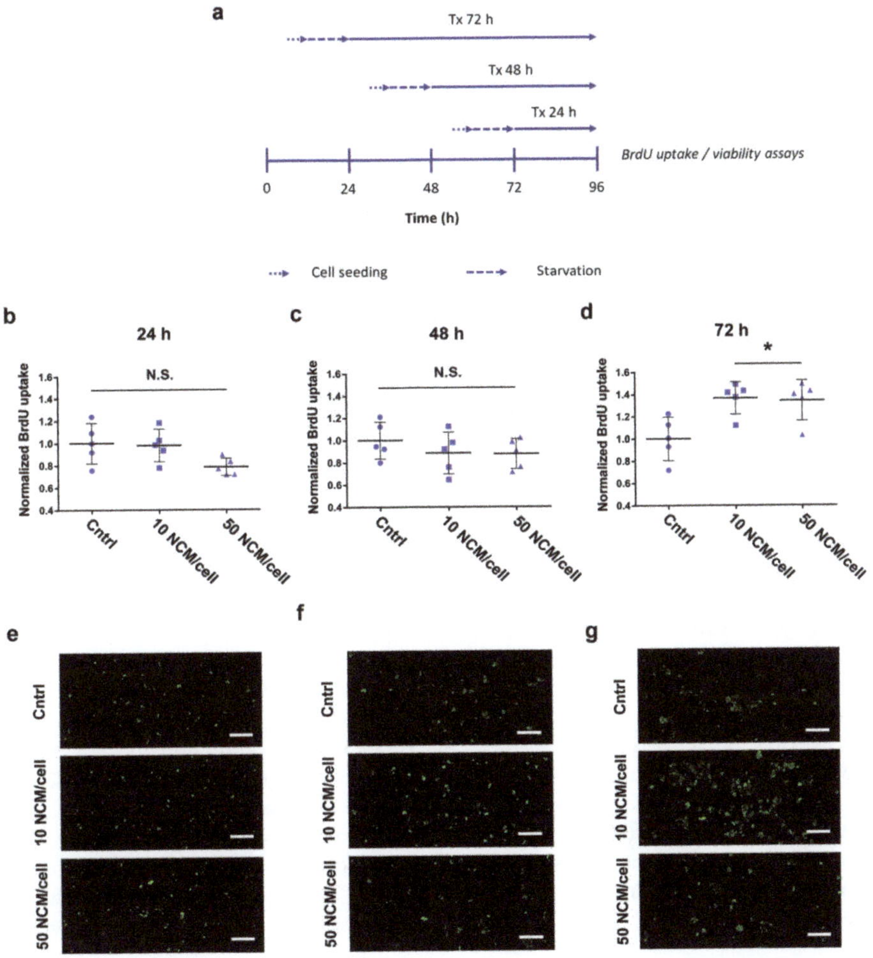

Figure 3. NCM proliferative response in HaCaT. (**a**) Experimental design to assess BrdU uptake (**b–d**) and cell viability (**e–g**) after treatment with NCMs at different doses and exposure times; (**b–d**) BrdU uptake in HaCaT cells after 24 h (**b**), 48 h (**c**) and 72 h (**d**) of treatment; (**e–g**) Representative confocal fluorescence images of cells probed with the live/dead viability kit (Green, living cells; Red, dead cells) 24 h (**e**), 48 h (**f**) and 72 h (**g**) after treatment with NCMs.*, $p < 0.05$; N.S., nonsignificant ($p > 0.05$). Scale bars, 200 μm. Cntrl, control with no NCM exposure.

3.4. Phagocytosis Determination

The M0, M1 and M2 macrophages were observed under inverted contrast phase microscope after 48 h of incubation with 5 and 10 NCM/cells to determine NCM interaction with macrophage subsets. As shown in Figure S3, NCMs were always located in the area occupied by macrophages, and not in their surrounding area.

To further confirm that NCMs were located inside cells, M0 macrophages were observed under SEM. The experiment was performed using 5 NCM/cell in order to facilitate visualization. Results showed a perfect colocalization of NCMs with macrophages (Figure 4a), and none located in the external surface. In addition, the cell membrane surrounding the NCMs could also be shown (Figure 4b), suggesting that they had been internalized by the cells. This fact was further confirmed through flow cytometry since an increase in cell complexity was found (Figure S4).

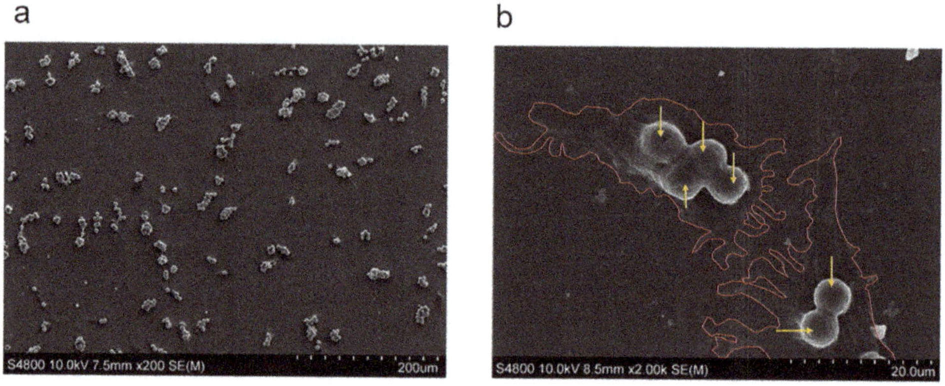

Figure 4. SEM images showing M0 macrophage after incubation with 5 NCM/cell. NCMs are colocalized with macrophages. (**a**) ×200; (**b**) ×2000. Edges of the cells (red line) and NCM (orange arrows) are shown.

3.5. Polarization Assay

The ability of NCMs to bias macrophages to a noninflammatory stage was assessed by flow cytometry. Macrophages were identified based on forward and side scatter (FSC and SSC, respectively) and CD14 presence. Analysis of the macrophage surface-marker expression after 48 h of incubation with NCMs is shown in Figures 5 and 6 for the M0 and M1 macrophages, respectively. Results showed that in the M0 macrophages, CD206 (typical M2 marker) was significantly upregulated, and CD64 (typical M1 marker) was downregulated, especially when the highest concentration of NCMs was used. Similar results were obtained for the M1 macrophages, and changes in the surface markers were even more pronounced in these cells. In this case, the expression of CD83 was also evaluated, showing a downregulation at the highest dose of NCMs. In most cases, changes in the surface-marker expression were dose-dependent, with the 10 NCM/cell ratio being the concentration able to induce the highest changes.

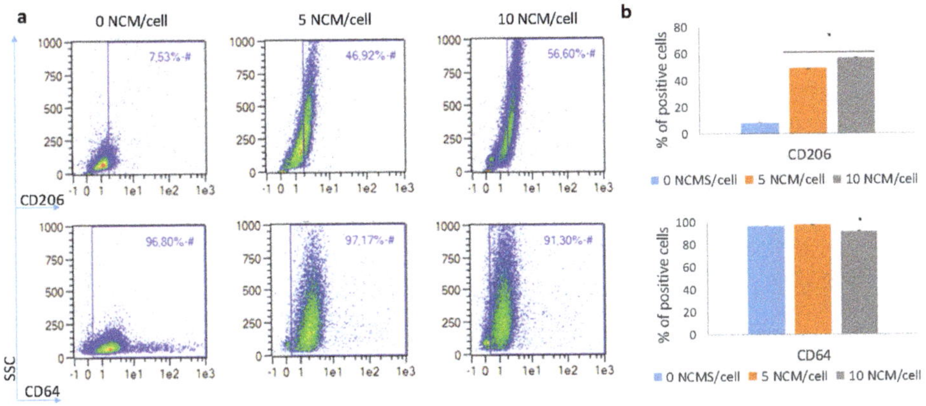

Figure 5. Surface marker changes when M0 macrophages were incubated with 5 and 10 NCM/cell. (**a**) Representative flow cytometry density plots. (**b**) Percentage of positive cells for each marker. *$p < 0.05$.

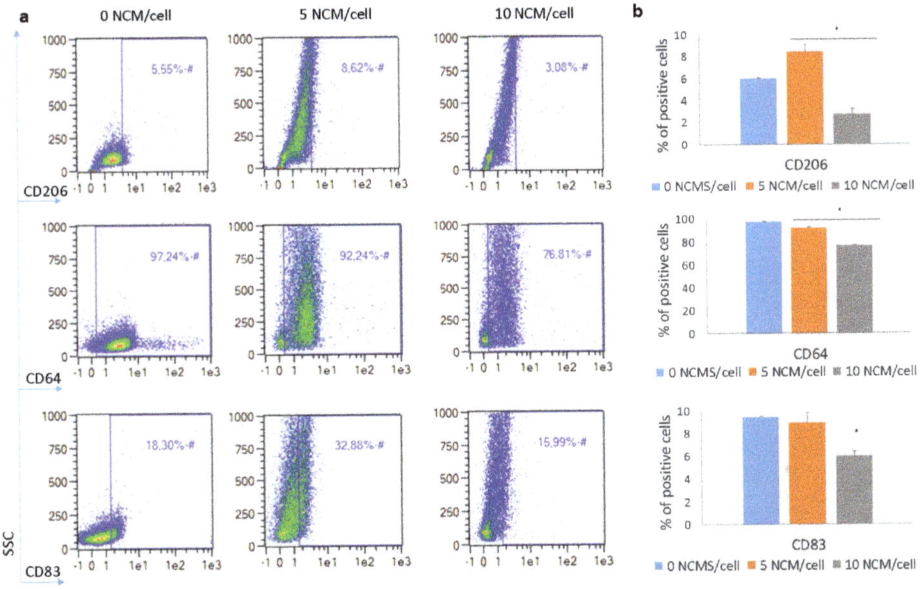

Figure 6. Surface marker changes when M1 macrophages were incubated with 5 and 10 NCM/cell. (**a**) Representative flow cytometry density plots. (**b**) Percentage of positive cells for each marker. *$p < 0.05$.

4. Discussion

In this work, we evaluated the potential of NCMs to enhance the wound-healing processes in terms of (i) compatibility of NCMs with relevant skin cells, (ii) their cell adhesive properties, (iii) their capacity to induce proliferative responses in target cells and (iv) their ability to switch macrophages to a noninflammatory stage.

Results from the cytotoxicity assay demonstrated good cell viability for most NCM concentrations tested, indicating their biocompatibility. However, at the highest NCM concentrations (≥ 100, 75 and 25 NCM/cell for HaCat, HDFa and macrophages, respectively) cell viability decreased. The selected

NCM concentrations for further studies were 50 and 10 NCM/cell for HaCat and HDFa, and 10 and 5 NCM/cell for macrophages.

FYG-NCMs showed cell-adhesive properties in both HaCaT and HDFa. On the one hand, polystyrene has already been demonstrated to possess physical-chemical properties suitable for cell attachment, migration, proliferation and differentiation, since it has been specifically tested as a material for wound healing [19,20], among others. On the other hand, it is well-known that polymers are a cornerstone of regenerative medicine, directing interactions at the tissue–material interface [21]. Cell attachment to NCMs can be of noteworthy importance for the mechanism of action of the NCMs, since that contact may trigger cell proliferation and thus, wound healing [22]. In fact, studies suggest that the in vivo efficacy of wound-healing products can be directly related to their ability to be adhered to cells [23–25].

The NCMs demonstrated their capability to induce an improved proliferative response in the two cell lines studied. We subjected cells treated with NCMs to BrdU pulses of 2 h after the different incubation times with the aim of scanning when (or if) proliferative responses were promoted by NCMs. HDFa showed an increased DNA synthesis after 24 h of treatment at low doses (10 NCM/cell). The inhibitory effect, observed when too many adhesion molecules are present, is in agreement with previous studies carried out by either the current authors or other groups when working with 3D cultures modified with increasing concentrations of cell-adhesion ligands. These studies argued that the strong adhesion forces derived from an excessive number of bound receptors might hinder cell division [26–29]. On the other hand, HaCaT cells presented a delayed response, requiring 72 h of treatment, after which we observed a significantly increased cell proliferation both at high and low doses (50 and 10 NCM/cell). These results are in agreement with previous findings demonstrating that NCMs influenced the activity and proliferation of various cell types normally present in wounds [17]. It seems that NCMs' specific surface area and geometry allow their interaction with cells through various mechanisms. First, exposure of NCMs to a biological environment results in the rapid adsorption of proteins to its surface [15]. In the same way, fibroblasts and keratinocytes deposit extracellular matrix-forming proteins (e.g., fibronectin, laminin and vitronectin), which are also adsorbed by NCMs and play a pivotal role in cell attachment [17,30]. We hypothesize that adsorbed proteins may interact with cellular receptors, especially with integrins; thus, triggering the activation of particular signal transduction pathways involved in cellular processes such as proliferation or migration [31,32]. Therefore, the nature and extent of this biologic response will largely depend on the integrin profile expressed by each particular cell type [33] and the layer of adsorbed proteins presented by the biomaterial surface [34]. In addition, further still-unraveled mechanisms may be responsible for cell attachment and subsequent biologic responses [35].

Regarding macrophages, we suggest that they are probably taken up by NCMs. This fact could be critical for the NCM effect, since particle accumulation in macrophages is thought to be advantageous for switching cell phenotype [36].

The polarization assay confirmed that NCMs may influence a macrophage's phenotype and bias it towards a noninflammatory state. This, in turn, can lead to resolution of the inflammation process. In both M0 and M1 macrophages, the expression of CD206 marker was increased, a typical M2 marker indicative of the resolution of the inflammation [11]. Similarly, CD64 was downregulated, especially when the higher concentration of NCMs was used, in accordance with its lower expression in M2 macrophages [37]. In addition, the expression of CD83 was also assessed in M1 macrophages. Although this marker is not expressed in most macrophages, it can be found in M1 ones (as well as in mature dendritic cells) [38]. This marker was downregulated, especially when the highest dose of NCMs was used, indicating the loss of the M1 pro-inflammatory phenotype. Altogether, analysis of the surface-marker expression indicated that NCMs tended to favor a noninflammatory milieu, i.e., cells skewed their phenotype towards an M2 in the presence of NCMs. This fact may be important to explain the effectiveness of the treatment observed in humans [39]. However, the exact mechanism by which these NCMs skew macrophages towards M2 has not been determined. The most plausible explanation is that the biomaterial itself produces an immunomodulatory immune response, instead of activating the immune response. In fact, studies have demonstrated that macrophages in contact with several biomaterials produce lower levels of proinflammatory cytokines, such as IL-1β, CXCL8(IL-8), IL-12 and TNF-α, and higher levels of immunosuppressive cytokines, such as IL-10 [11,40,41]. Although the mechanism is not clear, NCM characteristics, such as physical properties (geometry, topography and porosity) and biochemical properties (surface chemistry, ligand functionalization and degradation mode) have been determined as critical factors in the host response to the material [42].

Thus, we can postulate that in vivo, NCMs mechanically promote (i) switching of macrophages towards M2 and (ii) the induction of fibroblast and keratinocyte proliferation.

With the aim of switching macrophage phenotype in chronic wounds, several approaches have been evaluated, including the use of mesenchymal stromal cells, growth factors, biomaterials, heme oxygenase-1 induction and oxygen therapy, among others [43]. Among biomaterials, several micro/nanoparticles have been evaluated, including or not bioactive molecules [44]. In the case of NCMs, no drug has been encapsulated; thus, the effects are directly attributed to the presence of NCMs on the wound. Similar studies have been carried out with chitosan microparticles [45] and although M0 to M2 polarization was observed, these microparticles were not able to suppress pro-inflammatory factor release from M1. Silica nanoparticles have also been evaluated with the same purpose [46]. In that study, the ability of the macrophage subset to phagocyte the microparticles was evaluated, but not the capacity to switch their phenotype, nor the effects for wound healing. Taking into account these results, our study demonstrated that NCMs possess several advantages in comparison to similar products, as they can promote M2 phenotype of macrophages overcoming the inflammatory stage, a common characteristic of hard-to-heal wounds.

5. Conclusions

We have proved that the mechanism of action of NCMs to promote wound healing is mainly caused by the capability of skin cells to interact with NCMs, which in turn induces cell proliferation and macrophage differentiation. NCMs showed excellent cell-adhesive properties in keratinocytes and human fibroblasts, and were able to promote a prompt response in the proliferative capacity of human fibroblasts after 24 h of treatment, and after 72 h in the keratinocyte HaCaT cell line. Importantly, NCMs seemed to be taken up by macrophages and were able to modify their surface-marker expression, so that pro-inflammatory macrophage populations could switch to a noninflammatory phenotype. This finding is of noteworthy importance since one of the main problems of chronic wound healing is the presence of classically activated macrophages that impair tissue repair. Thus, this ability of NCMs can be crucial to overcoming the inflammatory stage of chronic wounds, such as the diabetic wounds which are so challenging in clinical settings.

Supplementary Materials: The following are available online at http://www.mdpi.com/2079-4991/10/6/1108/s1: Figure S1: Phase contrast images showing M0, M1 and M2 macrophage morphology, Figure S2: Cytotoxicity study for HaCaT, HDFa and macrophages after incubation with NCMs, Figure S3: Phase contrast images showing M0, M1 and M2 macrophage after 48 h of incubation with 5 and 10 NCM/cell, Figure S4: Representative density plots showing the different morphological features of M0, M1 and M2 macrophages when incubated with 5 and 10 NCM/cell.

Author Contributions: Conceptualization, G.G.; funding acquisition, S.V. and G.G.; investigation, E.S.-V., A.S. and C.V.; methodology, E.S.-V., A.S. and C.V.; project administration, G.G.; resources, S.V.; supervision, C.V.; validation, C.V.; writing—original draft, E.S.-V., A.S. and C.V.; writing—review and editing, C.V., M.I., R.M.H., L.C. and S.V. All authors have read and agreed to the published version of the manuscript.

Funding: The present work was partially funded by the Basque Government (Consolidated Groups, IT-907-16 and HAZITEK, ZE-2017/00014) and co-funded by the European Regional Development Fund (ERDF).

Acknowledgments: Authors are thankful for the technical support provided by the ICTS "NANBIOSIS" (Drug Formulation Unit, U10) of the CIBER-BBN at the University of Basque Country (UPV/EHU) in Vitoria-Gasteiz. We also thank Itxaso Garcia-Orue and Saioa Santos-Vizcaino for their technical assistance and invaluable advice.

Conflicts of Interest: Praxis Pharmaceutical possesses the sale license of PolyHeal® Micro and 10% of BioKeralty Research Institute AIE belongs to Praxis Pharmaceutical. No author had control on the results of the assays.

The authors have no other conflicts of interest that are directly relevant to the content of this manuscript, which remains their sole responsibility.

References

1. Zhao, R.; Liang, H.; Clarke, E.; Jackson, C.; Xue, M. Inflammation in chronic wounds. *Int. J. Mol. Sci.* **2016**, *17*, 2085. [CrossRef] [PubMed]
2. Eming, S.A.; Martin, P.; Tomic-Canic, M. Wound repair and regeneration: Mechanisms, signaling, and translation. *Sci. Transl. Med.* **2014**, *6*, 265sr6. [CrossRef] [PubMed]
3. Heher, P.; Muhleder, S.; Mittermayr, R.; Redl, H.; Slezak, P. Fibrin-based delivery strategies for acute and chronic wound healing. *Adv. Drug Deliv. Rev.* **2018**, *129*, 134–147. [CrossRef] [PubMed]
4. Han, G.; Ceilley, R. Chronic wound healing: A review of current management and treatments. *Adv. Ther.* **2017**, *34*, 599–610. [CrossRef] [PubMed]
5. Dickinson, L.E.; Gerecht, S. Engineered biopolymeric scaffolds for chronic wound healing. *Front. Physiol.* **2016**, *7*, 341. [CrossRef] [PubMed]
6. Frykberg, R.G.; Banks, J. Challenges in the treatment of chronic wounds. *Adv. Wound Care* **2015**, *4*, 560–582. [CrossRef] [PubMed]
7. Gordon, P.; Okai, B.; Hoare, J.I.; Erwig, L.P.; Wilson, H.M. SOCS3 is a modulator of human macrophage phagocytosis. *J. Leukoc. Biol.* **2016**, *100*, 771–780. [CrossRef]
8. Landen, N.X.; Li, D.; Stahle, M. Transition from inflammation to proliferation: A critical step during wound healing. *Cell Mol. Life Sci.* **2016**, *73*, 3861–3885. [CrossRef]
9. Mosser, D.M.; Edwards, J.P. Exploring the full spectrum of macrophage activation. *Nat. Rev. Immunol.* **2008**, *8*, 958–969. [CrossRef]
10. Zhu, Z.; Ding, J.; Ma, Z.; Iwashina, T.; Tredget, E.E. Systemic depletion of macrophages in the subacute phase of wound healing reduces hypertrophic scar formation. *Wound Repair Regen.* **2016**, *24*, 644–656. [CrossRef]
11. Krzyszczyk, P.; Schloss, R.; Palmer, A.; Berthiaume, F. The role of macrophages in acute and chronic wound healing and interventions to promote pro-wound healing phenotypes. *Front. Physiol.* **2018**, *9*, 419. [CrossRef] [PubMed]
12. Ogle, M.E.; Segar, C.E.; Sridhar, S.; Botchwey, E.A. Monocytes and macrophages in tissue repair: Implications for immunoregenerative biomaterial design. *Exp. Biol. Med. (Maywood)* **2016**, *241*, 1084–1097. [CrossRef] [PubMed]
13. Brodbeck, W.G.; Nakayama, Y.; Matsuda, T.; Colton, E.; Ziats, N.P.; Anderson, J.M. Biomaterial surface chemistry dictates adherent monocyte/macrophage cytokine expression in vitro. *Cytokine* **2002**, *18*, 311–319. [CrossRef] [PubMed]
14. Govrin, J.; Leonid, K.; Luger, E.; Tamir, J.; Zeilig, G.; Shafir, R. New method for treating hard-to-heal wounds: Clinical experience with charged polystyrene microspheres. *Wounds UK* **2010**, *6*, 52–61.
15. Lazaro-Martinez, J.L.; Garcia-Alvarez, Y.; Alvaro-Alfonso, F.J.; Garcia-Morales, E.; Sanz-Corbalan, I.; Molines-Barroso, R.J. Hard-to-heal diabetic foot ulcers treated using negatively charged polystyrene microspheres: A prospective case series. *J. Wound Care* **2019**, *28*, 104–109. [CrossRef]
16. Weissman, O.; Winkler, E.; Teot, L.; Remer, E.; Faber, N.; Bank, J.; Hundeshagen, G.; Zilinsky, I.; Haik, J. Treatment of wounds following breast reduction and mastopexy with subsequent wound dehiscence with charged polystyrene microspheres. *Wounds* **2014**, *26*, 37–42.
17. Mobed-Miremadi, M.; Grandio, D.; Kunkel, J. Polystyrene-based wound healing systems. In *Wound Healing Biomaterials*; Ågren, M.S., Ed.; Woodhead Publishing: Cambridge, UK, 2016; pp. 309–334.
18. Shoham, Y.; Kogan, L.; Weiss, J.; Tamir, E.; Krieger, Y.; Barnea, Y.; Regev, E.; Vigoda, D.; Haikin, N.; Inbal, A.; et al. Wound 'dechronification' with negatively-charged polystyrene microspheres: A double-blind RCT. *J. Wound Care* **2013**, *22*, 144–155. [CrossRef]
19. Feng, Y.; Borrelli, M.; Meyer-Ter-Vehn, T.; Reichl, S.; Schrader, S.; Geerling, G. Epithelial wound healing on keratin film, amniotic membrane and polystyrene in vitro. *Curr. Eye Res.* **2014**, *39*, 561–570. [CrossRef]
20. Drukala, J.; Bandura, L.; Cieslik, K.; Korohoda, W. Locomotion of human skin keratinocytes on polystyrene, fibrin, and collagen substrata and its modification by cell-to-cell contacts. *Cell Transplant.* **2001**, *10*, 765–771. [CrossRef]

21. Sands, R.W.; Mooney, D.J. Polymers to direct cell fate by controlling the microenvironment. *Curr. Opin. Biotechnol.* **2007**, *18*, 448–453. [CrossRef]
22. Khan, S.; Ul-Islam, M.; Ikram, M.; Islam, S.U.; Ullah, M.W.; Israr, M.; Jang, J.H.; Yoon, S.; Park, J.K. Preparation and structural characterization of surface modified microporous bacterial cellulose scaffolds: A potential material for skin regeneration applications in vitro and in vivo. *Int. J. Biol. Macromol.* **2018**, *117*, 1200–1210. [CrossRef] [PubMed]
23. Wang, Y.; Chen, Z.; Luo, G.; He, W.; Xu, K.; Xu, R.; Lei, Q.; Tan, J.; Wu, J.; Xing, M. In-situ-generated vasoactive intestinal peptide loaded microspheres in mussel-inspired polycaprolactone nanosheets creating spatiotemporal releasing microenvironment to promote wound healing and angiogenesis. *ACS Appl. Mater. Interfaces* **2016**, *8*, 7411–7421. [CrossRef] [PubMed]
24. Cereceres, S.; Touchet, T.; Browning, M.B.; Smith, C.; Rivera, J.; Höök, M.; Whitfield-Cargile, C.; Russell, B.; Cosgriff-Hernandez, E. Chronic wound dressings based on collagen-mimetic proteins. *Adv. Wound Care (New Rochelle)* **2015**, *4*, 444–456. [CrossRef] [PubMed]
25. Garcia-Orue, I.; Gainza, G.; Gutierrez, F.B.; Aguirre, J.J.; Evora, C.; Pedraz, J.L.; Hernandez, R.M.; Delgado, A.; Igartua, M. Novel nanofibrous dressings containing rhEGF and Aloe vera for wound healing applications. *Int. J. Pharm.* **2017**, *523*, 556–566. [CrossRef] [PubMed]
26. Garate, A.; Santos, E.; Pedraz, J.L.; Hernandez, R.M.; Orive, G. Evaluation of different RGD ligand densities in the development of cell-based drug delivery systems. *J. Drug Target.* **2015**, *23*, 808–812. [CrossRef]
27. Neff, J.A.; Tresco, P.A.; Cadwell, K.D. Surface modification for controlled studies of cell-ligand interactions. *Biomaterials* **1999**, *20*, 2377–2393. [CrossRef]
28. Santos, E.; Garate, A.; Pedraz, J.L.; Orive, G.; Hernandez, R.M. The synergistic effects of the RGD density and the microenvironment on the behavior of encapsulated cells: In vitro and in vivo direct comparative study. *J. Biomed. Mater. Res.* **2014**, *102*, 3965–3972. [CrossRef]
29. Comisar, W.A.; Kazmers, N.H.; Mooney, D.J.; Linderman, J.J. Engineering RGD nanopatterned hydrogels to control preosteoblast behavior: A combined computational and experimental approach. *Biomaterials* **2007**, *28*, 4409–4417. [CrossRef]
30. Ghadi, R.; Jain, A.; Khan, W.; Domb, A.J. Microparticulate polymers and hydrogels for wound healing. In *Wound Healing Biomaterials*; Ågren, M.S., Ed.; Woodhead Publishing: Cambridge, UK, 2016; pp. 203–225.
31. Khatua, D.; Kwak, B.; Shin, K.; Song, J.M.; Kim, J.S.; Choi, J.H. Influence of charge densities of randomly sulfonated polystyrene surfaces on cell attachment and proliferation. *J. Nanosci. Nanotechnol.* **2011**, *11*, 4227–4230. [CrossRef]
32. Carré, A.; Lacarrière, V. How substrate properties control cell adhesion. A physical–chemical approach. *J. Adhes. Sci. Technol.* **2010**, *24*, 815–830. [CrossRef]
33. Gonzalez-Pujana, A.; Santos-Vizcaino, E.; Garcia-Hernando, M.; Hernaez-Estrada, B.; de Pancorbo, M.M.; Benito-Lopez, F.; Igartua, M.; Basabe-Desmonts, L.; Hernandez, R.M. Extracellular matrix protein microarray-based biosensor with single cell resolution: Integrin profiling and characterization of cell-biomaterial interactions. *Sens. Actuators B Chem.* **2019**, *299*, 126954–126965. [CrossRef]
34. Aiyelabegan, H.T.; Sadroddiny, E. Fundamentals of protein and cell interactions in biomaterials. *Biomed. Pharmacother.* **2017**, *88*, 956–970. [CrossRef] [PubMed]
35. Hoshiba, T.; Yoshikawa, C.; Sakakibara, K. Characterization of initial cell adhesion on charged polymer substrates in serum-containing and serum-free media. *Langmuir* **2018**, *34*, 4043–4051. [CrossRef] [PubMed]
36. Chellat, F.; Merhi, Y.; Moreau, A.; Yahia, L. Therapeutic potential of nanoparticulate systems for macrophage targeting. *Biomaterials* **2005**, *26*, 7260–7275. [CrossRef] [PubMed]
37. Glim, J.E.; Niessen, F.B.; Everts, V.; van Egmond, M.; Beelen, R.H. Platelet derived growth factor-CC secreted by M2 macrophages induces alpha-smooth muscle actin expression by dermal and gingival fibroblasts. *Immunobiology* **2013**, *218*, 924–929. [CrossRef]
38. Prechtel, A.T.; Steinkasserer, A. CD83: An update on functions and prospects of the maturation marker of dendritic cells. *Arch. Dermatol. Res.* **2007**, *299*, 59–69. [CrossRef]
39. Guest, J.F.; Sladkevicius, E.; Panca, M. Cost-effectiveness of using Polyheal compared with surgery in the management of chronic wounds with exposed bones and/or tendons due to trauma in France, Germany and the UK. *Int. Wound J.* **2015**, *12*, 70–82. [CrossRef]
40. Ngobili, T.A.; Daniele, M.A. Nanoparticles and direct immunosuppression. *Exp. Biol. Med.* **2016**, *241*, 1064–1073. [CrossRef]

41. Gan, J.; Liu, C.; Li, H.; Wang, S.; Wang, Z.; Kang, Z.; Huang, Z.; Zhang, J.; Wang, C.; Lv, D.; et al. Accelerated wound healing in diabetes by reprogramming the macrophages with particle-induced clustering of the mannose receptors. *Biomaterials* **2019**, *219*. [CrossRef]
42. Nosenko, M.A.; Moysenovich, A.M.; Zvartsev, R.V.; Arkhipova, A.Y.; Zhdanova, A.S.; Agapov, I.I.; Vasilieva, T.V.; Bogush, V.G.; Debabov, V.G.; Nedospasov, S.A.; et al. Novel biodegradable polymeric microparticles facilitate scarless wound healing by promoting re-epithelialization and inhibiting fibrosis. *Front. Immunol.* **2018**, *9*. [CrossRef]
43. Kotwal, G.J.; Chien, S. Macrophage differentiation in normal and accelerated wound Healing. *Results Probl. Cell Differ.* **2017**, *62*, 353–364. [CrossRef] [PubMed]
44. Mihai, M.M.; Dima, M.B.; Dima, B.; Holban, A.M. Nanomaterials for wound healing and infection control. *Materials* **2019**, *12*, 2176. [CrossRef] [PubMed]
45. Fong, D.; Ariganello, M.B.; Girard-Lauziere, J.; Hoemann, C.D. Biodegradable chitosan microparticles induce delayed STAT-1 activation and lead to distinct cytokine responses in differentially polarized human macrophages in vitro. *Acta Biomater.* **2015**, *12*, 183–194. [CrossRef] [PubMed]
46. Hoppstädter, J.; Seif, M.; Dembek, A.; Cavelius, C.; Huwer, H.; Kraegeloh, A.; Kiemer, A.K. M2 polarization enhances silica nanoparticle uptake by macrophages. *Front. Pharmacol.* **2015**, *6*, 55. [CrossRef] [PubMed]

nanomaterials

MDPI

Review

Zebrafish Models for the Safety and Therapeutic Testing of Nanoparticles with a Focus on Macrophages

Alba Pensado-López [1,2], Juan Fernández-Rey [1,2], Pedro Reimunde [3,4], José Crecente-Campo [2], Laura Sánchez [1,*,†] and Fernando Torres Andón [2,*,†]

1 Department of Zoology, Genetics and Physical Anthropology, Campus de Lugo, Universidade de Santiago de Compostela, 27002 Lugo, Spain; alba.pensado.lopez@rai.usc.es (A.P.-L.); juanmanuel.fernandez.rey@rai.usc.es (J.F.-R.)
2 Center for Research in Molecular Medicine & Chronic Diseases (CIMUS), Campus Vida, Universidade de Santiago de Compostela, 15706 Santiago de Compostela, Spain; jose.crecente@usc.es
3 Department of Physiotherapy, Medicine and Biomedical Sciences, Universidade da Coruña, Campus de Oza, 15006 A Coruña, Spain; pedro.reimunde@udc.es
4 Department of Neurosurgery, Hospital Universitario Lucus Augusti, 27003 Lugo, Spain
* Correspondence: lauraelena.sanchez@usc.es (L.S.); fernando.torres.andon@usc.es (F.T.A.)
† These authors have contributed equally to this work.

Abstract: New nanoparticles and biomaterials are increasingly being used in biomedical research for drug delivery, diagnostic applications, or vaccines, and they are also present in numerous commercial products, in the environment and workplaces. Thus, the evaluation of the safety and possible therapeutic application of these nanomaterials has become of foremost importance for the proper progress of nanotechnology. Due to economical and ethical issues, in vitro and in vivo methods are encouraged for the testing of new compounds and/or nanoparticles, however in vivo models are still needed. In this scenario, zebrafish (*Danio rerio*) has demonstrated potential for toxicological and pharmacological screenings. Zebrafish presents an innate immune system, from early developmental stages, with conserved macrophage phenotypes and functions with respect to humans. This fact, combined with the transparency of zebrafish, the availability of models with fluorescently labelled macrophages, as well as a broad variety of disease models offers great possibilities for the testing of new nanoparticles. Thus, with a particular focus on macrophage–nanoparticle interaction in vivo, here, we review the studies using zebrafish for toxicological and biodistribution testing of nanoparticles, and also the possibilities for their preclinical evaluation in various diseases, including cancer and autoimmune, neuroinflammatory, and infectious diseases.

Keywords: zebrafish; nanomaterial; nanoparticle; drug delivery; macrophage; immune system; innate immunity

Citation: Pensado-López, A.; Fernández-Rey, J.; Reimunde, P.; Crecente-Campo, J.; Sánchez, L.; Torres Andón, F. Zebrafish Models for the Safety and Therapeutic Testing of Nanoparticles with a Focus on Macrophages. *Nanomaterials* **2021**, *11*, 1784. https://doi.org/10.3390/nano11071784

Academic Editor: Robyn L. Tanguay

Received: 11 June 2021
Accepted: 7 July 2021
Published: 9 July 2021

1. Introduction

Recent advances in nanotechnology offer the possibility to engineer a wide variety of new nanoparticles and biomaterials with potential application in medicine, but also with commercial interest, providing solutions for numerous sectors in society (i.e., electricity, cosmetics, food packaging, etc.) [1,2]. There is considerable evidence that nano- and microscale materials have unique biological interactions when compared with molecules or bulk materials [3]. Thus, safety assessment results are, of course, of paramount importance [4]. In the case of medical applications, nanomaterials are designed for drug delivery, imaging, diagnosis, sensing, and/or therapeutic purposes. Thus, the benefit/risk for the use of nanotechnologies in this case acquires a different dimension similar to the pharmacological/toxicological profile of other drugs [5]. For these studies, in silico and in vitro methods, including cell- and organ-based assays, are encouraged. However, animal tests are still needed [4,6].

In this context, the zebrafish (*Danio rerio*) has become a well-established model for the toxicological and pharmacological screening of new drugs [7] and nanomaterials [8]. Rapid embryo development, small size and transparency, genetic and physiological conservation, ethical and economic advantages have made zebrafish stand out from all other in vivo models [9]. Furthermore, the innate branch of the immune system, including macrophage functions, is well-conserved between humans and the zebrafish, presenting a powerful model for the study of immunotoxicity and also diseases causing and/or caused by inflammatory disorders (i.e., cancer, autoimmune diseases or infectious diseases) [10,11]. Several zebrafish models with fluorescently labeled macrophages have been developed and optimized for studies with a particular focus on the role of macrophages in the toxicological or therapeutic effects of new compounds and nanomaterials. Thus, it is our purpose in this review to collect the information available related to the safety and biomedical testing of new nanomaterials using zebrafish models, with a particular focus on their interaction with macrophages, starting with toxicological and/or biodistribution experimentation, followed by preclinical testing of nanoparticles for therapeutic purposes.

2. Zebrafish Innate Immune System: Role of Macrophages

The zebrafish immune system is able to develop both innate and adaptive responses. Despite differences in anatomical sites and time points with respect to mammals. Key cell types, molecular pathways, genetic programs, and transcription factors are highly conserved [12]. Whereas the innate immune system components are already present in early zebrafish embryo stages, the development of adaptive responses does not occur until 2–4 weeks post-fertilization (wpf), and complete immunocompetence is not achieved until 4–6 wpf [13]. Zebrafish innate immune system is composed of similar types of cells than mammals, being macrophages the first leukocytes in development and key players in directing the host immune response [14]. The origin of primitive macrophages in zebrafish occurs at 14–15 h post-fertilization (hpf). These cells migrate to the yolk sac, differentiate, and enter the circulation from 25 hpf [15,16]. The caudal hematopoietic tissue (CHT) at two days post-fertilization (dpf), equivalent to fetal liver or placenta in mammals, acts as a transient hematopoietic site and is a source of embryonic macrophages and neutrophils [17,18]. The thymus produces mature T-cells and the kidney, functional ortholog of mammalian bone marrow, produces myeloid, erythroid, thromboid, and lymphoid cells throughout adulthood [19,20].

Macrophages are phagocytic cells from the innate immune system which can display a wide variety of functions due to their plasticity, versatility and continuous adaptation and response to specific stimuli [21]. In mammals, macrophages have been classically classified according to their polarization extremes observed in the initiation or in the resolution of inflammatory processes [22]. And these cells have been respectively denominated as M1, classically activated or pro-inflammatory macrophages, versus the M2, alternatively activated or wound-healing macrophages [23,24] (Figure 1). These populations have been characterized in terms of gene expression, the pattern of surface molecules, and the production of biological mediators and metabolites [25,26]. An imbalance between M1 and M2 macrophages has been found in pathological tissues and correlated with a worse prognosis of the disease (i.e., high numbers of M1-like macrophages in arthritis or infiltration of M2-like macrophages in solid tumors) [21,27]. Furthermore, taking into account this knowledge, the reprogramming of M1-like macrophages towards M2-like anti-inflammatory effectors appears to be a reasonable strategy for the treatment of some autoimmune diseases [23], while the stimulation of M2-like immunosuppressive macrophages towards M1-like pro-inflammatory-anti-tumor effector cells is a promising approach for the treatment of cancer [21,25,28–31].

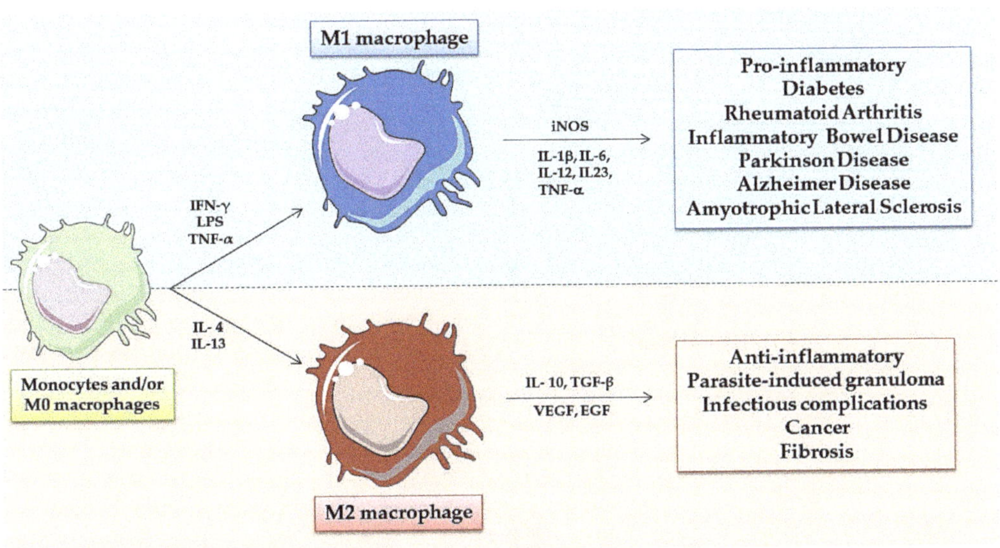

Figure 1. Macrophages originate from monocytes or tissue-resident macrophages. In response to different microenvironmental stimuli macrophages polarize towards an M1-like or M2-like phenotype, and the excessive accumulation of macrophages with a particular phenotype has been correlated with a poor prognosis in some diseases (on the right). In pathological tissues, these macrophages frequently contribute to the development and progression of the disease, thus their reprogramming towards an opposite polarization status has been recognized as an important therapeutic strategy.

In 2015, Nguyen-Chi et al. provided a seminal report on the polarization of macrophages in zebrafish, showing a great similarity of the M1-like and M2-like phenotypes with respect to mammals [32]. They used the Tg(*mpeg1*:mCherryF) transgenic zebrafish line, which enables to track macrophages [33,34], and generated the Tg (*tnfa*:eGFP-F) line to label M1-macrophages expressing tumor necrosis factor-α (TNF-α). Following fin wounding-induced inflammation or *Escherichia coli* inoculation in zebrafish larvae, they observed a recruitment of macrophages to the wound after amputation or to the muscle after bacteria-inoculation. To characterize the M1/M2 polarization, they mated both lines to generate the Tg(*tnfa*:eGFP-F/*mpeg1*:mCherryF), sorted mCherry+/eGFP+ and mCherry+ cells during the early and late phases of inflammation, and compared their RNA expression patterns, observing high levels of *tnfb*, *il1b* and *il6* pro-inflammatory markers of M1-like macrophages in double-labeled cells, while high levels of *tgfb1*, *ccr2* and *cxcr4b* anti-inflammatory markers were found in the M2-like macrophages only labeled with mCherry [24,32]. Similar results were obtained by Sanderson et al. using the Tg(*irg1*:EGFP)/Tg(*mpeg1*:mCherry) transgenic line, in which irg1 specifically labeled M1-like macrophages upon LPS inoculation or M2-like macrophages upon injection of human metastatic breast cancer cells [35]. Other zebrafish-macrophage-fluorescent reporter lines, such as Tg(*mpeg1*:eGFP)^{gl22} [33] or Tg(*mpeg1*:mCherry)^{UMSF001} [36], have enabled to track the precise behavior and physiology of these cells in vivo, during inflammatory, cancer or infectious processes, thus providing a highly valuable tool to study their role in the context of these pathologies, and also for the screening of new macrophage-targeted therapeutic approaches, including nanoparticles.

3. Toxicological and Biodistribution Evaluation of Nanoparticles Using Zebrafish: Focus on Macrophages

3.1. Toxicological Studies

The zebrafish is commonly used as an in vivo model for the toxicological evaluation of new compounds and nanomaterials, due to its reduced cost, ease of husbandry, and high fecundity rates [37,38]. Zebrafish and mammals present concordance in toxicological assays ranging from 64% to 100% [39]. Due to its short-life cycle, zebrafish can be used to evaluate intergenerational toxicity by exposing a generation (F0) to a compound and studying the effects on the next generations (F1, F2, etc.) [40,41]. Reproductive impairment can also be studied by assessing sperm motility, egg depositions, and steroid hormone levels [42,43].

The usual methods of exposure to new compounds or nanomaterials are microinjection and immersion [44,45]. A widely used harmonized approach is the OECD Fish Embryo Acute Toxicity (FET) Test [46]. The OECD guidelines present immersion exposure as the preferred method and propose that tests should be performed within the first 120 hpf (5 dpf) limit [47,48]. Nishimura et al. reviewed the methodology used in several zebrafish-based developmental toxicity tests and indicated that 5 hpf is the preferred time to start the exposure to a new sample, because at this point embryos are in the late blastula stage and dechorionation can be safely performed [49]. Variations of the FET test have served other researchers to develop assays destined to screen large libraries of compounds or to evaluate organ-specific drug toxicities. For example, Cornet et al. took advantage of the brief zebrafish development to combine in one test the study of cardio-, neuro-, and hepato-toxicity effects in the same individual, enabling recompilation of organ-specific toxicity data for 24 compounds [50]. In a different study, 91 compounds, including pesticides, drugs, and flame retardants, were screened for teratological and behavioral effects, by immersing dechorionated zebrafish embryos in solutions of the different chemicals [51]. In combination with in silico and in vitro assays, zebrafish models were used for the screening of compounds with anti-inflammatory activity from a library of more than 1200 chemicals [52].

Nanotoxicological studies are commonly divided into two fields: environmental health and nanomedicine safety [8]. In both fields, similar types of in vitro and in vivo assays are performed, which in the case of zebrafish models take into account endpoints such as death, hatching rate, developmental malformations, behavioral changes and gene-profiling to assess toxicity [8,53,54]. The main factors influencing nanotoxicological effects, such as composition, particle size, particle shape and surface charge [54], have been investigated in zebrafish [55–57]. Zeng et al. studied the effects of Ag nanoparticles (NPs) on zebrafish and found a decreased activity of enzymes implicated in oxidative stress, such as superoxide dismutase, hydrogen peroxide, and malondiadehyde [55]. Another study evaluated how the size of AgNPs could affect toxicity, revealing a higher sensitivity of zebrafish to 20 nm AgNPs versus 100 nm AgNPs [56]. To assess the effects of shape, Abramenko et al. followed OECD guidelines and observed that Ag nanoplates induce higher toxicity than spherical AgNPs [57]. The toxicity of AgNPs on neural development was also evaluated through the study of *gfap* and *ngn1* genetic profiling [58]. The safety of other inorganic based NPs (Au, Mg, Si, Zn) has been studied in zebrafish following similar methodologies [59–63]. Synergistic toxicity of methylmercury, SiNPs and AuNPs including surfactants have also been evaluated in zebrafish, proving it as a useful model to explore the toxicological effects of different compounds in the same organism [64,65]. A more comprehensive toxicological methodology, using zebrafish, and focused on 21 endpoints, was used for the screening of several NPs, leading to the conclusion that surface charge is a major determinant for NP-toxicity [66].

Numerous organic-based nanomaterials have been also tested in zebrafish [67–70]. The toxicity of polyamidoamine and polypropylenimin dendrimers was tested in zebrafish following the FET method, and with a parallel test in dechorionated embryos, showing for both dendrimers a lower toxicity in chorionated embryos [67]. In a different study, nanographene oxide with an external layer of polyethilenglycol was microinjected in zebrafish to evaluate its toxicity profile and effect on angiogenesis [68]. In another study, Teijeiro-Valiño et al. examined the toxicity of polymeric nanocapsules with an outer shell of hyaluronic acid and protamine [69].

The interaction of NPs with macrophages was investigated using zebrafish models, having important implications in the biocompatibility-toxicity, as well as in the biodistribution of the NPs (reviewed in the next section) [70–74]. On one hand, NPs may trigger direct cell toxicity through different molecular mechanisms [75], on the other hand numerous NPs can also trigger inflammatory responses when they are recognized as foreign agents by immune cells (i.e., macrophages) [5]. In response to NPs, the immune cells commonly produce soluble mediators, such as cytokines, chemokines, and complement factors, which result in the recruitment of more cells and development of acute or chronic inflammatory responses [76]. We should also remember that, in some cases, the inflammatory cells are capable of the biodegradation of NPs, e.g., through oxidative stress or enzymatic degradation (i.e., myeloperoxidase or eosinophil peroxidase) [77]. The balance of these responses is of foremost importance for immunotoxicological studies. As an example, graphene oxide immunotoxicity was evaluated by measuring glutathione, malondialdehyde, superoxide dismutase, catalase, and genetic profiling in adult zebrafish. TNF-α, IL-1β and IL-6 expression levels were significantly increased in a dose-dependent manner [74]. Similarly, it has been reported that several types of metallic NPs, such as gold NPs (AuNPs), silver NPs (AgNPs), or zinc oxide NPS (ZnO-NPs), may induce oxidative stress and disrupt signaling pathways related to innate immune responses [78–80]. Other studies involving drugs, nanocarriers, and macrophages practiced their experiments on zebrafish [81,82]. For example, poly(lactic-co-glycolic acid) NPs (PLGA-NPs) loaded with thioridazine were evaluated for toxicity and their therapeutic efficacy was tested in murine macrophages, human macrophages and zebrafish models [81]. These immunotoxicological studies, using zebrafish as in vivo model, demonstrate the relevance of safety assessment for nanomaterials with potential application in a variety of industrial sectors (i.e., cosmetics, paints, food package, etc.), and they also provide pharmacological/toxicological information of interest for their application with medical purposes.

3.2. Biodistribution

Nanotechnology is commonly used to improve the biodistribution/pharmacokinetics of drugs. Thus, biodistribution moves from being determined by the drug's physicochemical characteristics to be dictated by the NP's-features. Besides, by tuning the physicochemical properties of the NPs, a preferential accumulation in specific organs and/or cell populations can be achieved [83]. Taking this into consideration, zebrafish is gaining importance in the nanomedicine field as a simple and reliable model to screen biodistribution of drugs and/or NPs. The transparency of the embryos [84] and the availability of transgenic lines offer the possibility to study in biodistribution studies the role of the interaction of NPs at the cellular level, for example, by using macrophage-labelled embryos [85]. In this context, different scenarios can happen depending on the aimed cellular and/or molecular target: macrophages can be the final target for the nanomedicine, such as in the case of autoimmune or infectious diseases, and nano-vaccines [86], or they can be a cellular population to be avoided, due to the undesirable clearance of the therapeutic entity mediated by these phagocytic cells, such as in the case of drugs targeted towards cancer cells or others [72]. Of note, in the context of cancer both approaches, targeting and/or avoiding macrophages, could be intended to improve the efficacy of certain drugs, directed towards macrophages (i.e., immunotherapy) or to cancer cells (i.e., chemotherapy), respectively [87].

The overall biodistribution of a NP is governed by the combined effect of the administration route, the dose and the nanostructure's composition and properties (Figure 2). As previously described for the toxicity, the size, shape, charge and flexibility are also critical parameters that determine the final fate of the NPs [83,88]. The circulation time of NPs administered intravenously (i.v.) depends, mainly, on their interaction with immune and/or endothelial cells [89]. In fact, the majority of the NPs i.v. administered are cleared in the liver, by macrophages or by sinusoidal cells [85,90]. Part of these NPs are also captured by circulating monocytes/macrophages, and/or other immune cells, such as neutrophils, before reaching their target tissue, as it was recently shown for gelatine nanospheres [86] and liposomes [91]. In zebrafish, liposomes of 60 nm showed a decreased macrophage uptake as compared to larger 120 nm liposomes, which were more accumulated in the spleen [91]. Apart from immune cells, uptake by endothelial cells can also be responsible for the limited circulation time of certain NPs. For example, polystyrene (PS) NPs of 1000 nm were found adhered to the endothelium some minutes after the injection. On the contrary, with a lower adherence to the endothelium, 200 nm PS NPs showed a more prolonged circulation time. Our group evaluated the diffusion of NCs of different sizes and surface charges in zebrafish embryos [70]. These NPs are versatile nanosystems with applications in different fields, such as cancer, vaccination, and ocular diseases [92–95]. Both positively and negatively charged NCs of 70 nm spread faster and at a higher extent than medium size NCs (200 nm) after i.v. injection in zebrafish. Chitosan NCs (positively charged) were found to be attached to the endothelial cells of the blood vessels at a higher degree than inulin NCs (negatively charged). As a whole, zebrafish injected with the 70 nm chitosan NCs showed the highest intensity, due to the fluorescent-NCs, in the circulatory system, and also higher accumulation in other tissues, such as the brain and visceral organs. All NCs showed certain degree of co-localization with GFP-labelled macrophages. However, the positively charged NCs showed the highest accumulation in these cells. In relation to their particle size, 200 nm NCs interacted with macrophages from early time points (0.5 h), whereas 70 nm NCs presented less interaction at 0.5 h, but their accumulation in these cells increased with time. From this and other studies, it can be concluded that larger particles are commonly attached or captured by macrophages and/or endothelial cells, thus showing shorter circulation times.

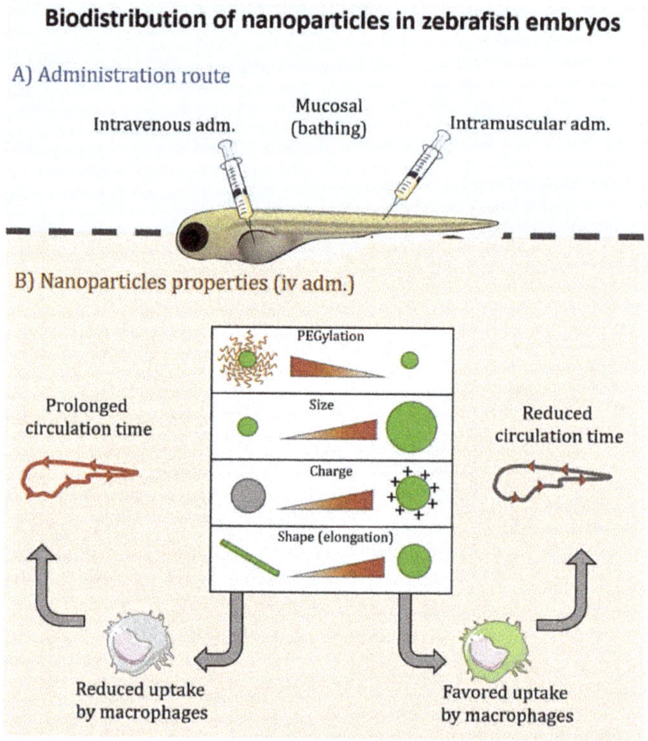

Figure 2. Biodistribution of nanoparticles in zebrafish is related to their interaction with macrophages. The biodistribution of nanoparticles in zebrafish embryos is mainly dictated by (**A**) the administration route and (**B**) the physicochemical properties of the nanoparticles. Among the characteristics that most impact the circulation time after intravenous administration are the degree of PEGylation, the particle size, the surface charge and the shape of the particles. By tuning these properties, the uptake by macrophages can be minimized and the circulation time can be prolonged.

Particle shape and flexibility have also an impact on NPs biodistribution. Generally elongated and rod-shaped NPs present a prolonged time in circulation compared with spherical particles, especially if they are flexible [96]. This effect was observed in different animal models (i.e., mice or pigs) [97], and also zebrafish [98]. In this case, the non-spherical NPs were poorly taken up by macrophages because of hydrodynamic shearing. However, other authors found that spherical NPs present prolonged circulation time versus NPs with fibrillar morphologies upon i.v. administration in zebrafish [99]. Overall, it is important to highlight that the final biodistribution and toxicological behaviour of a NP is orchestrated by the interplay between its different physicochemical properties (i.e., size, charge, and shape), and focusing only in one parameter can be misleading.

The composition of the NP's surface and/or its functionalization with specific molecules is also a key factor affecting its biodistribution. For instance, liposomes presented substantially higher circulation time after i.v. administration in zebrafish than PS NPs of similar size (nm) [72]. The different circulation patterns can be explained by the high affinity of PS NPs for the endothelium, while liposomes showed a slow macrophage-mediated clearance. With respect to decoration of NPs surface, polyethylene glycol (PEG) and other molecules have been used to avoid macrophage interaction, while ligands for specific receptors on macrophages-surface or other cells have been investigated. Functionalization with PEG chains is commonly implemented to "mask" a therapeutic agent from the immune system, reducing immunogenicity and antigenicity. PEGylated nanosystems show longer circulation times after i.v. administration than non-PEGylated ones, by reducing their interaction with opsonins and making NPs "invisible" to the immune system [72,89]. As an example, liposomes commonly cleared from the circulation by macrophages, when PEGylated, increased their circulation time, and their elimination by macrophages, although still occurring, is delayed [89]. In the case of PEGylated PS NPs, the increase in their circulation time has been attributed not only to their reduced capture by macrophages, but also to their reduced interaction with the endothelial cells [72]. The degree of PEGylation and its molecular weight also impacts on NPs biodistribution, showing decreased clearance by macrophages for liposomes decorated with a higher density of PEGs or increased molecular weight [91]. Other polymers with "shielding behaviour" have been used, such as polysarcosine or poly(N,N-dimethylacrylamide), showing an increase in NP-circulation time in zebrafish models [89].

Zebrafish models have also been used to study NP-biodistribution through other routes of administration. Upon intramuscular (i.m.) injection in zebrafish, NPs generally only spread along the muscle tissue close to the injection site, at least for short times [86]. As time goes by, the NPs are commonly internalized by macrophages to be cleared [86]. In our previously mentioned work, after i.m. injection, the 70 nm NCs disseminated further than 200 nm NCs, spreading through all the myomere and limited by myosepta [70]. Positively charged NCs (chitosan based) recruited more macrophages than negatively charged (inulin based) NCs, following a similar pattern to the i.v. route. To study the mucosal administration of new therapies using zebrafish, NPs can be simply incubated in water. Verrier and colleagues found that 200 nm PLA-NPs were able to cross the epithelial barrier of different mucosae (nasal, gills, gut, and skin) and be accumulated in antigen presenting cells, such as dendritic cells, macrophages and B cells in the gills and skin [100]. Interestingly, the NPs were able to enter the bloodstream through the gills, and to then reach internal organs, such as the liver and kidney. Our group showed the importance of surface composition in the ability of NCs to diffuse through the chorion before the zebrafish hatching [69]. The presence of a PEGylated surfactant is supposed to favour the diffusion of these NCs through the thick chorion barrier. Using hatched embryos, we demonstrated that hyaluronic acid NCs are not able to cross the epidermis. However, protamine-hyaluronic acid NCs were internalized and reached the yolk sac, the stomach, the esophagus and the olfactory pit. In this case, protamine, a well-known cell penetrating peptide, could be important to facilitate the internalization and transport through the zebrafish skin epithelium [69]. The particle size also influences de biodistribution by the mucosal routes.

For instance, after incubation with zebrafish in water, coumarin nanocrystals of 70 nm showed better permeability across the chorion, blood brain barrier, blood retinal barrier and gastrointestinal barrier than their counterparts of 200 nm. Besides, the smaller nanocrystals accumulated at a higher extent in internal organs via lipid raft-mediated endocytosis [101]. The importance of the particle shape was demonstrated by Vijver and his group [102]. After waterborne exposure of zebrafish embryos to gold NPs of different shapes, the macrophage's abundance was higher for urchin-shaped NPs compared to the spherical ones.

4. Preclinical Testing of Nanoparticles Using Zebrafish Models of Disease: Relevance of Macrophages

4.1. Cancer

Due to its unique features, zebrafish tumor models, mainly induced by transgenesis or xenotransplantation, are increasingly being used for cancer research and discovery of new antitumoral drugs [103]. Xenografts are routinely performed by implantation of human or murine cancer cells into different anatomical sites of zebrafish embryos (yolk sac, duct of Cuvier or perivitelline space) to obtain heterotopic or eventually orthotopic in vivo tumor models. The injection of labeled cancer cells in "transparent zebrafish" allows to track their survival, progression, migration, and interaction with the host microenvironment [104,105]. For the transgenic models, genetically modified zebrafish lines, mainly based on the expression of human oncogenes driven by tissue-specific or ubiquitous promoters (e.g., $BRAF^{V600E}$, $HRAS^{G12V}$ or $KRAS^{G12V}$) have been used [106–108]. While the transgenic models are commonly preferred for the mechanistic understanding of tumor development and/or interaction of cancer cells with the tumor microenvironment (TME), xenografts are more used for drug screenings. As the generation of stable transgenic zebrafish lines requires several months, it is technically challenging and less cost-effective when compared to the simple injection of tumor cells in xenografts [109]. In addition, xenograft models have been recently used to understand the metabolic and/or stem cell properties of cancer cells and they also offer the possibility to study patient-derived cancer cells in vivo [110,111].

The study of macrophages in tumors is nowadays a very active field of research. Tumors are complex tissues, comprising a heterogeneous population of cells plus the extracellular matrix they produce, which constitute the TME [112–115]. The cellular fraction is composed of malignant cancer cells, as well as endothelial cells, cancer-associated fibroblasts, and tumor-associated macrophages (TAMs), with the latter being the latest the most abundant cell type [116]. In human tumors, TAMs originate mostly from circulating precursor monocytes, but resident macrophages can be originally present in the tissue, later developing in a tumor [117]. TAM infiltration in tumor tissues has been shown to support tumor growth, angiogenesis, invasion and metastasis, and their high density in tumors has been correlated with tumor progression and resistance to therapies [118]. The secretion of CSF-1, CCL2 and VEGF, by cancer cells, induce the recruitment of macrophages towards the TME, and the Th2 cytokines IL-4, IL-13, IL-10 and TGF-β, metabolic signals (i.e., lactic acid and hypoxia) produced also by Treg and TAMs are key drivers of immunosuppression [116]. With the aim to better mimic human tumors, including the TME, zebrafish xenografts are being continuously improved, using reporter lines for analysis of vasculature [119], neutrophils [120] and/or macrophages [32,33,35]. Orthotopic xenotransplantation, consisting in the injection of tumor cells in the equivalent anatomical site, and the use of patient-derived xenografts (PDX), allows the preservation of tumor cells' original phenotype, and represents a further step to recapitulate the TME and tumor cell-host interactions [121]. The knowledge and practice acquired using these models will not only be useful for a better understanding of tumors, but also determinant for the development and evaluation of new antitumoral therapies [122], including nanotechnological strategies.

An enormous variety of nano-oncologicals (nanostructures for the treatment of cancer) have been developed and evaluated with the main purpose to improve the delivery of pharmacological molecules to the TME and reduce off-target effects [123–125]. NPs have been designed to improve the efficacy of classical chemotherapies, immunomodulatory drugs, but also delicate molecules such as nucleic acids, and even new cellular therapies [126,127]. Main therapeutic strategies to target and impact on TAMs include: (i) inhibition of TAM recruitment to the tumor, (ii) direct killing of TAMs, (iii) re-education of TAM from their M2-like protumoral phenotype into a M1-like antitumoral phenotype [87]; offering promising opportunities to switch the tumor-promoting immune suppressive microenvironment, characteristic of tumors rich in macrophages, to one that kills tumor cells, is anti-angiogenic and promotes adaptive immune responses [87,128].

In this context, zebrafish models offer the possibility to test the antitumoral effect of new nano-oncologicals, not only at the level of tumor growth in vivo [109], but also at the cellular level within the tumor (i.e., cancer cells or TAMs in vivo). Relevant examples of nano-oncologicals tested in zebrafish are reviewed below and summarized in Table 1.

Table 1. Evaluation of nanoparticle-based approaches for cancer treatment using xenograft zebrafish models.

Nanosystem	Drug	Mechanism	Tumor Type/ Cell Line	Zebrafish Stage	Injection Site	NPs Delivery	Remarkable Results	Reference
PtPP-HA	Kiteplatin pyrophosphate	Apoptosis through DNA platination	Breast cancer/ MDA-MB-231-GFP	48 hpf	Duct of Cuvier	Co-injection with cells	Decrease in breast cancer cells survival	[129]
Zinc oxide NPs	-	Apoptosis and ROS induction	Gingival squamous cell carcinoma/Ca9-22-DiL	48 hpf	Yolk sac	Immersion/48 hpf	Dose-dependent antitumoral activity	[130]
PMOsPOR-NH_2/ TPE-PDT	-	Porphyrin photosensitivity and ROS production	Breast Cancer/ MDA-MB-231-GFP	30 hpf	Duct of Cuvier	Pre-treatment of cancer cells	Complete extinction of cancer cells	[131]
PORBSNs/TPE-PDT	-	Porphyrin photosensitivity and ROS production	Breast cancer/ MDA-MB-231-GFP	24-30 hpf	Perivitelline space	Intravenously/4 dpi	Decrease of the tumor area	[132]
PAMAM-GC/ DOX/γ-radiation	DOX	GC radiosensitivity increases DOX release	Uterine cervical carcinoma/HeLa- CSFE	48 hpf	Yolk sac	Immersion/1 dpi	Synergistic antitumoral effect for the combination of GC/DOX and radiotherapy	[133]
PAMAM-DOX-siHIF	DOX/siHIF	NPs responsiveness to hypoxia and increased drug release	Breast cancer/ MCF-7-CM-DiL	48 hpf	Perivitelline space	Intracardiac injection/1 dpi	Feasibility of the cooperative strategy for in vivo applications	[134]
Nanogel^{DOX}	DOX	Hydrazone sensitivity to pH accelerate drug release	Melanoma/ B6-RFP or GPF	48 hpf	Neural tube	Intravenously/1 dpi	Selective accumulation of the NPs in the tumor and reduction in tumor growth	[135]
Tf-DOX-ReSi-Au	DOX	Enhanced tumor targeting by interaction between Tf and Tf receptor	Colorectal cancer/ HCT116-GFP	48 hpf	Yolk sac	Retro-orbital injection/1 dpi	Antitumoral activity without DOX-related cardiotoxic effects	[136]
PEG liposomes	-	-	Melanoma/Melmet 5-dsRed Kidney/HEK293-mCherry	48 hpf	Duct of Cuvier	Intravenously/2 dpi	NPs accumulation in human tumor structure, low macrophage uptake and high survival rate	[72]
PEG-PDPA-DOX	DOX	Polymersomes release the drug only at low pH	Melanoma/ B6-RFP or GPF	72 hpf	Neural tube	Intravenously/1 dpi	Selective accumulation of NPs in the tumor area, increased cancer cell apoptosis and reduced proliferation	[137]

dpi: days post-injection; DOX: doxorubicin; PAMAM-DOX-siHIF: G4.5 polyamidoamine dendrimers loaded with DOX and hypoxia-inducible factor 1a siRNA; PAMAM-GC/DOX: G4.5 polyamidoamine dendrimers with L-cysteine and loaded with DOX; PEG-PDPA-DOX: Poly(ethylene glycol)-block-poly(2-(diisopropyl amino) ethyl methacrylate) NPs loaded with DOX; PMOsPOR-NH2: porous porphyrin-based organosilica NPs; PORBSNs: non-porous porphyrin-based bridged silsesquioxane NPs; PtPP-HA: kiteplatin-pyrophosphate-loaded hydroxyapatite NPs; Tf-DOX-ReSi-Au: Redox-responsive silica-gold nanocomposites functionalized with transferrin and loaded with DOX; TPE-PDT: two-photon-excited photodynamic therapy.

Nadar and colleagues investigated the ability of drug-loaded hydroxyapatite NPs to release active therapeutics in vivo [129]. To this end, they used a zebrafish xenograft model with MDA-MB-231 breast cancer cells to test the antitumoral efficacy of kiteplatin-pyrophosphate-loaded hydroxyapatite NPs (PtPP-HA). Two days after the co-injection of cancer cells and the platinum-loaded HA NPs into 48 hpf zebrafish blood circulation, they found a significant decrease in survival of breast cancer cells [129]. Different types of metal oxide-NPs, not loaded with additional pharmacological molecules, have also been tested for antitumoral efficacy. ZnO-NPs were evaluated using a gingival squamous cell carcinoma xenograft model, showing antitumoral activity via induction of reactive oxygen species (ROS) and reduction of anti-oxidative enzymes with consequent oxidative damage to cells and tissues [130,138,139]. DiL-labeled Ca9-22 cells were implanted into the yolk sac of 48 hpf Tg(*fli1*:EGFP) embryos and fluorescence monitoring showed no effect on survival but dose-dependent inhibition of tumor growth [130]. The physicochemical properties of nanomaterials have also been exploited for photodynamic therapy (PDT) and tested in zebrafish. For instance, Jimenez et al. developed, and tested in zebrafish tumor xenografts, porous porphyrin-based organosilica NPs (PMOsPOR-NH2) [131]. At 2 dpi, treated-embryos were subjected to two-photon-excited photodynamic therapy (TPE-PDT) and a complete extinction of GFP-cancer cells was observed. Additionally, to analyze the efficiency of gene delivery, the same NPs were complexed with anti-GFP siRNA and co-injected together with GFP mRNA at one-cell stage, leading to a reduction in GFP expression a few hours later, thus also revealing the potential use of these NPs for gene therapy. Similarly, small-seized non-porous porphyrin-based bridged silsesquioxane NPs (PORBSNs) functionalized with PEG and mannose (20–30 nm) were developed for i.v. injection and tested in zebrafish with MDA-MB-231-GFP cells subjected to TPE-PDT, showing decreased tumor growth after irradiation [132]. Moreover, with targeting purposes, Peng et al. synthesized fluorescent cellulose acetate NPs functionalized with folate groups for their preferential accumulation in epithelial cancer cells overexpressing folic acid receptors [140]. These NPs can be tuned within the entire UV-VIS-NIR spectrum and were capable to target tumors in vivo. To test the combinatorial antitumoral efficacy of chemotherapy and radiotherapy using NPs, Wu et al. synthesized G4.5 polyamidoamine (PAMAM) dendrimers conjugated with L-cysteine (GC), acting the later as radiosensitizer, and further loaded with doxorubicin (PAMAM-GC/DOX) [133]. Cervical carcinoma HeLa cancer cells labeled with carboxyfluorescein succinimidyl ester (CFSE) were injected into the yolk sac at 2 dpf. Embryos were immersed in PAMAM-GC/DOX and further exposed to γ-radiation at 3 dpf. Synergistic antitumoral effect for the combination chemotherapy and radiotherapy with NPs was confirmed, versus only radiation or free DOX with or without irradiation. Likewise, PAMAM dendrimers, functionalized with PEG using a hypoxia-induced sensitive linker, were loaded with DOX and hypoxia-inducible factor 1a siRNA (PAMAM-DOX-siHIF) [134]. The antitumor activity of free DOX, PAMAM+DOX, and PAMAM-DOX+si-HIF was tested upon implantation of MCF-7-CM-DiL breast cancer cells into the perivitelline space of 48 hpf Tg(*fli1*:EGFP) embryos, and intracardiac injection of free DOX, PAP+DOX and PAP-DOX+si-HIF at 1 dpi, showing the best results for the "triple-therapeutic combination" (PAMAM-DOX+si-HIF). Despite these promising results in zebrafish, we still foresee some limitations for the translation of some results to the clinic, in part due to the differences in zebrafish anatomy versus mammals, because of the need for deeper penetration of radiotherapy in hidden tumors. However, a positive experience was recently reported by Costa et al., showing the utility of zebrafish to distinguish radiosensitive from radioresistant tumors using colorectal cancer cell lines and patient biopsies, and clinical response was correlated with induction of apoptosis in zebrafish [141].

Several redox- and pH-responsive-NPs have been developed, to favor the control delivery of drugs in the reducing and acidic TME, and several zebrafish models were optimized for the testing of these NPs. Transgenic mifepristone-inducible liver tumor zebrafish line expressing the enhanced green fluorescence protein (EGFP)-Kras^{v12} oncogene [142], as a model of hepatocellular carcinoma with elevated glutathione and liver acidity, was used [143,144]. While embryos treated with free DOX died at 2–3 dpi, lower toxicity and sustained regression of tumor size was observed for the DOX-loaded-NPs, demonstrating improved drug release to liver tumor cells and lower systemic toxicity [145]. A pH-sensitive hydrazone-linked DOX nanogel (Nanogel^{DOX}) was i.v. injected in zebrafish, previously implanted with B6 mouse melanoma cells into the neural tube at 48 hpf, showing significant reduction in tumor growth versus no effect for free DOX. [135]. Redox-responsive silica-gold nanocomposites functionalized with transferrin and loaded with DOX (Tf-DOX-ReSi-Au) were injected in a zebrafish colorectal cancer model, showing positive antitumoral activity without the typical DOX-related cardiotoxic adverse effects [136]. Others have tested the capacity of fluorescent-NPs to detect cancer cells in vivo, using similar zebrafish tumor models [146,147].

To understand the interaction between immune and tumor cells, several zebrafish xenograft models have been developed. These models have allowed to study the role of immune cells in tumor vascularization and invasion [148], the dynamic interaction between immune and cancer cells [149], or the positive correlation between the number of immune cells recruited to the tumor site and the degree of angiogenesis [150,151]. Póvoa et al. showed distinct engraftment profiles from the same patient at different stages of tumor progression in colorectal zebrafish xenograft models and explored the innate immune contribution to this process [152]. While cells derived from the primary tumor were able to recruit macrophages and neutrophils, thus being rapidly cleared (regressors), those cancer cells derived from a lymph node metastasis polarized macrophages towards a M2-like protumoral phenotype, engrafting very efficiently (progressors). Interestingly, mixing both types of cells resulted in decreased regressors clearance, reduced numbers of innate cells and increased M2-like polarization. Furthermore, depletion of macrophages resulted in a significant increase in the engraftment of regressors. These results provide the first experimental evidence of therapeutic manipulation of macrophages in zebrafish tumor models [152]. Detailed studies, using NPs for reprogramming TAMs into antitumoral M1-like macrophages, have still not been performed using zebrafish models of cancer. Nevertheless, a few investigations have explored the circulation time of NPs, their accumulation at the tumor site and their specific uptake by macrophages in tumors using these models. Evensen et al. were the first to image the accumulation of NPs to human tumor-like structures in a zebrafish xenograft model [72]. Comparing labeled polystyrene NPs and liposomes, with or without PEGylation, upon injection into the posterior cardinal vein of 2 dpf embryos, they noted that PEG-liposomes displayed the longest circulation time due to their lower affinity to the endothelium, the lowest macrophage uptake, and the highest survival rate. Using xenografts, with melanoma and kidney cancer cells, the PEG-liposomes showed a specific and rapid accumulation into the tumor and outside the vasculature after only 2–5 h post- injection (hpi) [72]. Kocere and colleagues demonstrated the selective accumulation of Cy5-labelled poly(ethylene glycol)-block-poly(2-(diisopropyl amino) ethyl methacrylate) (PEG-PDPA) NPs in TAMs using a melanoma xenograft model [137]. By injection of B6 mouse melanoma cells (labeled with GFP or RFP) in the neural tube of 3 dpf transgenic embryos ((Tg(*fli1a*:EGFP, Tg(*mpeg1*:mcherry), Tg(*mpx*:GFP)) [33,119,153], they were able to observe tumor growth, angiogenesis, and accumulation of macrophages, but not neutrophils, within the tumor at 10 dpf. Additionally, xenografts in 3 dpf Tg(*mpeg1*:GAL4/UAS:*NTR*-mCherry) embryos, which express a nitroreductase in macrophages in presence of metronidazole causing their selective apoptosis, revealed a slightly increased tumor growth when macrophages were absent. The injection of PEG-PDPA NPs, showed selective accumulation of NPs and increased number of macrophages at the tumor site. Moreover, a small fraction of NPs was internalized by cancer cells and TAMs. These DOX-loaded-PEG-PDPA NPs were i.v. injected in the melanoma model at 1 dpi, showing reduced toxicity, decreased proliferation, and increased apoptosis of cancer cells six days after treatment [137].

As a whole, these studies provide a consistent knowledge and experience for the development of several types of tumors in zebrafish and the testing of nano-oncologicals with different features. Zebrafish models provide excellent opportunities for genetic modifications and for in vivo evaluation/tracking of innate immune cells, being these key aspects for the testing of NPs. A major limitation for the use of zebrafish embryos to test antitumoral therapies is their lack of adaptive immune system. This challenge has partially been addressed through the suppression of the adult immune system, either by γ-irradiation, dexamethasone treatment [154–156] or more recently using adult immunocompromised strains [157–159], followed by the injection of human or murine immune cells (i.e., T cells). These adult zebrafish xenografts enable a closer resemblance of cell–tumor microenvironment interactions, a longer tumor engraftment and a clinically-relevant dose response [160,161]. Remarkably, Yan et al. created an optically clear, homozygous mutants (*prkdc−/−*, *il2rga−/−*) which lacks T, B, and natural killer (NK) cells. These animals survived at 37 °C (optimal for mammal cells), robustly engrafted a variety of human tumor cells and subsequently responded to drug treatments. Importantly, similar histological and molecular features in both fish and mouse xenografts were confirmed and pharmacokinetics of antitumoral treatments, such as olaparib and temozolomide, were comparable to that found in both mouse preclinical models and humans. Nevertheless, this adult immunocompromised strain must be improved, as several cancer cell types failed to engraft into the model and pre-treating fish with clodronate liposomes to deplete macrophages was required [159]. Additional disadvantages of zebrafish models are that some strains do not breed, develop gill inflammation, and likely autoimmunity [158], or they could be quite prone to infection and require specialized food and antibiotic treatment [162], thus raising the cost of maintenance. Despite these challenges, the results demonstrate that zebrafish tumor models are important tools with high potential to improve the translation of nano-oncologicals towards the clinic.

4.2. *Autoimmune Diseases*

4.2.1. Inflammatory Bowel Disease

Inflammatory bowel diseases (IBDs) refer to chronic inflammatory disorders of the gastrointestinal tract which comprise both Crohn's disease and ulcerative colitis. Although their etiology is not clear, they are thought to be a result of host genetic susceptibility and environmental factors (e.g., diet) [163,164], which lead to altered interactions between gut microbiota and the intestinal immune system [165]. Intestinal homeostasis is partly maintained by resident macrophages with enhanced phagocytic and bactericidal activity and decreased production of pro-inflammatory cytokines [166]. Nevertheless, when gut dysbiosis and further disruption of normal mucosal immunity occur, monocytes are continuously recruited to become inflammatory macrophages, they participate in the inflammatory response and contribute to chronic intestine inflammation [167]. In this context, zebrafish models are useful to study the relationship between immune system and inflammation. For instance, Coronado et al. treated fish with a previously established inflammatory diet [168] and found a strong increase in the number of neutrophils, macrophages and T helper cells recruited to the gut [169]. Looking into the genetic susceptibility, Kaya et al. were able to validate the implication of GPR35-expressing macrophages in intestinal immune homeostasis and inflammation by generating a zebrafish mutant line [170]. Other researchers have shown the potential of zebrafish for the screening of drugs to treat IBDs [171–173]. With regard to NPs, to date, we only found one study where the administration of copper NPs to zebrafish resulted in intestinal developmental defects, through ER stress and ROS generation, showing similar alterations to IBD patients (Table 2) [174]. Thus, these studies provide the starting point for the study of IBD pathology and testing of NPs which might offer new solutions to patients suffering these intestinal disorders.

4.2.2. Type I Diabetes Mellitus

Type 1 diabetes mellitus (T1DM) is an autoimmune disease caused by immune-mediated progressive destruction of the pancreatic β-cells, driven by the interaction of multiple environmental and genetic factors. The pathogenesis of T1DM is characterized by the infiltration of islet antigen-specific T cells and pro-inflammatory APCs associated with impairment of Foxp3+ Tregs. The destruction of β-cells leads to the loss of ability to produce insulin and in turn, to chronic hyperglycemia [175,176]. T1DM treatment is mainly based on lifelong insulin replacement therapy and several nanoparticles have been designed to improve its administration [177,178]. Others have explored the inhibition of the destructive autoimmune response against insulin-producing β-cells, for example by regulating T-cell autoreactivity as a therapeutic approach [179,180]. In zebrafish models, to mimic T1DM, the destruction of β-cells has been achieved by either surgery [181], chemical destruction [182], or genetic ablation [183], followed by their subsequent regeneration ability allowing to study the mechanisms of β-cells regeneration and also the testing of antidiabetic drugs [184,185]. A number of chemical screens to induce β-cell generation in zebrafish have been reported [186–188] and the antidiabetic effect of different bioactive molecules and NPs has been tested (Table 2).

Silver nanoparticles loaded with *Eysenhardtia polystachya* (EP/AgNPs), with a spherical shape and diameter of 5–21 nm, were tested on glucose-induced diabetic adult zebrafish and the results confirmed the effectiveness of NPs in ameliorating hyperglycemia [189]. The utility of quercetin NPs (NQs) in ameliorating diabetic retinopathy, a common complication derived from diabetes was shown by Wang et al. [190]. Chemically induced diabetes and diabetic retinopathy were established in adult zebrafish, and further treatment with NQs led to a reduction in glucose blood levels as wells as to the improvement of different morphological, behavioral, and biochemical parameters linked to diabetic retinopathy [190]. Others have evaluated the biocompatibility/toxicological profile of different types of NPs with potential antidiabetic activity, such as peptide-major histocompatibility complexes-NPs or curcumin encapsulated in polycaprolactone-grafted oligocarrageenan nanomicelles [191,192]. These studies provide a solid basis for the further use of zebrafish models to screen new antidiabetic nanotechnological approaches.

4.2.3. Rheumatoid Arthritis

Rheumatoid arthritis (RA) is a chronic inflammatory and autoimmune disease characterized by synovial and joint swelling, pain, and bone destruction [193]. The pathogenesis of RA is a multistep process, initially starting outside the joints by the aberrant activation of antigen-presenting cells, triggered by genetic or environmental causes, which leads to the activation of a pro-inflammatory cascade, production of autoantibodies as well as altered T-cell and B-cell cross-activation [194,195]. These events lead to monocyte recruitment to the diseased tissue and activation and polarization of macrophages towards a M1-like pro-inflammatory phenotype, boosting the inflammatory cascade [196]. Current RA-treatments include nonsteroidal anti-inflammatory drugs (NSAIDs), corticosteroids, disease-modifying antirheumatic drugs, and different natural substances to reduce joint inflammation [197]. With the aim to mimic human disease, improve its understanding and test new therapies, several animal models have been developed [198,199], and zebrafish models could be also implemented as a useful tool. Zebrafish have served as a model to evaluate the anti-inflammatory properties of different synthetic and natural compounds, although no reports on nanomaterials are available yet. *Clerodendrum cyrtophyllum* Turcz is a commonly used plant in Vietnam for treating RA. Ngyuyen et al. confirmed the anti-inflammatory properties of ethanol extracts of this plant in a copper-induced inflammation zebrafish model, via downregulation of inflammation mediators and pro-inflammatory cytokines (e.g., *cox-2* or *il-1β*) [200]. Similarly, Jiang et al. demonstrated anti-inflammatory effects of isothiocyanate prodrugs in a zebrafish neutrophilic inflammation model, as the number of migrating neutrophils in treated zebrafish was smaller than in the control group [201]. Wang et al. demonstrated the inhibition of cyclooxygenase, as the anti-inflammatory mechanisms of action of *Gentiana dahurica* roots, in a zebrafish model of induced production of cyclooxygenases 1 and 2 [202]. Genetic approaches using zebrafish were applied to study the role of *c5orf30*, whose variants have been associated with RA. Upon tail transection in the *c5orf30* knockdown fish an increased recruitment of macrophages to the wound site was observed, confirming the anti-inflammatory role of *c5orf30*, with implications in RA [203]. With reference to early diagnosis, Feng et al. designed and synthesized fluorescent probes for the quantitative detection of hypochlorous acid, a biomarker of RA, and confirmed their efficiency in an LPS-induced inflammatory model of adult zebrafish [204]. Additionally, zebrafish has served as a platform to evaluate the toxicity of new treatments with potential application in RA [205,206]. Although mammalian models of RA are needed before the clinical translation of new therapeutic approaches, these zebrafish models provide a valuable tool for the initial screening of innovative nanotechnological approaches to treat RA.

4.2.4. Neuroinflammatory and Neurodegenerative Diseases

Several zebrafish models have been established and optimized for the understanding of neuroinflammatory or neurodegenerative diseases [207,208]. In parallel, different types of NPs have been engineered for the treatment and/or diagnosis of neuro-related disorders [209,210]. Interestingly, zebrafish models have also been used to study the neurotoxic or neuroprotective effects of a wide variety of NPs and biomaterials [207]. Below, we provide some examples of investigations using zebrafish models and NPs to improve drug targeting and/or efficacy in the context of neuroinflammatory and neurodegenerative diseases (Table 2).

Neuroprotective effects of NPs in Parkinson's disease (PD) using zebrafish models have been observed, commonly mediated by the antioxidant and/or neuro-antiinflammatory activity of these NPs. Bacopa monnieri platinum NPs (BmE-PtNPs) demonstrated the same activity of Complex I, as that of oxidizing NADH to NAD(+), suggesting that BmE-PtNPs could be a potential medicinal substance for oxidative stress mediated disease with suppressed mitochondrial complex I as it happens in PD. Hence, in 1-methyl-4-phenyl-1,2,3,6-tetrahydropyridine (MPTP)-induced experimental Parkinsonism in zebrafish model, BmE-PtNPs pretreatment significantly reversed the toxic effects of MPTP by increasing the levels of dopamine, its metabolites, GSH, and activities of GPx, catalase, SOD and complex I, and reducing levels of MDA along with enhanced locomotor activity [211]. Schisantherin A (SA) is a promising anti-Parkinsonism Chinese herbal medicine and SA nanocrystals (SA-NC) were used to reverse the MPTP-induced dopaminergic neuronal loss and locomotion deficiency in zebrafish. This strong neuroprotective effect of SA-NC may be partially mediated by the activation of the protein kinase B (Akt)/glycogen synthase kinase-3β (Gsk3β) pathway [212]. On the other hand, it has been shown that, after exposure of different concentrations of titanium dioxide NPs (TiO2 NPs) to zebrafish embryos from fertilization to 96 hpf, the hatching time of zebrafish was decreased accompanied by an increase in malformation rate, while no significant increases in mortality relative to controls were observed [213]; moreover, accumulation of TiO2 NPs was found in the brain of zebrafish larvae, resulting in loss of dopaminergic neurons, ROS generation and cell death in hypothalamus. Meanwhile, q-PCR analysis showed that TiO2 NPs exposure increased the *pink1*, *parkin*, *α-syn*, and *uchl1* gene expressions, which are related with the formation of Lewy bodies [213]. Data from zebrafish behavioral phenotype revealed observable effects of silica nanoparticles (SiNPs) on disturbing light/dark preference, dampening exploratory behavior and inhibiting memory capability; furthermore, the relationship between neurotoxic symptom and the transcriptional alteration of autophagy- and parkinsonism-related genes was showed [62]. Similarly, another study showed that 15-nm silica SiNPs produced significant changes in advanced cognitive neurobehavioral patterns (color preference) and caused PD-like behavior compared with 50-nm SiNPs. Analyses at the tissue, cell and molecular levels corroborated the behavioral observations [214]. Both studies demonstrated that nanosilica acted on the retina and dopaminergic neurons to change color preference and to cause PD-like behavior [62,214]. Puerarin has emerged as a promising herb-derived anti-Parkinsonism compound and puerarin nanocristals (PU-NCs) demonstrated no obvious toxic effects on zebrafish, as evidenced by the unaltered morphology, hatching, survival rate, body length, and heart rate; fluorescence resonance energy transfer

(FRET) imaging revealed that intact nanocrystals were found in the intestine and brain of adult zebrafish [215,216]. Moreover, other NPs with alleged neuroprotective effects for treating PD, such as polymeric NPs of Ginkgolide B, have shown correct bioavailability and cerebral accumulation in zebrafish models [217].

Similarly, as with PD, some authors have shown neuroprotective and neuroregenerative effects of different NPs in Alzheimer's disease (AD) zebrafish models. Thereby, it has been shown that casein coated-gold nanoparticles (βCas AuNPs) in systemic circulation translocate across the blood brain barrier (BBB) of zebrafish larvae, sequester intracerebral Aβ42 and its elicited toxicity in a nonspecific chaperone-like manner. This was evidenced by behavioral pathology, ROS, and neuronal dysfunction biomarkers assays, complemented by brain histology and inductively coupled plasma-mass spectroscopy. The capacity of βCas AuNPs in recovering the mobility and cognitive function of adult zebrafish exposed to Aβ was demonstrated [218]. Other study evaluated the role of solid lipid NPs of quercetin (SLN-Q), a flavonoid with multiple pharmacological actions like vascular integrity and regulatory action on the BBB, using pentylenetetrazole (PTZ) induced cognitive impairment of *Danio rerio* species [219]. The intraperitoneal pretreatment of SLN-Q showed an attenuating effect in PTZ induced neurocognitive impairments, along with amelioration of biochemical changes (acetylcholinesterase activity, lipid peroxidation, and reduced glutathione levels), showing differences with fish treated with donepezil. Some authors have demonstrated with confocal image analyses that amphiphilic yellow-emissive carbon dots (Y-CDs) crossed the BBB of five-day old wild-type zebrafish, most probably by passive diffusion due to the amphiphilicity of Y-CDs; furthermore, Y-CDs were internalized by the cells, inhibiting the overexpression of human amyloid precursor protein (APP) and β-amyloid (Aβ) which is a major factor responsible for AD pathology [220].

Amyotrophic Lateral Sclerosis (ALS), a fatal neurodegenerative disease affecting the upper and lower motor neurons in the motor cortex and spinal cord, could be ameliorated by reducing the levels of superoxide dismutase I (SOD1). Thus, calcium phosphate lipid coated nanoparticles (CaP-lipid NPs) were developed and tested in zebrafish for the delivery of SOD1 antisense oligonucleotides (ASO) with success, and their preferential accumulation in the brain, blood stream, and spinal cord was observed [221].

In addition, the toxic profile of several NPs with potential interest for neurological diseases was also evaluated using zebrafish models. As examples, Carbamazepine or Tacrine were co-administered with PAMAM dendrimers and neurotoxicity, cardiotoxicity, or hepatotoxicity were evaluated in zebrafish larvae [222,223]. These reports provide satisfactory experience in the study of neuro-related disorders using zebrafish models and a good basis for their use as a screening platform to support new nanotechnologies for the treatment of these diseases.

Table 2. Summary of nanoparticles tested in zebrafish models of autoimmune diseases: inflammatory bowel disease, type I diabetes mellitus, parkinson's disease, alzheimer's disease, amyotrophic lateral sclerosis.

Disease	Disease Induction	Zebrafish Stage	Nanosystem	NPs Delivery	Remarkable Results	Reference
Inflammatory Bowel Disease	Copper NPs- induced intestinal developmental defects	From 0 hpf	Copper NPs	Immersion	CuNPs cause intestinal developmental defects via inducing ER stress and ROS generation, which corresponds with elevated serum copper levels in IBD patients	[174]
Type 1 diabetes mellitus	Glucose-induced diabetic zebrafish	Adult	EP/AgNPs	Immersion	Hyperglycemia amelioration	[189]
Type 1 diabetes mellitus	STZ- induced diabetic retinopathy	Adult	Quercetin NPs	Intraperitoneal injection	Reduction of glycemia and improvement of morphological, behavioral and biochemical parameters linked to retinopathy	[190]
Type 1 diabetes mellitus	-	From 4 hpf	pMHC-NPs	Immersion	Neither off-target toxicity, nor morphological abnormalities	[191]
Parkinson's Disease	MPTP-induced parkinsonism	Adult	BmE-PtNPs	Intraperitoneal injection	Significant reversion of toxic effects of MPTP by increasing the levels of dopamine, GSH, GPx, catalase, SOD and complex I, and reducing levels of MDA	[211]
Parkinson's Disease	MPTP-induced parkinsonism	From 72 hpf	Schisantherin nanocrystals	Immersion	Reversed dopaminergic neuronal loss and locomotion deficiency by the activation of the Akt/Gsk3β pathway	[212]
Parkinson's Disease	-	From 0 hpf	Titanium dioxide NPs	Immersion	Loss of dopaminergic neurons, ROS generation and cell death in hypothalamus. Increased Lewy bodies-related markers.	[213]
Parkinson's Disease	-	Adult	Silica NPs	Immersion	Changes in dopaminergic neurons with disturbed light/dark preference, dampened exploratory behavior, inhibited memory capability and PD-like behavior	[62,214]
Parkinson's Disease	-	From 6 hpf	Puerarin Nanocristals	Immersion	Promising anti-Parkinsonism NCs. Unaltered morphology, hatching, survival rate, body length and heart rate	[215,216]
Parkinson's Disease	-	From 120 hpf	Ginkgolide B-PEG-PCL NPs	Immersion	Correct bioavailability and cerebral accumulation in zebrafish models	[217]
Alzheimer's Disease	Aβ- induced toxicity	Adult	Casein coated-gold NPs	Retro-orbital injection	Inhibition of Aβ toxicity and recover of the mobility and cognitive function	[218]
Alzheimer's Disease	PTZ- induced cognitive impairment	Adult	Solid lipid NPs of Quercetin	Intraperitoneal injection	Attenuation of PTZ-induced neurocognitive impairments and amelioration of biochemical changes	[219]
Amyotrophic Lateral Sclerosis	-	From 96 hpf	ASO- CaP-lipid NPs	Brain, spinal cord, intravenous and retro-orbital injection	Successful delivery and preferential accumulation in brain, bloodstream and spinal cord	[221]

APP: Human amyloid precursor protein; ASO-CaP-lipid NPs: SOD1 antisense oligonucleotide-calcium phosphate lipid coated NPs; Aβ: β-amyloid; BmE-PtNPs: Bacopa monnieri platinum NPs; EP/AgNPs: *Eysenhardtia polystachya*-loaded silver NPs; ER: Endoplasmic reticulum; GSH: Glutathione; GSH-Px: Glutathione peroxidase; MDA: Malondialdehyde; MPTP: 1-methyl-4-phenyl-1,2,3,6-tetrahydropyridine; STZ: Streptozotocin; PEG-PCL NPs: Poly(ethylene glycol)-co-poly(ε-caprolactone); pMHC-NPs: Peptide-major histocompatibility complexes NPs; PTZ: Pentylenetetrazole; SOD: Superoxide dismutase.

4.3. Infectious Diseases

Zebrafish models have been largely used to study infectious diseases, taking advantage of its transparency, possibilities to study both innate and adaptive immunity, and feasibility for the highly controlled administration of pathogens, commonly through microinjection. Prospective treatments are mostly administered by microinjection too, although other routes such as intubation have been described [224]. Most of the studies reviewed in this section have been performed using zebrafish in the first month of life, which does not present a completely developed adaptive immune system but allows for the separate study of macrophages and neutrophils during pathogenic infection [225,226]. Transgenic lines that attach fluorescent proteins to robust macrophages markers, such as *mpeg1* or *csf1ra*, have been used [227]. As an example, Palha et al. infected Tg(*fnφ1*:mCherry) zebrafish larvae with two Chikungunya virus strains, one of which expressed GFP, allowing to follow infection progress and its quantification by flow cytometry. This work, using zebrafish, demonstrated similarities with the process in mammals and a critical role of the IFN response to control the infection. Furthermore, the differential role of macrophages and neutrophils was investigated using a transgenic metronidazole-inducible cell ablation system to deplete macrophages. Neutrophil depletion was studied in *csf3r* knockdown larvae that were highly susceptible to Chikungunya virus, exhibiting a high increase of virus transcripts and mortality [228]. In another study, selective depletion of macrophages by incubation in metronidazole reduced the virulence of infection caused by the *Burkholderia cepacia* complex, revealing the important role of these cells in the infectious process [229]. The easiness for monitoring macrophages in zebrafish allowed extensive studies of tuberculosis and facilitated the observation of granulomas caused by *Mycobacterium marinum* [230–232]. Clay et al. took advantage of the transparency of the zebrafish to report a dichotomous role of macrophages in early *M. marinum* infection. First, they performed dual fluorescent antibody detection of L-plastin and myeloperoxidase to confirm that only macrophages and not neutrophils phagocytose bacteria. Most bacteria were found in macrophages (L-plastin positive but MPO-negative). Second, they assessed whether macrophages upregulate inflammatory cytokines as a response to *M. marinum*. They injected separately the bacteria and similar-sized fluorescent beads into the hindbrain, demonstrating that macrophages migrated to the area in response to *M. marinum* but not in response to the beads. Macrophage-defective zebrafish embryos were created by the injection of morpholinos against the *pu.1* gene to evaluate the role of macrophages on mycobacterial growth. Finally, the Tg(*fli1*:EGFP) transgenic line and *pu.1* morphants were used to study bacteria dissemination through the vascular system and the role of macrophages. By injecting red fluorescent bacteria into the bloodstream, they found that control embryos had a higher number of extravascular bacteria than *pu.1* morphants and bacteria injected in the hindbrain could only disseminate out of this space in the control zebrafish with macrophages [231]. Similarly, Davis and Ramakrishnan exploited zebrafish transparency to assess the role of macrophages in tuberculous infection through three-dimensional differential interference contrast microscopy (3D DIC) and fluorescence in vivo microscopy. Embryos were infected with wild type and attenuated *M. marinum*, lacking the ESX-1/RD1 secretion system locus, throughout their experiments. Upon injection of the bacteria into the hindbrain ventricle and daily monitoring, infected macrophages recruited uninfected macrophages in a RD1-dependent manner. Further, the combination of 3D DIC with time-lapse microscopy showed that uninfected macrophages become infected quicker when they are recruited by RD1-competent bacteria. Zebrafish transparency also enabled close observation of the macrophage's morphology both in WT and RD1 defective bacteria, which proved to be different. Finally, after proving that macrophages become infected when phagocyting dead infected macrophages, granuloma dissemination initiated by macrophages from primary granulomas was also observed. To assess the migration of infected macrophages, they used a bacteria strain that constitutively expresses the Kaede photoactivable protein [232]. Other pathogens relevant for humans (*Candida albicans*, *Herpes simplex*, *Pseudomonas aeruginosa*, *Staphylococcus aureus*, *Streptococcus pneumonia*) [233–236] and fish (*Vibrio anguillarum, Aeromonas salmonicida, Yersinia ruckeria*, etc.) [237–239] have also been studied using zebrafish models [240,241]. In relation with the study of tuberculosis, Oksanen et al. demonstrated that zebrafish is a useful model for preclinical DNA vaccine development. They vaccinated zebrafish with a combination of plasmids encoding for Ag85B, CFP-10, and ESAT-6, well known mycobacterial antigens, through intramuscular microinjection. Three weeks after immunisation, zebrafish were challenged with a high dose of *M. marinum* (20,500 CFU) by microinjection. Vaccinated fish showed increased survival and the analysis of the bacterial load by qPCR revealed that unvaccinated zebrafish had a higher load than the vaccinated group [242]. Taken together these studies are proof of the versatility of zebrafish to study pathogen infection and dissemination in vivo. Genetic-wise, besides an already existing repertoire of transgenic lines, Clay et al. proved *D. rerio* can be tailored to the needs of the researchers for the study of macrophages by the knockdown of key regulator genes [231].

Several nanotechnology-based-approaches have been developed for vaccination, prophylactic and therapeutic purposes, in the context of infectious diseases, and tested in zebrafish models (Table 3). With prophylactic purposes, Torrealba et al. generated inclusion bodies (IBs) containing TNFα or CCL4 [243]. The resulting nanostructures (IBs) showed good stability under different pH conditions (2.5 and 8). While $IB^{TNF\alpha}$ were cylindrical with a diameter between 380–900 nm and an average length of 1134.6 $\pm$ 196.6 nm, the IB^{CCL4} showed spherical shape with a diameter between 220–850 nm. Both IBs were added to the cell culture of ATTC® CRL-2643 (zebrafish liver cells) and RT-HKM (trout macrophages) to evaluate their uptake, showing positive results for both cell types. Further, treatment of RT-HKM with $IB^{TNF\alpha}$ stimulated the expression of pro-inflammatory cytokines. In vivo, zebrafish were immunised with $IB^{TNF\alpha}$, IB^{CCL4}, or $IB^{iRFP\text{-}H6}$ (an IB containing a control protein) by microinjection and later challenged with *P. aeruginosa*. Zebrafish injected intraperitoneally with both types of IBs exhibited reduced mortality after a challenge with *P. aeruginosa*. Similar inclusion bodies were also used to encapsulate proteins of pancreatic necrosis virus (IPNV), haemorrhagic septicaemia virus (VHSV) and viral nervous necrosis virus (VNNV) for the development of oral prophylactics [224]. IPNV-IBs were barrel shaped and porous with an average width and length of 607 and 734 nm, respectively. VHSV-IBs were round with a width and length of 488 and 608 nm. VNNV-IBs presented an irregular shape with spherical protrusions and a mean diameter of 422 nm. Gene expression analysis of trout macrophages stimulated in vitro with IPNV-IBs and VHSV-IBs showed upregulation of pro-inflammatory markers: *vig1*, *gig2*, *stat1b*, *mx*, *irf7*, and *ccl4*. In vivo uptake of the fluorescently labelled IBs was evaluated by intubating zebrafish adults with the IBs solutions and later analysing gut cells by flow cytometry. Uptake of VHSV-IBs or VNNV-IBs was observed by all fish, while IPNV-IBs were only taken up by 75% of fish. In another study, various recombinant vaccines based on glycoprotein G of viral haemorrhagic septicaemia virus encapsulated in NPs were developed. NPs were produced by complexing poly(I:C) with chitosan, size ranged from 100 to 550 nm with an average diameter of 368 $\pm$ 1.3 nm and an average surface charge of +36.2 mV. Fish vaccinated with NPs containing poly(I:C) showed lower mortality rates than non-vaccinated fish or fish vaccinated with NPs without poly(I:C) [244]. Chitosan was also used as a polymer to coat *Piscirickettsia salmonis* membrane nanovesicles for immunisation. The chitosan-coated NPs showed an average diameter of 182.2 $\pm$ 4.3 nm and a Z-potential of 31.2 $\pm$ 1.8 mV. Immunisation was successful and the upregulation of immune related genes (*IL-8*, *IL-1β*, *IL-10*, and *IL-6*) was reported by analysis of kidney samples [245]. In essence, these articles provide evidence for the use of adult zebrafish as a valid model for immunological studies and as an economic platform for the testing of nano-based approaches designed to improve fish survival, which is of particular interest in aquaculture.

Table 3. Summary of nanoparticles tested in zebrafish models of infectious diseases.

Disease Induction	Zebrafish Stage	Nanosystem	NPs Delivery	Immune Cells Behavior	Remarkable Results	Reference
Pseudomonas aeruginosa infection	Adult	Nanostructured cytokines ($IB^{TNF\alpha}$, IB^{CCL4})	Intraperitoneal injection	Interaction of IBs with immune cells	Prophylactic potential in vivo	[243]
-	Adult	IPNV, VHSV and VNNV-encapsulated IBs	Oral intubation	-	Successful NPs uptake in gut cells after oral administration	[224]
VHSV infection	Adult	Viral glycoprotein G encapsulated in chitosan-poly(I:C) NPs	Intraperitoneal injection	Upregulation of antiviral cytokines	Significant protection against VHSV through induction of anti-viral state	[244]
Piscirickettsia salmonis infection	Adult	Chitosan-coated MVs from *P. salmonis*	Intraperitoneal injection	Upregulation of immune related genes	Successful immunisation. Potential use of chitosan-coated MVs for vaccination	[245]
Streptococcus pneumonia infection	From 48 hpf	Auranofin-PLGA-NPs	Immersion	-	Auranofin-NPs capability of decreasing the bacterial population compared to free drug	[246]

IBs: Inclusion bodies; IPNV: Pancreatic necrosis virus; VHSV: Viral hemorrhagic septicemia virus; VNNV: Viral nervous necrosis virus; MVs: Membrane nanovesicles; PLGA-NPs: Poly(lactic-co-glycolic acid) NPs; LPS: Lipopolysaccharide.

In the search for anti-bacterial compounds to deal with antibiotic resistance, Díez-Martínez et al. assayed the anti-bacterial effect of Auranofin, an FDA-approved drug for the treatment of rheumatoid arthritis, free and encapsulated in nanocapsules of poly(lactic-co-glycolic acid) (PLGA-NPs) in vivo using a zebrafish infection model of *Streptococcus pneumoniae*. PLGA-NPs loaded with Auranofin were spherical with a diameter of 60 nm and a negative surface charge (−30mV). Then, 48 hpf zebrafish embryos were infected by immersion with the pathogen and later treated with free auranofin or auranofin-PLGA-NPs, again by immersion. Encapsulated auranofin was more efficient at rescuing infected embryos in a dose dependent manner than the free drug. Moreover, when compared with encapsulated ampicillin, auranofin PLGA-NPs were still more efficient at increasing survival rates of infected fish [246]. As a cheap, high-throughput model organism, zebrafish could greatly contribute to the initial development of new approaches in the fight against antimicrobial resistance.

Taken together, these findings demonstrate that zebrafish models are very useful for the study of infectious diseases and for the testing of new therapeutic approaches, including NPs. As described above, the evaluation of macrophage and/or neutrophil behavior in this context is of foremost interest, and zebrafish models offer an appropriate environment to study the role of these innate immune cells along the course of the disease and in response to treatment.

5. Conclusions

In the last years, the use of zebrafish models in biomedical research has increased substantially to study the cellular and/or molecular basis of human diseases, and for the faster and more economic testing of new compounds, drugs, biomaterials, and nanoparticles. In Figure 3, we can clearly observe the rising number of studies published each year, including zebrafish or nanomaterials, related to toxicity, biodistribution, macrophages, cancer, infectious diseases, or other autoimmune disorders. Manuscripts with a focus on toxicity, macrophages, and cancer are the most frequent, and their number has been consistently increasing in the last decade. Only a few nanomaterials have still been tested in zebrafish models, but the number of this type of studies is also clearly increasing.

In addition to economic and ethical issues, zebrafish models provide excellent opportunities for genetic modifications and for in vivo evaluation/tracking of innate immune cells, such as macrophages. Such unique features make zebrafish amenable to a multitude of methodologies and the establishment of disease models which have already proven viable to study the interaction of macrophages with nanoparticles. These technical advances have been used for a precise toxicological and/or biodistribution testing of nanomaterials with safety or medical purposes. Following a similar trend, we foresee an increase in the testing of nanotechnological approaches for the treatment of cancer, infectious disease, or other autoimmune disorders, using zebrafish models of disease, and providing further information about the role of macrophages in the initiation, progression, and remission of the disease over the course of the treatment. Ultimately, we expect that these studies will contribute to the safe use of nanotechnologies and to their translation towards the clinic, providing new solutions for patients.

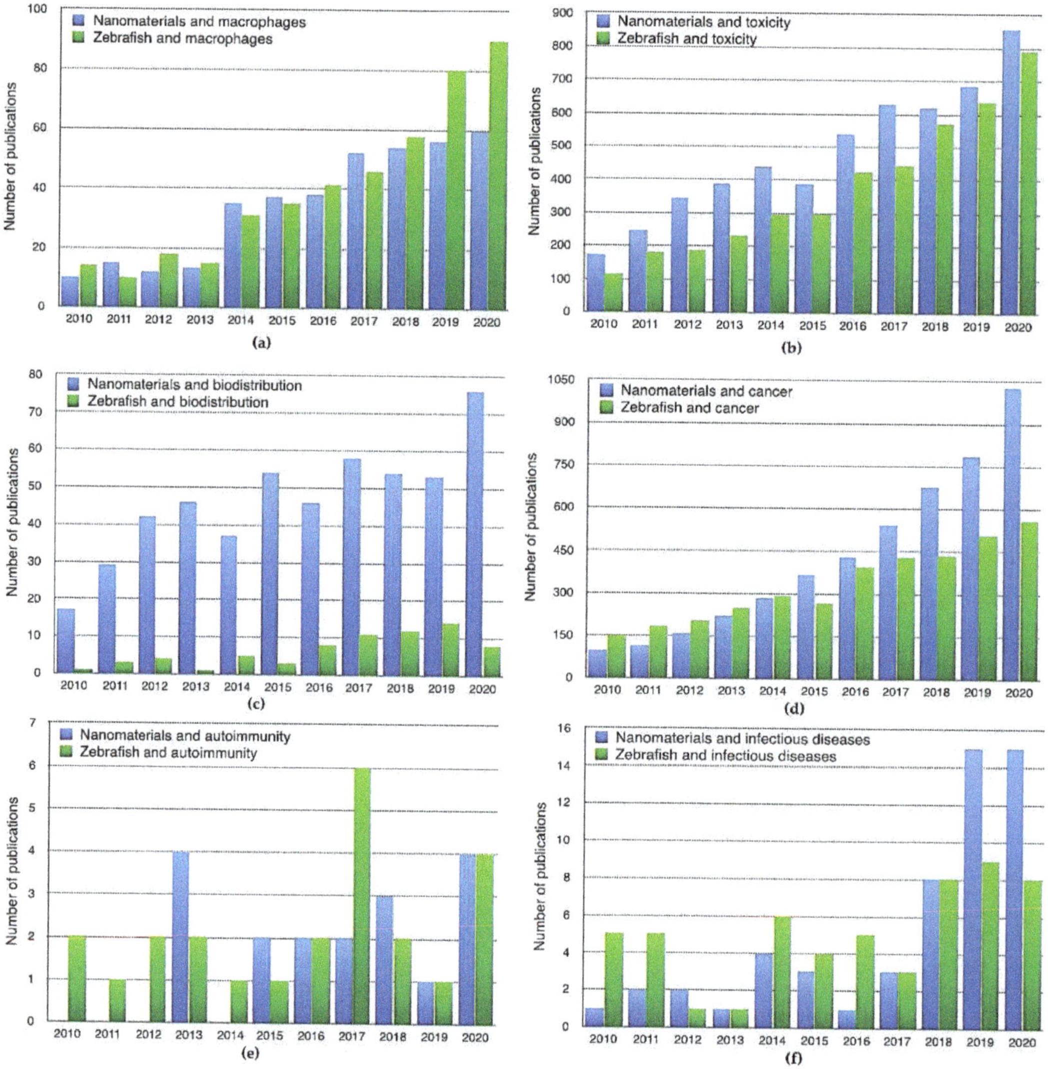

Figure 3. Number of publications each year in Pubmed for indicated terms from 2010 to 2020: (**a**) Nanomaterials and macrophages/Zebrafish and macrophages; (**b**) Nanomaterials and toxicity/Zebrafish and toxicity; (**c**) Nanomaterials and biodistributrion/Zebrafish and biodistribution; (**d**) Nanomaterials and cancer/Zebrafish and cancer; (**e**) Nanomaterials and autoimmunity/Zebrafish and autoimmunity; (**f**) Nanomaterials and infectious diseases/Zebrafish and infectious diseases.

Author Contributions: J.F.-R., P.R. and J.C.-C. have contributed to writing and elaboration of Figures 2 and 3, A.P.-L. to writing and elaboration of Figure 1, the tables, review and editing. L.S. and F.T.A. to the writing, review, and editing. All authors have read and agreed to the published version of the manuscript.

Funding: A.P.-L. is supported by the Xunta de Galicia Pre-doctoral Fellowship (ED481A-2018/095); F.T.A. is recipient of a grant by the AECC ("Asociación Española Contra el Cáncer", Spain). J.F.-R. was supported by a scholarship awarded by "Fundación Barrié".

Acknowledgments: The images used for the different figures were reproduced from Servier Medical Art under a Creative Commons Attribution 3.0 Unported License (https://creativecommons.org/licenses/by/3.0).

Conflicts of Interest: The authors declare no conflict of interest. The authors certify that they have no affiliations with or involvement in any organization or entity with any financial interest or non-financial interest in the subject matter or materials discussed in this manuscript.

Abbreviations

AD	Alzheimer's disease
AgNPs	Silver NPs
ALS	Amyotrophic Lateral Sclerosis
APCs	Antigen-presenting cells
APP	Human amyloid precursor protein
ASO-CaP-lipid NPs	SOD1 antisense oligonucleotide-calcium phosphate lipid coated NPs
AuNPs	Gold NPs
Aβ	β-amyloid
BBB	Blood-brain-barrier
BmE-PtNPs	Bacopa monnieri platinum NPs
CFSE	Carboxyfluorescein succinimidyl ester
CHT	Caudal hematopoietic tissue
cox-2	Cyclooxygenase-2
CuNPs	Copper nanoparticles
DOX	Doxorubicin
dpf	Days post-fertilization
dpi	days post-injection
EGF	Epithelial growth factor
EP/AgNPs	*Eysenhardtia polystachya*-loaded silver NPs
ER	Endoplasmic reticulum
FET	Fish Embryo Acute Toxicity
GFP	Green fluorescent protein
GSH	Glutathione
GSH-Px	Glutathione peroxidase
hpf	Hours post-fertilization
hpi	Hours post-injection
HSCs	Hematopoietic stem cells
i.m.	Intramuscular
i.v.	Intravenously
IBD	Inflammatory bowel disease
IBs	Inclusion bodies
IFN-γ	Interferon-γ
IL	Interleukin
IPNV	Pancreatic necrosis virus
LPS	Lipopolysaccharide
MDA	Malondialdehyde
MPTP	1-methyl-4-phenyl-1,2,3,6-tetrahydropyridine
mRNA	Messenger RNA
MVs	Membrane nanovesicles
NCs	Nanocapsules
NK	Natural killer
NPs	Nanoparticles
NQs	Quercetin NPs
NSAIDs	Nonsteroidal anti-inflammatory drugs
PAMAM	Polyamidoamine
PD	Parkinson's disease
PDT	Photodynamic therapy
PDX	Patient-derived xenografts

PEG	Polyethylene glycol
PEG-PCL NPs	Poly(ethylene glycol)-co-poly(ε-caprolactone) NPs
PEG-PDPA NPs	Poly(ethylene glycol)-block-poly(2-(diisopropyl amino) ethyl methacrylate) NPs
PLA NPs	Poly(Lactic Acid) NPs
PLGA-NPs	Poly(lactic-co-glycolic acid) NPs
pMHC-NPs	Peptide-major histocompatibility complexes NPs
PMOsPOR-NH_2	Porous porphyrin-based organosilica NPs
PORBSNs	Non-porous porphyrin-based bridged silsesquioxane NPs
PS	Polystyrene
PtPP-HA	Kiteplatin-pyrophosphate-loaded hydroxyapatite NPs
PTZ	Pentylenetetrazole
PU-NCs	Puerarin nanocristals
RA	Rheumatoid arthritis
RFP	Red fluorescent protein
ROS	Reactive oxygen species
SA-NCs	Schisantherin nanocrystals
siHIF	Hypoxia-inducible factor 1a siRNA
SiNPs	Silica NPs
SLN-Q	Solid lipid NPs of quercetin
SOD	Superoxide dismutase
STZ	Streptozotocin
T1DM	Type 1 diabetes mellitus
TAMs	Tumor-associated macrophages
Tf-DOX-ReSi-Au	Redox-responsive silica-gold NPs functionalized with transferrin- DOX
TGF-β	Transforming growth factor-β
TiO2 NPs	Titanium dioxide NPs
TME	Tumor microenvironment
TNF-α	Tumor necrosis factor-α
TPE-PDT	Two-photon-excited photodynamic therapy
VEGF	Vascular endothelial growth factor
VHSV	Viral hemorrhagic septicemia virus
VNNV	Viral nervous necrosis virus
wpf	Weeks post-fertilization
Y-CDs	Amphiphilic yellow-emissive carbon dots
ZnO-NPs	Zinc oxide NPs
βCas AuNPs	Casein coated-gold NPs

References

1. Pelaz, B.; Alexiou, C.; Alvarez-Puebla, R.A.; Alves, F.; Andrews, A.M.; Ashraf, S.; Balogh, L.P.; Ballerini, L.; Bestetti, A.; Brendel, C.; et al. Diverse Applications of Nanomedicine. *ACS Nano* **2017**, *11*, 2313–2381. [CrossRef]
2. Ramsden, J. *Nanotechnology: An Introduction*; William Andrew: Norwich, NY, USA, 2016.
3. Faria, M.; Björnmalm, M.; Thurecht, K.J.; Kent, S.J.; Parton, R.G.; Kavallaris, M.; Johnston, A.P.R.; Gooding, J.J.; Corrie, S.R.; Boyd, B.J.; et al. Minimum information reporting in bio–nano experimental literature. *Nat. Nanotechnol.* **2018**, *13*, 777–785. [CrossRef] [PubMed]
4. Fadeel, B.; Farcal, L.; Hardy, B.; Vázquez-Campos, S.; Hristozov, D.; Marcomini, A.; Lynch, I.; Valsami-Jones, E.; Alenius, H.; Savolainen, K. Advanced tools for the safety assessment of nanomaterials. *Nat. Nanotechnol.* **2018**, *13*, 537–543. [CrossRef] [PubMed]
5. Andón, F.T.; Fadeel, B. Nanotoxicology: Towards safety by design. In *Nano-Oncologicals: New Targeting and Delivery Approaches*; Alonso, M.J., Garcia-Fuentes, M., Eds.; Springer International Publishing: Cham, Germany, 2014; pp. 391–424. [CrossRef]
6. Wang, H.; Brown, P.C.; Chow, E.C.Y.; Ewart, L.; Ferguson, S.S.; Fitzpatrick, S.; Freedman, B.S.; Guo, G.L.; Hedrich, W.; Heyward, S.; et al. 3D Cell Culture Models: Drug Pharmacokinetics, Safety Assessment, and Regulatory Consideration. *Clin. Transl. Sci.* **2021**. [CrossRef]
7. Fazio, M.; Ablain, J.; Chuan, Y.; Langenau, D.M.; Zon, L.I. Zebrafish patient avatars in cancer biology and precision cancer therapy. *Nat. Rev. Cancer* **2020**, *20*, 263–273. [CrossRef] [PubMed]

8. Jia, H.R.; Zhu, Y.X.; Duan, Q.Y.; Chen, Z.; Wu, F.G. Nanomaterials meet zebrafish: Toxicity evaluation and drug delivery applications. *J. Control. Release* **2019**, *311*, 301–318. [CrossRef]
9. Zon, L.I. Zebrafish: A new model for human disease. *Genome Res.* **1999**, *9*, 99–100.
10. Xie, Y.; Meijer, A.H.; Schaaf, M.J.M. Modeling inflammation in zebrafish for the development of anti-inflammatory drugs. *Front. Cell Dev. Biol.* **2021**, *8*. [CrossRef]
11. Astin, J.; Keerthisinghe, P.; Du, L.; Sanderson, L.; Crosier, K.; Crosier, P.; Hall, C. Innate immune cells and bacterial infection in zebrafish. In *Methods in Cell Biology*; Elsevier: Amsterdam, The Netherlands, 2017; Volume 138, pp. 31–60.
12. Renshaw, S.A.; Trede, N.S. A model 450 million years in the making: Zebrafish and vertebrate immunity. *Dis. Models Mech.* **2012**, *5*, 38–47. [CrossRef] [PubMed]
13. Lam, S.; Chua, H.; Gong, Z.; Lam, T.; Sin, Y. Development and maturation of the immune system in zebrafish, *Danio rerio*: A gene expression profiling, in situ hybridization and immunological study. *Dev. Comp. Immunol.* **2004**, *28*, 9–28. [CrossRef]
14. de Jong, J.L.; Zon, L.I. Use of the zebrafish system to study primitive and definitive hematopoiesis. *Annu. Rev. Genet.* **2005**, *39*, 481–501. [CrossRef] [PubMed]
15. Paik, E.J.; Zon, L.I. Hematopoietic development in the zebrafish. *Int. J. Dev. Biol.* **2010**, *54*, 1127–1137. [CrossRef] [PubMed]
16. Herbomel, P.; Thisse, B.; Thisse, C. Ontogeny and behaviour of early macrophages in the zebrafish embryo. *Development* **1999**, *126*, 3735–3745. [CrossRef] [PubMed]
17. Gore, A.V.; Pillay, L.M.; Venero Galanternik, M.; Weinstein, B.M. The zebrafish: A fintastic model for hematopoietic development and disease. *Wiley Interdiscip. Rev. Dev. Biol.* **2018**, *7*, e312. [CrossRef] [PubMed]
18. Murayama, E.; Kissa, K.; Zapata, A.; Mordelet, E.; Briolat, V.; Lin, H.F.; Handin, R.I.; Herbomel, P. Tracing hematopoietic precursor migration to successive hematopoietic organs during zebrafish development. *Immunity* **2006**, *25*, 963–975. [CrossRef]
19. Liang, D.; Jia, W.; Li, J.; Li, K.; Zhao, Q. Retinoic acid signaling plays a restrictive role in zebrafish primitive myelopoiesis. *PLoS ONE* **2012**, *7*, e30865. [CrossRef]
20. Chen, A.T.; Zon, L.I. Zebrafish blood stem cells. *J. Cell. Biochem.* **2009**, *108*, 35–42. [CrossRef]
21. Locati, M.; Curtale, G.; Mantovani, A. Diversity, Mechanisms, and Significance of Macrophage Plasticity. *Annu. Rev. Pathol.* **2020**, *15*, 123–147. [CrossRef]
22. Varol, C.; Mildner, A.; Jung, S. Macrophages: Development and Tissue Specialization. *Annu. Rev. Immunol.* **2015**, *33*, 643–675. [CrossRef]
23. Funes, S.C.; Rios, M.; Escobar-Vera, J.; Kalergis, A.M. Implications of macrophage polarization in autoimmunity. *Immunology* **2018**, *154*, 186–195. [CrossRef]
24. Mantovani, A.; Sozzani, S.; Locati, M.; Allavena, P.; Sica, A. Macrophage polarization: Tumor-associated macrophages as a paradigm for polarized M2 mononuclear phagocytes. *Trends Immunol.* **2002**, *23*, 549–555. [CrossRef]
25. Murray, P.J. Macrophage Polarization. *Annu. Rev. Physiol.* **2017**, *79*, 541–566. [CrossRef]
26. Bronte, V.; Brandau, S.; Chen, S.H.; Colombo, M.P.; Frey, A.B.; Greten, T.F.; Mandruzzato, S.; Murray, P.J.; Ochoa, A.; Ostrand-Rosenberg, S.; et al. Recommendations for myeloid-derived suppressor cell nomenclature and characterization standards. *Nat. Commun.* **2016**, *7*, 12150. [CrossRef]
27. Sica, A.; Erreni, M.; Allavena, P.; Porta, C. Macrophage polarization in pathology. *Cell. Mol. Life Sci. CMLS* **2015**, *72*, 4111–4126. [CrossRef]
28. Zhang, X.; Mosser, D.M. Macrophage activation by endogenous danger signals. *J. Pathol.* **2008**, *214*, 161–178. [CrossRef]
29. Mosser, D.M.; Edwards, J.P. Exploring the full spectrum of macrophage activation. *Nat. Rev. Immunol.* **2008**, *8*, 958–969. [CrossRef] [PubMed]
30. Martinez, F.O.; Gordon, S. The M1 and M2 paradigm of macrophage activation: Time for reassessment. *F1000Prime Rep.* **2014**, *6*, 13. [CrossRef] [PubMed]
31. Allavena, P.; Anfray, C.; Ummarino, A.; Andón, F.T. Therapeutic manipulation of tumor-associated macrophages: Facts and hopes from a clinical and translational perspective. *Clin. Cancer Res.* **2021**, *27*, 3291–3297. [CrossRef] [PubMed]
32. Nguyen-Chi, M.; Laplace-Builhe, B.; Travnickova, J.; Luz-Crawford, P.; Tejedor, G.; Phan, Q.T.; Duroux-Richard, I.; Levraud, J.P.; Kissa, K.; Lutfalla, G.; et al. Identification of polarized macrophage subsets in zebrafish. *eLife* **2015**, *4*, e07288. [CrossRef] [PubMed]
33. Ellett, F.; Pase, L.; Hayman, J.W.; Andrianopoulos, A.; Lieschke, G.J. mpeg1 promoter transgenes direct macrophage-lineage expression in zebrafish. *Blood* **2011**, *117*, e49–e56. [CrossRef]
34. Nguyen-Chi, M.; Phan, Q.T.; Gonzalez, C.; Dubremetz, J.F.; Levraud, J.P.; Lutfalla, G. Transient infection of the zebrafish notochord with *E. coli* induces chronic inflammation. *Dis. Models Mech.* **2014**, *7*, 871–882. [CrossRef] [PubMed]
35. Sanderson, L.E.; Chien, A.T.; Astin, J.W.; Crosier, K.E.; Crosier, P.S.; Hall, C.J. An inducible transgene reports activation of macrophages in live zebrafish larvae. *Dev. Comp. Immunol.* **2015**, *53*, 63–69. [CrossRef]
36. Bernut, A.; Herrmann, J.L.; Kissa, K.; Dubremetz, J.F.; Gaillard, J.L.; Lutfalla, G.; Kremer, L. Mycobacterium abscessus cording prevents phagocytosis and promotes abscess formation. *Proc. Natl. Acad. Sci. USA* **2014**, *111*, E943–E952. [CrossRef]
37. Johnston, H.J.; Verdon, R.; Gillies, S.; Brown, D.M.; Fernandes, T.F.; Henry, T.B.; Rossi, A.G.; Tran, L.; Tucker, C.; Tyler, C.R.; et al. Adoption of in vitro systems and zebrafish embryos as alternative models for reducing rodent use in assessments of immunological and oxidative stress responses to nanomaterials. *Crit. Rev. Toxicol.* **2018**, *48*, 252–271. [CrossRef]

38. Brannen, K.C.; Chapin, R.E.; Jacobs, A.C.; Green, M.L. Alternative models of developmental and reproductive toxicity in pharmaceutical risk assessment and the 3Rs. *ILAR J.* **2016**, *57*, 144–156. [CrossRef]
39. Sipes, N.S.; Padilla, S.; Knudsen, T.B. Zebrafish: As an integrative model for twenty-first century toxicity testing. *Birth Defects Res. Part C Embryo Today Rev.* **2011**, *93*, 256–267. [CrossRef]
40. Cheng, H.; Yan, W.; Wu, Q.; Liu, C.; Gong, X.; Hung, T.C.; Li, G. Parental exposure to microcystin-LR induced thyroid endocrine disruption in zebrafish offspring, a transgenerational toxicity. *Environ. Pollut.* **2017**, *230*, 981–988. [CrossRef] [PubMed]
41. Han, Z.; Li, Y.; Zhang, S.; Song, N.; Xu, H.; Dang, Y.; Liu, C.; Giesy, J.P.; Yu, H. Prenatal transfer of decabromodiphenyl ether (BDE-209) results in disruption of the thyroid system and developmental toxicity in zebrafish offspring. *Aquat. Toxicol. (Amst. Neth.)* **2017**, *190*, 46–52. [CrossRef] [PubMed]
42. Newman, T.A.C.; Carleton, C.R.; Leeke, B.; Hampton, M.B.; Horsfield, J.A. Embryonic oxidative stress results in reproductive impairment for adult zebrafish. *Redox Biol.* **2015**, *6*, 648–655. [CrossRef] [PubMed]
43. Cao, F.; Zhu, L.; Li, H.; Yu, S.; Wang, C.; Qiu, L. Reproductive toxicity of azoxystrobin to adult zebrafish (*Danio rerio*). *Environ. Pollut.* **2016**, *219*, 1109–1121. [CrossRef] [PubMed]
44. Kim, J.Y.; Kim, S.J.; Bae, M.A.; Kim, J.R.; Cho, K.H. Cadmium exposure exacerbates severe hyperlipidemia and fatty liver changes in zebrafish via impairment of high-density lipoproteins functionality. *Toxicol. Vitr.* **2018**, *47*, 249–258. [CrossRef]
45. Qin, X.; Laroche, F.F.J.; Peerzade, S.; Lam, A.; Sokolov, I.; Feng, H. In Vivo Targeting of Xenografted Human Cancer Cells with Functionalized Fluorescent Silica Nanoparticles in Zebrafish. *J. Vis. Exp.* **2020**, *159*, e61187. [CrossRef]
46. Rothenbücher, T.S.P.; Ledin, J.; Gibbs, D.; Engqvist, H.; Persson, C.; Hulsart-Billström, G. Zebrafish embryo as a replacement model for initial biocompatibility studies of biomaterials and drug delivery systems. *Acta Biomater.* **2019**, *100*, 235–243. [CrossRef]
47. No, O.T. 236: Fish embryo acute toxicity (FET) test. *OECD Guidel. Test. Chem. Sect.* **2013**, *2*, 1–22.
48. OJEU. Directive 2010/63/EU of the European Parliament and of the Council on the protection of animals used for scientific purposes. *Off. J. Eur. Union* **2010**, *276*, 33–79.
49. Nishimura, Y.; Inoue, A.; Sasagawa, S.; Koiwa, J.; Kawaguchi, K.; Kawase, R.; Maruyama, T.; Kim, S.; Tanaka, T. Using zebrafish in systems toxicology for developmental toxicity testing. *Congenit. Anom.* **2016**, *56*, 18–27. [CrossRef] [PubMed]
50. Cornet, C.; Calzolari, S.; Miñana-Prieto, R.; Dyballa, S.; van Doornmalen, E.; Rutjes, H.; Savy, T.; D'Amico, D.; Terriente, J. ZeGlobalTox: An Innovative Approach to Address Organ Drug Toxicity Using Zebrafish. *Int. J. Mol. Sci.* **2017**, *18*, 864. [CrossRef]
51. Dach, K.; Yaghoobi, B.; Schmuck, M.R.; Carty, D.R.; Morales, K.M.; Lein, P.J. Teratological and Behavioral Screening of the National Toxicology Program 91-Compound Library in Zebrafish (*Danio rerio*). *Toxicol. Sci.* **2019**, *167*, 77–91. [CrossRef] [PubMed]
52. Marrero-Ponce, Y.; Siverio-Mota, D.; Gálvez-Llompart, M.; Recio, M.C.; Giner, R.M.; García-Domènech, R.; Torrens, F.; Arán, V.J.; Cordero-Maldonado, M.L.; Esguera, C.V.; et al. Discovery of novel anti-inflammatory drug-like compounds by aligning in silico and in vivo screening: The nitroindazolinone chemotype. *Eur. J. Med. Chem.* **2011**, *46*, 5736–5753. [CrossRef] [PubMed]
53. Chakraborty, C.; Sharma, A.R.; Sharma, G.; Lee, S.S. Zebrafish: A complete animal model to enumerate the nanoparticle toxicity. *J. Nanobiotechnol.* **2016**, *14*, 65. [CrossRef] [PubMed]
54. Bai, C.; Tang, M. Toxicological study of metal and metal oxide nanoparticles in zebrafish. *J. Appl. Toxicol. JAT* **2020**, *40*, 37–63. [CrossRef]
55. Zeng, J.; Xu, P.; Chen, G.; Zeng, G.; Chen, A.; Hu, L.; Huang, Z.; He, K.; Guo, Z.; Liu, W.; et al. Effects of silver nanoparticles with different dosing regimens and exposure media on artificial ecosystem. *J. Environ. Sci. (China)* **2019**, *75*, 181–192. [CrossRef] [PubMed]
56. Liu, H.; Wang, X.; Wu, Y.; Hou, J.; Zhang, S.; Zhou, N.; Wang, X. Toxicity responses of different organs of zebrafish (*Danio rerio*) to silver nanoparticles with different particle sizes and surface coatings. *Environ. Pollut.* **2019**, *246*, 414–422. [CrossRef] [PubMed]
57. Abramenko, N.B.; Demidova, T.B.; Abkhalimov, E.V.; Ershov, B.G.; Krysanov, E.Y.; Kustov, L.M. Ecotoxicity of different-shaped silver nanoparticles: Case of zebrafish embryos. *J. Hazard. Mater.* **2018**, *347*, 89–94. [CrossRef] [PubMed]
58. Xin, Q.; Rotchell, J.M.; Cheng, J.; Yi, J.; Zhang, Q. Silver nanoparticles affect the neural development of zebrafish embryos. *J. Appl. Toxicol. JAT* **2015**, *35*, 1481–1492. [CrossRef] [PubMed]
59. Brundo, M.V.; Pecoraro, R.; Marino, F.; Salvaggio, A.; Tibullo, D.; Saccone, S.; Bramanti, V.; Buccheri, M.A.; Impellizzeri, G.; Scuderi, V.; et al. Toxicity Evaluation of New Engineered Nanomaterials in Zebrafish. *Front. Physiol.* **2016**, *7*, 130. [CrossRef]
60. Ghobadian, M.; Nabiuni, M.; Parivar, K.; Fathi, M.; Pazooki, J. Toxic effects of magnesium oxide nanoparticles on early developmental and larval stages of zebrafish (*Danio rerio*). *Ecotoxicol. Environ. Saf.* **2015**, *122*, 260–267. [CrossRef]
61. Girigoswami, K.; Viswanathan, M.; Murugesan, R.; Girigoswami, A. Studies on polymer-coated zinc oxide nanoparticles: UV-blocking efficacy and in vivo toxicity. *Mater. Sci. Eng. C Mater. Biol. Appl.* **2015**, *56*, 501–510. [CrossRef]
62. Li, X.; Ji, X.; Wang, R.; Zhao, J.; Dang, J.; Gao, Y.; Jin, M. Zebrafish behavioral phenomics employed for characterizing behavioral neurotoxicity caused by silica nanoparticles. *Chemosphere* **2020**, *240*, 124937. [CrossRef]
63. Vranic, S.; Shimada, Y.; Ichihara, S.; Kimata, M.; Wu, W.; Tanaka, T.; Boland, S.; Tran, L.; Ichihara, G. Toxicological Evaluation of SiO_2 Nanoparticles by Zebrafish Embryo Toxicity Test. *Int. J. Mol. Sci.* **2019**, *20*, 882. [CrossRef]
64. Duan, J.; Hu, H.; Li, Q.; Jiang, L.; Zou, Y.; Wang, Y.; Sun, Z. Combined toxicity of silica nanoparticles and methylmercury on cardiovascular system in zebrafish (*Danio rerio*) embryos. *Environ. Toxicol. Pharmacol.* **2016**, *44*, 120–127. [CrossRef] [PubMed]
65. Ginzburg, A.L.; Truong, L.; Tanguay, R.L.; Hutchison, J.E. Synergistic Toxicity Produced by Mixtures of Biocompatible Gold Nanoparticles and Widely Used Surfactants. *ACS Nano* **2018**, *12*, 5312–5322. [CrossRef] [PubMed]

66. Harper, B.; Thomas, D.; Chikkagoudar, S.; Baker, N.; Tang, K.; Heredia-Langner, A.; Lins, R.; Harper, S. Comparative hazard analysis and toxicological modeling of diverse nanomaterials using the embryonic zebrafish (EZ) metric of toxicity. *J. Nanoparticle Res.* **2015**, *17*, 250. [CrossRef] [PubMed]
67. Bodewein, L.; Schmelter, F.; Di Fiore, S.; Hollert, H.; Fischer, R.; Fenske, M. Differences in toxicity of anionic and cationic PAMAM and PPI dendrimers in zebrafish embryos and cancer cell lines. *Toxicol. Appl. Pharmacol.* **2016**, *305*, 83–92. [CrossRef]
68. Jeong, J.; Cho, H.J.; Choi, M.; Lee, W.S.; Chung, B.H.; Lee, J.S. In vivo toxicity assessment of angiogenesis and the live distribution of nano-graphene oxide and its PEGylated derivatives using the developing zebrafish embryo. *Carbon* **2015**, *93*, 431–440. [CrossRef]
69. Teijeiro-Valiño, C.; Yebra-Pimentel, E.; Guerra-Varela, J.; Csaba, N.; Alonso, M.J.; Sánchez, L. Assessment of the permeability and toxicity of polymeric nanocapsules using the zebrafish model. *Nanomed. (Lond. Engl.)* **2017**, *12*, 2069–2082. [CrossRef]
70. Crecente-Campo, J.; Guerra-Varela, J.; Peleteiro, M.; Gutiérrez-Lovera, C.; Fernández-Mariño, I.; Diéguez-Docampo, A.; González-Fernández, Á.; Sánchez, L.; Alonso, M.J. The size and composition of polymeric nanocapsules dictate their interaction with macrophages and biodistribution in zebrafish. *J. Control. Release* **2019**, *308*, 98–108. [CrossRef]
71. Chang, H.; Yhee, J.Y.; Jang, G.H.; You, D.G.; Ryu, J.H.; Choi, Y.; Na, J.H.; Park, J.H.; Lee, K.H.; Choi, K.; et al. Predicting the in vivo accumulation of nanoparticles in tumor based on in vitro macrophage uptake and circulation in zebrafish. *J. Control. Release* **2016**, *244*, 205–213. [CrossRef]
72. Evensen, L.; Johansen, P.L.; Koster, G.; Zhu, K.; Herfindal, L.; Speth, M.; Fenaroli, F.; Hildahl, J.; Bagherifam, S.; Tulotta, C.; et al. Zebrafish as a model system for characterization of nanoparticles against cancer. *Nanoscale* **2016**, *8*, 862–877. [CrossRef]
73. Li, H.; Cao, F.; Zhao, F.; Yang, Y.; Teng, M.; Wang, C.; Qiu, L. Developmental toxicity, oxidative stress and immunotoxicity induced by three strobilurins (pyraclostrobin, trifloxystrobin and picoxystrobin) in zebrafish embryos. *Chemosphere* **2018**, *207*, 781–790. [CrossRef] [PubMed]
74. Chen, M.; Yin, J.; Liang, Y.; Yuan, S.; Wang, F.; Song, M.; Wang, H. Oxidative stress and immunotoxicity induced by graphene oxide in zebrafish. *Aquat. Toxicol. (Amst. Neth.)* **2016**, *174*, 54–60. [CrossRef]
75. Andón, F.T.; Fadeel, B. Programmed Cell Death: Molecular Mechanisms and Implications for Safety Assessment of Nanomaterials. *Acc. Chem. Res.* **2013**, *46*, 733–742. [CrossRef] [PubMed]
76. Bhattacharya, K.; Andón, F.T.; El-Sayed, R.; Fadeel, B. Mechanisms of carbon nanotube-induced toxicity: Focus on pulmonary inflammation. *Adv. Drug Deliv. Rev.* **2013**, *65*, 2087–2097. [CrossRef] [PubMed]
77. Andón, F.T.; Kapralov, A.A.; Yanamala, N.; Feng, W.; Baygan, A.; Chambers, B.J.; Hultenby, K.; Ye, F.; Toprak, M.S.; Brandner, B.D.; et al. Biodegradation of Single-Walled Carbon Nanotubes by Eosinophil Peroxidase. *Small* **2013**, *9*, 2721–2729. [CrossRef]
78. Truong, L.; Tilton, S.C.; Zaikova, T.; Richman, E.; Waters, K.M.; Hutchison, J.E.; Tanguay, R.L. Surface functionalities of gold nanoparticles impact embryonic gene expression responses. *Nanotoxicology* **2013**, *7*, 192–201. [CrossRef] [PubMed]
79. Krishnaraj, C.; Harper, S.L.; Yun, S.I. In Vivo toxicological assessment of biologically synthesized silver nanoparticles in adult Zebrafish (*Danio rerio*). *J. Hazard. Mater.* **2016**, *301*, 480–491. [CrossRef]
80. Brun, N.R.; Lenz, M.; Wehrli, B.; Fent, K. Comparative effects of zinc oxide nanoparticles and dissolved zinc on zebrafish embryos and eleuthero-embryos: Importance of zinc ions. *Sci. Total Environ.* **2014**, *476-477*, 657–666. [CrossRef]
81. Vibe, C.B.; Fenaroli, F.; Pires, D.; Wilson, S.R.; Bogoeva, V.; Kalluru, R.; Speth, M.; Anes, E.; Griffiths, G.; Hildahl, J. Thioridazine in PLGA nanoparticles reduces toxicity and improves rifampicin therapy against mycobacterial infection in zebrafish. *Nanotoxicology* **2016**, *10*, 680–688. [CrossRef]
82. Velikova, N.; Mas, N.; Miguel-Romero, L.; Polo, L.; Stolte, E.; Zaccaria, E.; Cao, R.; Taverne, N.; Murguía, J.R.; Martinez-Manez, R.; et al. Broadening the antibacterial spectrum of histidine kinase autophosphorylation inhibitors via the use of ε-poly-L-lysine capped mesoporous silica-based nanoparticles. *Nanomedicine* **2017**, *13*, 569–581. [CrossRef]
83. Blanco, E.; Shen, H.; Ferrari, M. Principles of nanoparticle design for overcoming biological barriers to drug delivery. *Nat. Biotechnol.* **2015**, *33*, 941–951. [CrossRef]
84. Lee, K.Y.; Jang, G.H.; Byun, C.H.; Jeun, M.; Searson, P.C.; Lee, K.H. Zebrafish models for functional and toxicological screening of nanoscale drug delivery systems: Promoting preclinical applications. *Biosci. Rep.* **2017**, *37*. [CrossRef]
85. Shwartz, A.; Goessling, W.; Yin, C. Macrophages in Zebrafish Models of Liver Diseases. *Front. Immunol.* **2019**, *10*, 2840. [CrossRef]
86. Zhang, X.; Song, J.; Klymov, A.; Zhang, Y.; de Boer, L.; Jansen, J.A.; van den Beucken, J.J.; Yang, F.; Zaat, S.A.; Leeuwenburgh, S.C. Monitoring local delivery of vancomycin from gelatin nanospheres in zebrafish larvae. *Int. J. Nanomed.* **2018**, *13*, 5377–5394. [CrossRef]
87. Andón, F.T.; Digifico, E.; Maeda, A.; Erreni, M.; Mantovani, A.; Alonso, M.J.; Allavena, P. Targeting tumor associated macrophages: The new challenge for nanomedicine. *Semin. Immunol.* **2017**, *34*, 103–113. [CrossRef]
88. Duan, X.; Li, Y. Physicochemical characteristics of nanoparticles affect circulation, biodistribution, cellular internalization, and trafficking. *Small* **2013**, *9*, 1521–1532. [CrossRef]
89. Dal, N.K.; Kocere, A.; Wohlmann, J.; Van Herck, S.; Bauer, T.A.; Resseguier, J.; Bagherifam, S.; Hyldmo, H.; Barz, M.; De Geest, B.G.; et al. Zebrafish Embryos Allow Prediction of Nanoparticle Circulation Times in Mice and Facilitate Quantification of Nanoparticle-Cell Interactions. *Small* **2020**, *16*, e1906719. [CrossRef] [PubMed]
90. Campbell, F.; Bos, F.L.; Sieber, S.; Arias-Alpizar, G.; Koch, B.E.; Huwyler, J.; Kros, A.; Bussmann, J. Directing Nanoparticle Biodistribution through Evasion and Exploitation of Stab2-Dependent Nanoparticle Uptake. *ACS Nano* **2018**, *12*, 2138–2150. [CrossRef] [PubMed]

91. Sieber, S.; Grossen, P.; Uhl, P.; Detampel, P.; Mier, W.; Witzigmann, D.; Huwyler, J. Zebrafish as a predictive screening model to assess macrophage clearance of liposomes in vivo. *Nanomedicine* **2019**, *17*, 82–93. [CrossRef] [PubMed]
92. Teijeiro-Valiño, C.; Novoa-Carballal, R.; Borrajo, E.; Vidal, A.; Alonso-Nocelo, M.; de la Fuente Freire, M.; Lopez-Casas, P.P.; Hidalgo, M.; Csaba, N.; Alonso, M.J. A multifunctional drug nanocarrier for efficient anticancer therapy. *J. Control. Release* **2019**, *294*, 154–164. [CrossRef] [PubMed]
93. Crecente-Campo, J.; Lorenzo-Abalde, S.; Mora, A.; Marzoa, J.; Csaba, N.; Blanco, J.; González-Fernández, Á.; Alonso, M.J. Bilayer polymeric nanocapsules: A formulation approach for a thermostable and adjuvanted E. coli antigen vaccine. *J. Control. Release* **2018**, *286*, 20–32. [CrossRef]
94. Vicente, S.; Peleteiro, M.; Gonzalez-Aramundiz, J.V.; Díaz-Freitas, B.; Martínez-Pulgarín, S.; Neissa, J.I.; Escribano, J.M.; Sanchez, A.; González-Fernández, A.; Alonso, M.J. Highly versatile immunostimulating nanocapsules for specific immune potentiation. *Nanomed. (Lond. Engl.)* **2014**, *9*, 2273–2289. [CrossRef]
95. de la Fuente, M.; Raviña, M.; Paolicelli, P.; Sanchez, A.; Seijo, B.; Alonso, M.J. Chitosan-based nanostructures: A delivery platform for ocular therapeutics. *Adv. Drug Deliv. Rev.* **2010**, *62*, 100–117. [CrossRef]
96. Truong, N.P.; Whittaker, M.R.; Mak, C.W.; Davis, T.P. The importance of nanoparticle shape in cancer drug delivery. *Expert Opin. Drug Deliv.* **2015**, *12*, 129–142. [CrossRef]
97. Wibroe, P.P.; Anselmo, A.C.; Nilsson, P.H.; Sarode, A.; Gupta, V.; Urbanics, R.; Szebeni, J.; Hunter, A.C.; Mitragotri, S.; Mollnes, T.E.; et al. Bypassing adverse injection reactions to nanoparticles through shape modification and attachment to erythrocytes. *Nat. Nanotechnol.* **2017**, *12*, 589–594. [CrossRef] [PubMed]
98. Sangabathuni, S.; Murthy, R.V.; Chaudhary, P.M.; Subramani, B.; Toraskar, S.; Kikkeri, R. Mapping the Glyco-Gold Nanoparticles of Different Shapes Toxicity, Biodistribution and Sequestration in Adult Zebrafish. *Sci. Rep.* **2017**, *7*, 4239. [CrossRef]
99. Saez Talens, V.; Arias-Alpizar, G.; Makurat, D.M.M.; Davis, J.; Bussmann, J.; Kros, A.; Kieltyka, R.E. Stab2-Mediated Clearance of Supramolecular Polymer Nanoparticles in Zebrafish Embryos. *Biomacromolecules* **2020**, *21*, 1060–1068. [CrossRef] [PubMed]
100. Rességuier, J.; Delaune, E.; Coolen, A.L.; Levraud, J.P.; Boudinot, P.; Le Guellec, D.; Verrier, B. Specific and Efficient Uptake of Surfactant-Free Poly(Lactic Acid) Nanovaccine Vehicles by Mucosal Dendritic Cells in Adult Zebrafish after Bath Immersion. *Front. Immunol.* **2017**, *8*, 190. [CrossRef] [PubMed]
101. Li, Y.; Miao, X.; Chen, T.; Yi, X.; Wang, R.; Zhao, H.; Lee, S.M.; Wang, X.; Zheng, Y. Zebrafish as a visual and dynamic model to study the transport of nanosized drug delivery systems across the biological barriers. *Colloids Surfaces B Biointerfaces* **2017**, *156*, 227–235. [CrossRef] [PubMed]
102. van Pomeren, M.; Peijnenburg, W.; Vlieg, R.C.; van Noort, S.J.T.; Vijver, M.G. The biodistribution and immuno-responses of differently shaped non-modified gold particles in zebrafish embryos. *Nanotoxicology* **2019**, *13*, 558–571. [CrossRef] [PubMed]
103. Brown, J.M.; Recht, L.; Strober, S. The promise of targeting macrophages in cancer therapy. *Clin. Cancer Res.* **2017**, *23*, 3241–3250. [CrossRef]
104. Nicoli, S.; Ribatti, D.; Cotelli, F.; Presta, M. Mammalian tumor xenografts induce neovascularization in zebrafish embryos. *Cancer Res.* **2007**, *67*, 2927–2931. [CrossRef]
105. Nicoli, S.; Presta, M. The zebrafish/tumor xenograft angiogenesis assay. *Nat. Protoc.* **2007**, *2*, 2918. [CrossRef] [PubMed]
106. Patton, E.E.; Widlund, H.R.; Kutok, J.L.; Kopani, K.R.; Amatruda, J.F.; Murphey, R.D.; Berghmans, S.; Mayhall, E.A.; Traver, D.; Fletcher, C.D.; et al. BRAF mutations are sufficient to promote nevi formation and cooperate with p53 in the genesis of melanoma. *Curr. Biol.* **2005**, *15*, 249–254. [CrossRef] [PubMed]
107. Michailidou, C.; Jones, M.; Walker, P.; Kamarashev, J.; Kelly, A.; Hurlstone, A.F. Dissecting the roles of Raf- and PI3K-signalling pathways in melanoma formation and progression in a zebrafish model. *Dis Model. Mech.* **2009**, *2*, 399–411. [CrossRef]
108. Park, S.W.; Davison, J.M.; Rhee, J.; Hruban, R.H.; Maitra, A.; Leach, S.D. Oncogenic KRAS induces progenitor cell expansion and malignant transformation in zebrafish exocrine pancreas. *Gastroenterology* **2008**, *134*, 2080–2090. [CrossRef]
109. Sieber, S.; Grossen, P.; Bussmann, J.; Campbell, F.; Kros, A.; Witzigmann, D.; Huwyler, J. Zebrafish as a preclinical in vivo screening model for nanomedicines. *Adv. Drug Deliv. Rev.* **2019**, *151*, 152–168. [CrossRef] [PubMed]
110. Valle, S.; Alcalá, S.; Martin-Hijano, L.; Cabezas-Sáinz, P.; Navarro, D.; Muñoz, E.R.; Yuste, L.; Tiwary, K.; Walter, K.; Ruiz-Cañas, L.; et al. Exploiting oxidative phosphorylation to promote the stem and immunoevasive properties of pancreatic cancer stem cells. *Nat. Commun.* **2020**, *11*, 5265. [CrossRef] [PubMed]
111. Pudelko, L.; Edwards, S.; Balan, M.; Nyqvist, D.; Al-Saadi, J.; Dittmer, J.; Almlöf, I.; Helleday, T.; Bräutigam, L. An orthotopic glioblastoma animal model suitable for high-throughput screenings. *Neuro-oncology* **2018**, *20*, 1475–1484. [CrossRef] [PubMed]
112. Quail, D.F.; Joyce, J.A. Microenvironmental regulation of tumor progression and metastasis. *Nat. Med.* **2013**, *19*, 1423–1437. [CrossRef] [PubMed]
113. Mantovani, A.; Allavena, P.; Sica, A.; Balkwill, F. Cancer-related inflammation. *Nature* **2008**, *454*, 436–444. [CrossRef]
114. Hanahan, D.; Weinberg, R.A. Hallmarks of cancer: The next generation. *Cell* **2011**, *144*, 646–674. [CrossRef]
115. Sounni, N.E.; Noel, A. Targeting the tumor microenvironment for cancer therapy. *Clin. Chem.* **2013**, *59*, 85–93. [CrossRef]
116. Mantovani, A.; Marchesi, F.; Malesci, A.; Laghi, L.; Allavena, P. Tumour-associated macrophages as treatment targets in oncology. *Nat. Rev. Clin. Oncol.* **2017**, *14*, 399–416. [CrossRef]
117. Movahedi, K.; Van Ginderachter, J.A. The Ontogeny and Microenvironmental Regulation of Tumor-Associated Macrophages. *Antioxid. Redox Signal.* **2016**, *25*, 775–791. [CrossRef] [PubMed]

118. Anfray, C.; Ummarino, A.; Andón, F.T.; Allavena, P. Current Strategies to Target Tumor-Associated-Macrophages to Improve Anti-Tumor Immune Responses. *Cells* **2019**, *9*, 46. [CrossRef] [PubMed]
119. Lawson, N.D.; Weinstein, B.M. In Vivo Imaging of Embryonic Vascular Development Using Transgenic Zebrafish. *Dev. Biol.* **2002**, *248*, 307–318. [CrossRef] [PubMed]
120. Renshaw, S.; Loynes, C.; Trushell, D.; Elworthy, S.; Ingham, P.; Whyte, M. A transgenic zebrafish model of neutrophilic inflammation. *Blood* **2007**, *108*, 3976–3978. [CrossRef]
121. Cabezas-Sáinz, P.; Pensado-López, A.; Sáinz, B., Jr.; Sánchez, L. Modeling Cancer Using Zebrafish Xenografts: Drawbacks for Mimicking the Human Microenvironment. *Cells* **2020**, *9*, 1978. [CrossRef]
122. Baxendale, S.; van Eeden, F.; Wilkinson, R. The power of zebrafish in personalised medicine. In *Personalised Medicine*; Springer: Berlin/Heidelberg, Germany, 2017; pp. 179–197.
123. Germain, M.; Caputo, F.; Metcalfe, S.; Tosi, G.; Spring, K.; Åslund, A.K.O.; Pottier, A.; Schiffelers, R.; Ceccaldi, A.; Schmid, R. Delivering the power of nanomedicine to patients today. *J. Control. Release* **2020**, *326*, 164–171. [CrossRef]
124. Shi, J.; Kantoff, P.W.; Wooster, R.; Farokhzad, O.C. Cancer nanomedicine: Progress, challenges and opportunities. *Nat. Rev. Cancer* **2017**, *17*, 20–37. [CrossRef]
125. Alonso, M.; Garcia-Fuentes, M. *Nano-Oncologicals: New Targeting and Delivery Approaches*; Springer: Berlin/Heidelberg, Germany, 2014. [CrossRef]
126. Goldberg, M.S. Improving cancer immunotherapy through nanotechnology. *Nat. Rev. Cancer* **2019**, *19*, 587–602. [CrossRef]
127. Lächelt, U.; Wagner, E. Nucleic acid therapeutics using polyplexes: A journey of 50 years (and beyond). *Chem. Rev.* **2015**, *115*, 11043–11078. [CrossRef]
128. Hu, G.; Guo, M.; Xu, J.; Wu, F.; Fan, J.; Huang, Q.; Yang, G.; Lv, Z.; Wang, X.; Jin, Y. Nanoparticles Targeting Macrophages as Potential Clinical Therapeutic Agents Against Cancer and Inflammation. *Front. Immunol.* **2019**, *10*, 1998. [CrossRef]
129. Nadar, R.A.; Asokan, N.; Degli Esposti, L.; Curci, A.; Barbanente, A.; Schlatt, L.; Karst, U.; Iafisco, M.; Margiotta, N.; Brand, M.; et al. Preclinical evaluation of platinum-loaded hydroxyapatite nanoparticles in an embryonic zebrafish xenograft model. *Nanoscale* **2020**, *12*, 13582–13594. [CrossRef] [PubMed]
130. Wang, S.W.; Lee, C.H.; Lin, M.S.; Chi, C.W.; Chen, Y.J.; Wang, G.S.; Liao, K.W.; Chiu, L.P.; Wu, S.H.; Huang, D.M.; et al. ZnO Nanoparticles Induced Caspase-Dependent Apoptosis in Gingival Squamous Cell Carcinoma through Mitochondrial Dysfunction and p70S6K Signaling Pathway. *Int. J. Mol. Sci.* **2020**, *21*, 1612. [CrossRef]
131. Mauriello Jimenez, C.; Aggad, D.; Croissant, J.G.; Tresfield, K.; Laurencin, D.; Berthomieu, D.; Cubedo, N.; Rossel, M.; Alsaiari, S.; Anjum, D.H. Porous Porphyrin-Based Organosilica Nanoparticles for NIR Two-Photon Photodynamic Therapy and Gene Delivery in Zebrafish. *Adv. Funct. Mater.* **2018**, *28*, 1800235. [CrossRef]
132. Dib, S.; Aggad, D.; Mauriello Jimenez, C.; Lakrafi, A.; Hery, G.; Nguyen, C.; Durand, D.; Morère, A.; El Cheikh, K.; Sol, V.; et al. Porphyrin-based bridged silsesquioxane nanoparticles for targeted two-photon photodynamic therapy of zebrafish xenografted with human tumor. *Cancer Rep.* **2019**, *2*, e1186. [CrossRef] [PubMed]
133. Wu, S.Y.; Chou, H.Y.; Yuh, C.H.; Mekuria, S.L.; Kao, Y.C.; Tsai, H.C. Radiation-Sensitive Dendrimer-Based Drug Delivery System. *Adv. Sci.* **2018**, *5*, 1700339. [CrossRef] [PubMed]
134. Xie, Z.; Guo, W.; Guo, N.; Huangfu, M.; Liu, H.; Lin, M.; Xu, W.; Chen, J.; Wang, T.; Wei, Q.; et al. Targeting tumor hypoxia with stimulus-responsive nanocarriers in overcoming drug resistance and monitoring anticancer efficacy. *Acta Biomater.* **2018**, *71*, 351–362. [CrossRef]
135. Van Driessche, A.; Kocere, A.; Everaert, H.; Nuhn, L.; Van Herck, S.; Griffiths, G.; Fenaroli, F.; De Geest, B.G. pH-Sensitive Hydrazone-Linked Doxorubicin Nanogels via Polymeric-Activated Ester Scaffolds: Synthesis, Assembly, and In Vitro and In Vivo Evaluation in Tumor-Bearing Zebrafish. *Chem. Mater.* **2018**, *30*, 8587–8596. [CrossRef]
136. Tu, W.M.; Huang, X.C.; Chen, Y.L.; Luo, Y.L.; Liau, I.; Hsu, H.Y. Longitudinal and quantitative assessment platform for concurrent analysis of anti-tumor efficacy and cardiotoxicity of nano-formulated medication in vivo. *Anal. Chim. Acta* **2020**, *1095*, 129–137. [CrossRef] [PubMed]
137. Kocere, A.; Resseguier, J.; Wohlmann, J.; Skjeldal, F.M.; Khan, S.; Speth, M.; Dal, N.J.K.; Ng, M.Y.W.; Alonso-Rodriguez, N.; Scarpa, E.; et al. Real-time imaging of polymersome nanoparticles in zebrafish embryos engrafted with melanoma cancer cells: Localization, toxicity and treatment analysis. *EBioMedicine* **2020**, *58*, 102902. [CrossRef] [PubMed]
138. Yu, C.I.; Chen, C.Y.; Liu, W.; Chang, P.C.; Huang, C.W.; Han, K.F.; Lin, I.P.; Lin, M.Y.; Lee, C.H. Sandensolide Induces Oxidative Stress-Mediated Apoptosis in Oral Cancer Cells and in Zebrafish Xenograft Model. *Mar. Drugs* **2018**, *16*, 387. [CrossRef] [PubMed]
139. Carmody, R.J.; Cotter, T.G. Signalling apoptosis: A radical approach. *Redox Rep.* **2001**, *6*, 77–90. [CrossRef]
140. Peng, B.; Almeqdadi, M.; Laroche, F.; Palantavida, S.; Dokukin, M.; Roper, J.; Yilmaz, O.H.; Feng, H.; Sokolov, I. Ultrabright fluorescent cellulose acetate nanoparticles for imaging tumors through systemic and topical applications. *Mater. Today* **2019**, *23*, 16–25. [CrossRef]
141. Costa, B.; Ferreira, S.; Póvoa, V.; Cardoso, M.J.; Vieira, S.; Stroom, J.; Fidalgo, P.; Rio-Tinto, R.; Figueiredo, N.; Parés, O.; et al. Developments in zebrafish avatars as radiotherapy sensitivity reporters-towards personalized medicine. *EBioMedicine* **2020**, *51*, 102578. [CrossRef]
142. Nguyen, A.T.; Emelyanov, A.; Koh, C.H.V.; Spitsbergen, J.M.; Parinov, S.; Gong, Z. An inducible kras(V12) transgenic zebrafish model for liver tumorigenesis and chemical drug screening. *Dis. Models Mech.* **2012**, *5*, 63–72. [CrossRef]

143. Huang, Z.Z.; Chen, C.; Zeng, Z.; Yang, H.; Oh, J.; Chen, L.; Lu, S.C. Mechanism and significance of increased glutathione level in human hepatocellular carcinoma and liver regeneration. *FASEB J.* **2001**, *15*, 19–21. [CrossRef]
144. Volk, T.; Jähde, E.; Fortmeyer, H.P.; Glüsenkamp, K.H.; Rajewsky, M.F. pH in human tumour xenografts: Effect of intravenous administration of glucose. *Br. J. Cancer* **1993**, *68*, 492–500. [CrossRef]
145. Ang, C.Y.; Tan, S.Y.; Teh, C.; Lee, J.M.; Wong, M.F.E.; Qu, Q.; Poh, L.Q.; Li, M.; Zhang, Y.; Korzh, V.; et al. Redox and pH Dual Responsive Polymer Based Nanoparticles for In Vivo Drug Delivery. *Small* **2017**, *13*, 1602379. [CrossRef]
146. Palantavida, S.; Guz, N.V.; Woodworth, C.D.; Sokolov, I. Ultrabright fluorescent mesoporous silica nanoparticles for prescreening of cervical cancer. *Nanomedicine* **2013**, *9*, 1255–1262. [CrossRef]
147. Peerzade, S.; Qin, X.; Laroche, F.J.F.; Palantavida, S.; Dokukin, M.; Peng, B.; Feng, H.; Sokolov, I. Ultrabright fluorescent silica nanoparticles for in vivo targeting of xenografted human tumors and cancer cells in zebrafish. *Nanoscale* **2019**, *11*, 22316–22327. [CrossRef] [PubMed]
148. He, S.; Lamers, G.E.; Beenakker, J.W.M.; Cui, C.; Ghotra, V.P.; Danen, E.H.; Meijer, A.H.; Spaink, H.P.; Snaar-Jagalska, B.E. Neutrophil-mediated experimental metastasis is enhanced by VEGFR inhibition in a zebrafish xenograft model. *J. Pathol.* **2012**, *227*, 431–445. [CrossRef]
149. Roh-Johnson, M.; Shah, A.N.; Stonick, J.A.; Poudel, K.R.; Kargl, J.; Yang, G.H.; di Martino, J.; Hernandez, R.E.; Gast, C.E.; Zarour, L.R.; et al. Macrophage-Dependent Cytoplasmic Transfer during Melanoma Invasion In Vivo. *Dev. Cell* **2017**, *43*, 549–562.e6. [CrossRef] [PubMed]
150. Britto, D.D.; Wyroba, B.; Chen, W.; Lockwood, R.A.; Tran, K.B.; Shepherd, P.R.; Hall, C.J.; Crosier, K.E.; Crosier, P.S.; Astin, J.W. Macrophages enhance Vegfa-driven angiogenesis in an embryonic zebrafish tumour xenograft model. *Dis. Models Mech.* **2018**, *11*, dmm035998. [CrossRef] [PubMed]
151. Seoane, S.; Martinez-Ordoñez, A.; Eiro, N.; Cabezas-Sainz, P.; Garcia-Caballero, L.; Gonzalez, L.O.; Macia, M.; Sanchez, L.; Vizoso, F.; Perez-Fernandez, R. POU1F1 transcription factor promotes breast cancer metastasis via recruitment and polarization of macrophages. *J. Pathol.* **2019**, *249*, 381–394. [CrossRef] [PubMed]
152. Póvoa, V.; Rebelo de Almeida, C.; Maia-Gil, M.; Sobral, D.; Domingues, M.; Martinez-Lopez, M.; de Almeida Fuzeta, M.; Silva, C.; Grosso, A.R.; Fior, R. Innate immune evasion revealed in a colorectal zebrafish xenograft model. *Nat. Commun.* **2021**, *12*, 1156. [CrossRef]
153. Lieschke, G.J.; Oates, A.C.; Crowhurst, M.O.; Ward, A.C.; Layton, J.E. Morphologic and functional characterization of granulocytes and macrophages in embryonic and adult zebrafish. *Blood* **2001**, *98*, 3087–3096. [CrossRef]
154. Stoletov, K.; Montel, V.; Lester, R.D.; Gonias, S.L.; Klemke, R. High-resolution imaging of the dynamic tumor cell vascular interface in transparent zebrafish. *Proc. Natl. Acad. Sci. USA* **2007**, *104*, 17406–17411. [CrossRef]
155. Heilmann, S.; Ratnakumar, K.; Langdon, E.M.; Kansler, E.R.; Kim, I.S.; Campbell, N.R.; Perry, E.B.; McMahon, A.J.; Kaufman, C.K.; van Rooijen, E.; et al. A Quantitative System for Studying Metastasis Using Transparent Zebrafish. *Cancer Res.* **2015**, *75*, 4272. [CrossRef]
156. Traver, D.; Winzeler, A.; Stern, H.M.; Mayhall, E.A.; Langenau, D.M.; Kutok, J.L.; Look, A.T.; Zon, L.I. Effects of lethal irradiation in zebrafish and rescue by hematopoietic cell transplantation. *Blood* **2004**, *104*, 1298–1305. [CrossRef] [PubMed]
157. Tang, Q.; Abdelfattah, N.S.; Blackburn, J.S.; Moore, J.C.; Martinez, S.A.; Moore, F.E.; Lobbardi, R.; Tenente, I.M.; Ignatius, M.S.; Berman, J.N. Optimized cell transplantation using adult rag2 mutant zebrafish. *Nat. Methods* **2014**, *11*, 821–824. [CrossRef] [PubMed]
158. Moore, J.C.; Tang, Q.; Yordán, N.T.; Moore, F.E.; Garcia, E.G.; Lobbardi, R.; Ramakrishnan, A.; Marvin, D.L.; Anselmo, A.; Sadreyev, R.I.; et al. Single-cell imaging of normal and malignant cell engraftment into optically clear prkdc-null SCID zebrafish. *J. Exp. Med.* **2016**, *213*, 2575–2589. [CrossRef] [PubMed]
159. Yan, C.; Brunson, D.C.; Tang, Q.; Do, D.; Iftimia, N.A.; Moore, J.C.; Hayes, M.N.; Welker, A.M.; Garcia, E.G.; Dubash, T.D.; et al. Visualizing Engrafted Human Cancer and Therapy Responses in Immunodeficient Zebrafish. *Cell* **2019**, *177*, 1903–1914.e14. [CrossRef] [PubMed]
160. Yan, C.; Yang, Q.; Do, D.; Brunson, D.C.; Langenau, D.M. Adult immune compromised zebrafish for xenograft cell transplantation studies. *EBioMedicine* **2019**, *47*, 24–26. [CrossRef]
161. Xiao, J.; Glasgow, E.; Agarwal, S. Zebrafish Xenografts for Drug Discovery and Personalized Medicine. *Trends Cancer* **2020**, *6*, 569–579. [CrossRef]
162. Yan, C.; Do, D.; Yang, Q.; Brunson, D.C.; Rawls, J.F.; Langenau, D.M. Single-cell imaging of human cancer xenografts using adult immunodeficient zebrafish. *Nat. Protoc.* **2020**, *15*, 3105–3128. [CrossRef]
163. Wawrzyniak, M.; Scharl, M. Genetics and epigenetics of inflammatory bowel disease. *Swiss Med. Wkly.* **2018**, *148*, w14671. [CrossRef]
164. Uhlig, H.H.; Powrie, F. Translating Immunology into Therapeutic Concepts for Inflammatory Bowel Disease. *Annu. Rev. Immunol.* **2018**, *36*, 755–781. [CrossRef]
165. Yoo, J.Y.; Groer, M.; Dutra, S.V.O.; Sarkar, A.; McSkimming, D.I. Gut Microbiota and Immune System Interactions. *Microorganisms* **2020**, *8*, 1587. [CrossRef]
166. Smythies, L.E.; Sellers, M.; Clements, R.H.; Mosteller-Barnum, M.; Meng, G.; Benjamin, W.H.; Orenstein, J.M.; Smith, P.D. Human intestinal macrophages display profound inflammatory anergy despite avid phagocytic and bacteriocidal activity. *J. Clin. Investig.* **2005**, *115*, 66–75. [CrossRef] [PubMed]

167. Wang, J.; Chen, W.D.; Wang, Y.D. The Relationship Between Gut Microbiota and Inflammatory Diseases: The Role of Macrophages. *Front. Microbiol.* **2020**, *11*, 1065. [CrossRef]
168. Hedrera, M.I.; Galdames, J.A.; Jimenez-Reyes, M.F.; Reyes, A.E.; Avendaño-Herrera, R.; Romero, J.; Feijóo, C.G. Soybean meal induces intestinal inflammation in zebrafish larvae. *PLoS ONE* **2013**, *8*, e69983. [CrossRef]
169. Coronado, M.; Solis, C.J.; Hernandez, P.P.; Feijóo, C.G. Soybean Meal-Induced Intestinal Inflammation in Zebrafish Is T Cell-Dependent and Has a Th17 Cytokine Profile. *Front. Immunol.* **2019**, *10*, 610. [CrossRef]
170. Kaya, B.; Doñas, C.; Wuggenig, P.; Diaz, O.E.; Morales, R.A.; Melhem, H.; Hernández, P.P.; Kaymak, T.; Das, S.; Hruz, P.; et al. Lysophosphatidic Acid-Mediated GPR35 Signaling in CX3CR1+ Macrophages Regulates Intestinal Homeostasis. *Cell Rep.* **2020**, *32*, 107979. [CrossRef] [PubMed]
171. Jardine, S.; Anderson, S.; Babcock, S.; Leung, G.; Pan, J.; Dhingani, N.; Warner, N.; Guo, C.; Siddiqui, I.; Kotlarz, D.; et al. Drug Screen Identifies Leflunomide for Treatment of Inflammatory Bowel Disease Caused by TTC7A Deficiency. *Gastroenterology* **2020**, *158*, 1000–1015. [CrossRef] [PubMed]
172. Sheng, Y.; Li, H.; Liu, M.; Xie, B.; Wei, W.; Wu, J.; Meng, F.; Wang, H.Y.; Chen, S. A Manganese-Superoxide Dismutase From Thermus thermophilus HB27 Suppresses Inflammatory Responses and Alleviates Experimentally Induced Colitis. *Inflamm. Bowel Dis.* **2019**, *25*, 1644–1655. [CrossRef]
173. Ge, H.; Tang, H.; Liang, Y.; Wu, J.; Yang, Q.; Zeng, L.; Ma, Z. Rhein attenuates inflammation through inhibition of NF-κB and NALP3 inflammasome in vivo and in vitro. *Drug Des. Dev. Ther.* **2017**, *11*, 1663–1671. [CrossRef] [PubMed]
174. Zhao, G.; Zhang, T.; Sun, H.; Liu, J.X. Copper nanoparticles induce zebrafish intestinal defects via endoplasmic reticulum and oxidative stress. *Metallomics* **2020**, *12*, 12–22. [CrossRef]
175. Eizirik, D.L.; Pasquali, L.; Cnop, M. Pancreatic β-cells in type 1 and type 2 diabetes mellitus: Different pathways to failure. *Nat. Rev. Endocrinol.* **2020**, *16*, 349–362. [CrossRef]
176. Cerna, M. Epigenetic Regulation in Etiology of Type 1 Diabetes Mellitus. *Int. J. Mol. Sci.* **2019**, *21*, 36. [CrossRef] [PubMed]
177. Hu, Q.; Luo, Y. Recent advances of polysaccharide-based nanoparticles for oral insulin delivery. *Int. J. Biol. Macromol.* **2018**, *120*, 775–782. [CrossRef]
178. Wong, C.Y.; Al-Salami, H.; Dass, C.R. Potential of insulin nanoparticle formulations for oral delivery and diabetes treatment. *J. Control. Release* **2017**, *264*, 247–275. [CrossRef] [PubMed]
179. Xu, X.; Bian, L.; Shen, M.; Li, X.; Zhu, J.; Chen, S.; Xiao, L.; Zhang, Q.; Chen, H.; Xu, K.; et al. Multipeptide-coupled nanoparticles induce tolerance in 'humanised' HLA-transgenic mice and inhibit diabetogenic CD8+ T cell responses in type 1 diabetes. *Diabetologia* **2017**, *60*, 2418–2431. [CrossRef] [PubMed]
180. Prasad, S.; Neef, T.; Xu, D.; Podojil, J.R.; Getts, D.R.; Shea, L.D.; Miller, S.D. Tolerogenic Ag-PLG nanoparticles induce tregs to suppress activated diabetogenic CD4 and CD8 T cells. *J. Autoimmun.* **2018**, *89*, 112–124. [CrossRef] [PubMed]
181. Delaspre, F.; Beer, R.L.; Rovira, M.; Huang, W.; Wang, G.; Gee, S.; Vitery, M.d.C.; Wheelan, S.J.; Parsons, M.J. Centroacinar Cells Are Progenitors That Contribute to Endocrine Pancreas Regeneration. *Diabetes* **2015**, *64*, 3499–3509. [CrossRef]
182. Castañeda, R.; Rodriguez, I.; Nam, Y.H.; Hong, B.N.; Kang, T.H. Trigonelline promotes auditory function through nerve growth factor signaling on diabetic animal models. *Phytomedicine* **2017**, *36*, 128–136. [CrossRef] [PubMed]
183. Ye, L.; Robertson, M.A.; Hesselson, D.; Stainier, D.Y.R.; Anderson, R.M. Glucagon is essential for alpha cell transdifferentiation and beta cell neogenesis. *Dev. (Camb. Engl.)* **2015**, *142*, 1407–1417. [CrossRef] [PubMed]
184. Zang, L.; Maddison, L.A.; Chen, W. Zebrafish as a Model for Obesity and Diabetes. *Front. Cell Dev. Biol.* **2018**, *6*, 91. [CrossRef]
185. Yang, B.; Covington, B.A.; Chen, W. In vivo generation and regeneration of β cells in zebrafish. *Cell Regen.* **2020**, *9*, 9. [CrossRef]
186. Lu, J.; Liu, K.-C.; Schulz, N.; Karampelias, C.; Charbord, J.; Hilding, A.; Rautio, L.; Bertolino, P.; Östenson, C.-G.; Brismar, K.; et al. IGFBP1 increases β-cell regeneration by promoting α- to β-cell transdifferentiation. *EMBO J.* **2016**, *35*, 2026–2044. [CrossRef] [PubMed]
187. Liu, K.C.; Leuckx, G.; Sakano, D.; Seymour, P.A.; Mattsson, C.L.; Rautio, L.; Staels, W.; Verdonck, Y.; Serup, P.; Kume, S.; et al. Inhibition of Cdk5 Promotes β-Cell Differentiation From Ductal Progenitors. *Diabetes* **2018**, *67*, 58–70. [CrossRef] [PubMed]
188. Wang, G.; Rajpurohit, S.K.; Delaspre, F.; Walker, S.L.; White, D.T.; Ceasrine, A.; Kuruvilla, R.; Li, R.J.; Shim, J.S.; Liu, J.O.; et al. First quantitative high-throughput screen in zebrafish identifies novel pathways for increasing pancreatic β-cell mass. *eLife* **2015**, *4*, e08261. [CrossRef]
189. Garcia Campoy, A.H.; Perez Gutierrez, R.M.; Manriquez-Alvirde, G.; Muñiz Ramirez, A. Protection of silver nanoparticles using Eysenhardtia polystachya in peroxide-induced pancreatic β-Cell damage and their antidiabetic properties in zebrafish. *Int. J. Nanomed.* **2018**, *13*, 2601–2612. [CrossRef] [PubMed]
190. Wang, S.; Du, S.; Wang, W.; Zhang, F. Therapeutic investigation of quercetin nanomedicine in a zebrafish model of diabetic retinopathy. *Biomed. Pharmacother.* **2020**, *130*, 110573. [CrossRef]
191. Singha, S.; Shao, K.; Yang, Y.; Clemente-Casares, X.; Solé, P.; Clemente, A.; Blanco, J.; Dai, Q.; Song, F.; Liu, S.W.; et al. Peptide–MHC-based nanomedicines for autoimmunity function as T-cell receptor microclustering devices. *Nat. Nanotechnol.* **2017**, *12*, 701–710. [CrossRef]
192. Youssouf, L.; Bhaw-Luximon, A.; Diotel, N.; Catan, A.; Giraud, P.; Gimié, F.; Koshel, D.; Casale, S.; Bénard, S.; Meneyrol, V.; et al. Enhanced effects of curcumin encapsulated in polycaprolactone-grafted oligocarrageenan nanomicelles, a novel nanoparticle drug delivery system. *Carbohydr. Polym.* **2019**, *217*, 35–45. [CrossRef]

193. Tateiwa, D.; Yoshikawa, H.; Kaito, T. Cartilage and Bone Destruction in Arthritis: Pathogenesis and Treatment Strategy: A Literature Review. *Cells* **2019**, *8*, 818. [CrossRef]
194. Anfray, C.; Mainini, F.; Andón, F.T. Chapter 11—Nanoparticles for immunotherapy. In *Frontiers of Nanoscience*; Parak, W.J., Feliu, N., Eds.; Elsevier: Amsterdam, The Netherlands, 2020; Volume 16, pp. 265–306.
195. Gambari, L.; Grassi, F.; Roseti, L.; Grigolo, B.; Desando, G. Learning from Monocyte-Macrophage Fusion and Multinucleation: Potential Therapeutic Targets for Osteoporosis and Rheumatoid Arthritis. *Int. J. Mol. Sci.* **2020**, *21*, 6001. [CrossRef]
196. Yang, X.; Chang, Y.; Wei, W. Emerging role of targeting macrophages in rheumatoid arthritis: Focus on polarization, metabolism and apoptosis. *Cell Prolif.* **2020**, *53*, e12854. [CrossRef]
197. Li, P.; Zheng, Y.; Chen, X. Drugs for Autoimmune Inflammatory Diseases: From Small Molecule Compounds to Anti-TNF Biologics. *Front. Pharmacol.* **2017**, *8*, 460. [CrossRef] [PubMed]
198. Yang, Y.; Guo, L.; Wang, Z.; Liu, P.; Liu, X.; Ding, J.; Zhou, W. Targeted silver nanoparticles for rheumatoid arthritis therapy via macrophage apoptosis and Re-polarization. *Biomaterials* **2020**, *264*, 120390. [CrossRef] [PubMed]
199. Wu, H.; Su, S.; Wu, Y.; Wu, Y.; Zhang, Z.; Chen, Q. Nanoparticle-facilitated delivery of BAFF-R siRNA for B cell intervention and rheumatoid arthritis therapy. *Int. Immunopharmacol.* **2020**, *88*, 106933. [CrossRef] [PubMed]
200. Nguyen, T.H.; Le, H.D.; Kim, T.N.T.; The, H.P.; Nguyen, T.M.; Cornet, V.; Lambert, J.; Kestemont, P. Anti-Inflammatory and Antioxidant Properties of the Ethanol Extract of Clerodendrum Cyrtophyllum Turcz in Copper Sulfate-Induced Inflammation in Zebrafish. *Antioxidants* **2020**, *9*, 192. [CrossRef] [PubMed]
201. Jiang, Y.; Li, H.Y.; Li, X.H.; Lu, J.; Zhang, Q.; Bai, C.G.; Chen, Y. Therapeutic effects of isothiocyanate prodrugs on rheumatoid arthritis. *Bioorganic Med. Chem. Lett.* **2018**, *28*, 737–741. [CrossRef] [PubMed]
202. Wang, Y.M.; Xu, M.; Wang, D.; Yang, C.R.; Zeng, Y.; Zhang, Y.J. Anti-inflammatory compounds of "Qin-Jiao", the roots of Gentiana dahurica (Gentianaceae). *J. Ethnopharmacol.* **2013**, *147*, 341–348. [CrossRef]
203. Dorris, E.R.; Tazzyman, S.J.; Moylett, J.; Ramamoorthi, N.; Hackney, J.; Townsend, M.; Muthana, M.; Lewis, M.J.; Pitzalis, C.; Wilson, A.G. The Autoimmune Susceptibility Gene C5orf30 Regulates Macrophage-Mediated Resolution of Inflammation. *J. Immunol. (Baltim. Md.)* **2019**, *202*, 1069–1078. [CrossRef]
204. Feng, H.; Zhang, Z.; Meng, Q.; Jia, H.; Wang, Y.; Zhang, R. Rapid Response Fluorescence Probe Enabled In Vivo Diagnosis and Assessing Treatment Response of Hypochlorous Acid-Mediated Rheumatoid Arthritis. *Adv. Sci. (Weinh. Baden-Wurtt. Ger.)* **2018**, *5*, 1800397. [CrossRef]
205. Sunke, R.; Bankala, R.; Thirupataiah, B.; Ramarao, E.V.V.S.; Kumar, J.S.; Doss, H.M.; Medishetti, R.; Kulkarni, P.; Kapavarapu, R.K.; Rasool, M.; et al. InCl3 mediated heteroarylation of indoles and their derivatization via CH activation strategy: Discovery of 2-(1H-indol-3-yl)-quinoxaline derivatives as a new class of PDE4B selective inhibitors for arthritis and/or multiple sclerosis. *Eur. J. Med. Chem.* **2019**, *174*, 198–215. [CrossRef]
206. Gao, X.Y.; Li, K.; Jiang, L.L.; He, M.F.; Pu, C.H.; Kang, D.; Xie, J. Developmental toxicity of auranofin in zebrafish embryos. *J. Appl. Toxicol. JAT* **2017**, *37*, 602–610. [CrossRef]
207. Stella, S.L., Jr.; Geathers, J.S.; Weber, S.R.; Grillo, M.A.; Barber, A.J.; Sundstrom, J.M.; Grillo, S.L. Neurodegeneration, Neuroprotection and Regeneration in the Zebrafish Retina. *Cells* **2021**, *10*, 633. [CrossRef]
208. Lee, J.G.; Cho, H.J.; Jeong, Y.M.; Lee, J.S. Genetic Approaches Using Zebrafish to Study the Microbiota-Gut-Brain Axis in Neurological Disorders. *Cells* **2021**, *10*, 566. [CrossRef] [PubMed]
209. Zhang, W.; Mehta, A.; Tong, Z.; Esser, L.; Voelcker, N.H. Development of Polymeric Nanoparticles for Blood-Brain Barrier Transfer-Strategies and Challenges. *Adv. Sci. (Weinh. Baden-Wurtt. Ger.)* **2021**, *8*, 2003937. [CrossRef]
210. Zorkina, Y.; Abramova, O.; Ushakova, V.; Morozova, A.; Zubkov, E.; Valikhov, M.; Melnikov, P.; Majouga, A.; Chekhonin, V. Nano Carrier Drug Delivery Systems for the Treatment of Neuropsychiatric Disorders: Advantages and Limitations. *Molecules* **2020**, *25*, 5294. [CrossRef]
211. Nellore, J.; Pauline, C.; Amarnath, K. Bacopa monnieri Phytochemicals Mediated Synthesis of Platinum Nanoparticles and Its Neurorescue Effect on 1-Methyl 4-Phenyl 1,2,3,6 Tetrahydropyridine-Induced Experimental Parkinsonism in Zebrafish. *J. Neurodegener. Dis.* **2013**, *2013*, 972391. [CrossRef] [PubMed]
212. Chen, T.; Li, C.; Li, Y.; Yi, X.; Lee, S.M.; Zheng, Y. Oral Delivery of a Nanocrystal Formulation of Schisantherin A with Improved Bioavailability and Brain Delivery for the Treatment of Parkinson's Disease. *Mol. Pharm.* **2016**, *13*, 3864–3875. [CrossRef]
213. Hu, Q.; Guo, F.; Zhao, F.; Fu, Z. Effects of titanium dioxide nanoparticles exposure on parkinsonism in zebrafish larvae and PC12. *Chemosphere* **2017**, *173*, 373–379. [CrossRef] [PubMed]
214. Li, X.; Liu, B.; Li, X.L.; Li, Y.X.; Sun, M.Z.; Chen, D.Y.; Zhao, X.; Feng, X.Z. SiO_2 nanoparticles change colour preference and cause Parkinson's-like behaviour in zebrafish. *Sci. Rep.* **2014**, *4*, 3810. [CrossRef]
215. Chen, T.; Liu, W.; Xiong, S.; Li, D.; Fang, S.; Wu, Z.; Wang, Q.; Chen, X. Nanoparticles Mediating the Sustained Puerarin Release Facilitate Improved Brain Delivery to Treat Parkinson's Disease. *ACS Appl. Mater. Interfaces* **2019**, *11*, 45276–45289. [CrossRef]
216. Xiong, S.; Liu, W.; Li, D.; Chen, X.; Liu, F.; Yuan, D.; Pan, H.; Wang, Q.; Fang, S.; Chen, T. Oral Delivery of Puerarin Nanocrystals To Improve Brain Accumulation and Anti-Parkinsonian Efficacy. *Mol. Pharm.* **2019**, *16*, 1444–1455. [CrossRef]
217. Zhao, Y.; Xiong, S.; Liu, P.; Liu, W.; Wang, Q.; Liu, Y.; Tan, H.; Chen, X.; Shi, X.; Wang, Q.; et al. Polymeric Nanoparticles-Based Brain Delivery with Improved Therapeutic Efficacy of Ginkgolide B in Parkinson's Disease. *Int. J. Nanomed.* **2020**, *15*, 10453–10467. [CrossRef] [PubMed]

218. Javed, I.; Peng, G.; Xing, Y.; Yu, T.; Zhao, M.; Kakinen, A.; Faridi, A.; Parish, C.L.; Ding, F.; Davis, T.P.; et al. Inhibition of amyloid beta toxicity in zebrafish with a chaperone-gold nanoparticle dual strategy. *Nat. Commun.* **2019**, *10*, 3780. [CrossRef] [PubMed]
219. Rishitha, N.; Muthuraman, A. Therapeutic evaluation of solid lipid nanoparticle of quercetin in pentylenetetrazole induced cognitive impairment of zebrafish. *Life Sci.* **2018**, *199*, 80–87. [CrossRef] [PubMed]
220. Zhou, Y.; Liyanage, P.Y.; Devadoss, D.; Rios Guevara, L.R.; Cheng, L.; Graham, R.M.; Chand, H.S.; Al-Youbi, A.O.; Bashammakh, A.S.; El-Shahawi, M.S.; et al. Nontoxic amphiphilic carbon dots as promising drug nanocarriers across the blood-brain barrier and inhibitors of β-amyloid. *Nanoscale* **2019**, *11*, 22387–22397. [CrossRef] [PubMed]
221. Chen, L.; Watson, C.; Morsch, M.; Cole, N.J.; Chung, R.S.; Saunders, D.N.; Yerbury, J.J.; Vine, K.L. Improving the Delivery of SOD1 Antisense Oligonucleotides to Motor Neurons Using Calcium Phosphate-Lipid Nanoparticles. *Front. Neurosci.* **2017**, *11*, 476. [CrossRef] [PubMed]
222. Igartúa, D.E.; Martinez, C.S.; Temprana, C.F.; Alonso, S.D.V.; Prieto, M.J. PAMAM dendrimers as a carbamazepine delivery system for neurodegenerative diseases: A biophysical and nanotoxicological characterization. *Int. J. Pharm.* **2018**, *544*, 191–202. [CrossRef] [PubMed]
223. Igartúa, D.E.; Martinez, C.S.; Del, V.A.S.; Prieto, M.J. Combined Therapy for Alzheimer's Disease: Tacrine and PAMAM Dendrimers Co-Administration Reduces the Side Effects of the Drug without Modifying its Activity. *AAPS PharmSciTech* **2020**, *21*, 110. [CrossRef] [PubMed]
224. Thwaite, R.; Ji, J.; Torrealba, D.; Coll, J.; Sabés, M.; Villaverde, A.; Roher, N. Protein Nanoparticles Made of Recombinant Viral Antigens: A Promising Biomaterial for Oral Delivery of Fish Prophylactics. *Front. Immunol.* **2018**, *9*, 1652. [CrossRef]
225. Sullivan, C.; Kim, C.H. Zebrafish as a model for infectious disease and immune function. *Fish. Shellfish. Immunol.* **2008**, *25*, 341–350. [CrossRef]
226. Levraud, J.P.; Palha, N.; Langevin, C.; Boudinot, P. Through the looking glass: Witnessing host-virus interplay in zebrafish. *Trends Microbiol.* **2014**, *22*, 490–497. [CrossRef]
227. Torraca, V.; Masud, S.; Spaink, H.P.; Meijer, A.H. Macrophage-pathogen interactions in infectious diseases: New therapeutic insights from the zebrafish host model. *Dis. Model. Mech.* **2014**, *7*, 785–797. [CrossRef]
228. Palha, N.; Guivel-Benhassine, F.; Briolat, V.; Lutfalla, G.; Sourisseau, M.; Ellett, F.; Wang, C.H.; Lieschke, G.J.; Herbomel, P.; Schwartz, O.; et al. Real-time whole-body visualization of Chikungunya Virus infection and host interferon response in zebrafish. *PLoS Pathog.* **2013**, *9*, e1003619. [CrossRef] [PubMed]
229. Mesureur, J.; Feliciano, J.R.; Wagner, N.; Gomes, M.C.; Zhang, L.; Blanco-Gonzalez, M.; van der Vaart, M.; O'Callaghan, D.; Meijer, A.H.; Vergunst, A.C. Macrophages, but not neutrophils, are critical for proliferation of Burkholderia cenocepacia and ensuing host-damaging inflammation. *PLoS Pathog.* **2017**, *13*, e1006437. [CrossRef] [PubMed]
230. Bouz, G.; Al Hasawi, N. The zebrafish model of tuberculosis-no lungs needed. *Crit. Rev. Microbiol.* **2018**, *44*, 779–792. [CrossRef]
231. Clay, H.; Davis, J.M.; Beery, D.; Huttenlocher, A.; Lyons, S.E.; Ramakrishnan, L. Dichotomous role of the macrophage in early Mycobacterium marinum infection of the zebrafish. *Cell Host Microbe* **2007**, *2*, 29–39. [CrossRef]
232. Davis, J.M.; Ramakrishnan, L. The role of the granuloma in expansion and dissemination of early tuberculous infection. *Cell* **2009**, *136*, 37–49. [CrossRef]
233. Chao, C.C.; Hsu, P.C.; Jen, C.F.; Chen, I.H.; Wang, C.H.; Chan, H.C.; Tsai, P.W.; Tung, K.C.; Wang, C.H.; Lan, C.Y.; et al. Zebrafish as a model host for Candida albicans infection. *Infect. Immun.* **2010**, *78*, 2512–2521. [CrossRef] [PubMed]
234. Burgos, J.S.; Ripoll-Gomez, J.; Alfaro, J.M.; Sastre, I.; Valdivieso, F. Zebrafish as a new model for herpes simplex virus type 1 infection. *Zebrafish* **2008**, *5*, 323–333. [CrossRef] [PubMed]
235. Phennicie, R.T.; Sullivan, M.J.; Singer, J.T.; Yoder, J.A.; Kim, C.H. Specific resistance to Pseudomonas aeruginosa infection in zebrafish is mediated by the cystic fibrosis transmembrane conductance regulator. *Infect. Immun.* **2010**, *78*, 4542–4550. [CrossRef] [PubMed]
236. Rounioja, S.; Saralahti, A.; Rantala, L.; Parikka, M.; Henriques-Normark, B.; Silvennoinen, O.; Rämet, M. Defense of zebrafish embryos against Streptococcus pneumoniae infection is dependent on the phagocytic activity of leukocytes. *Dev. Comp. Immunol.* **2012**, *36*, 342–348. [CrossRef]
237. Schmidt, J.G.; Korbut, R.; Ohtani, M.; Jørgensen, L.V.G. Zebrafish (*Danio rerio*) as a model to visualize infection dynamics of *Vibrio anguillarum* following intraperitoneal injection and bath exposure. *Fish Shellfish. Immunol.* **2017**, *67*, 692–697. [CrossRef]
238. Lin, B.; Chen, S.; Cao, Z.; Lin, Y.; Mo, D.; Zhang, H.; Gu, J.; Dong, M.; Liu, Z.; Xu, A. Acute phase response in zebrafish upon Aeromonas salmonicida and Staphylococcus aureus infection: Striking similarities and obvious differences with mammals. *Mol. Immunol.* **2007**, *44*, 295–301. [CrossRef]
239. Korbut, R.; Mehrdana, F.; Kania, P.W.; Larsen, M.H.; Frees, D.; Dalsgaard, I.; Jørgensen, L. Antigen Uptake during Different Life Stages of Zebrafish (*Danio rerio*) Using a GFP-Tagged Yersinia ruckeri. *PLoS ONE* **2016**, *11*, e0158968. [CrossRef] [PubMed]
240. Lohi, O.; Parikka, M.; Rämet, M. The zebrafish as a model for paediatric diseases. *Acta Paediatr. (Oslo Nor.)* **2013**, *102*, 104–110. [CrossRef] [PubMed]
241. Jørgensen, L.V.G. Zebrafish as a Model for Fish Diseases in Aquaculture. *Pathogens* **2020**, *9*, 609. [CrossRef]
242. Oksanen, K.E.; Halfpenny, N.J.; Sherwood, E.; Harjula, S.K.; Hammarén, M.M.; Ahava, M.J.; Pajula, E.T.; Lahtinen, M.J.; Parikka, M.; Rämet, M. An adult zebrafish model for preclinical tuberculosis vaccine development. *Vaccine* **2013**, *31*, 5202–5209. [CrossRef]

243. Torrealba, D.; Parra, D.; Seras-Franzoso, J.; Vallejos-Vidal, E.; Yero, D.; Gibert, I.; Villaverde, A.; Garcia-Fruitós, E.; Roher, N. Nanostructured recombinant cytokines: A highly stable alternative to short-lived prophylactics. *Biomaterials* **2016**, *107*, 102–114. [CrossRef] [PubMed]
244. Kavaliauskis, A.; Arnemo, M.; Speth, M.; Lagos, L.; Rishovd, A.L.; Estepa, A.; Griffiths, G.; Gjøen, T. Protective effect of a recombinant VHSV-G vaccine using poly(I:C) loaded nanoparticles as an adjuvant in zebrafish (*Danio rerio*) infection model. *Dev. Comp. Immunol.* **2016**, *61*, 248–257. [CrossRef]
245. Tandberg, J.; Lagos, L.; Ropstad, E.; Smistad, G.; Hiorth, M.; Winther-Larsen, H.C. The Use of Chitosan-Coated Membrane Vesicles for Immunization against Salmonid Rickettsial Septicemia in an Adult Zebrafish Model. *Zebrafish* **2018**, *15*, 372–381. [CrossRef] [PubMed]
246. Díez-Martínez, R.; García-Fernández, E.; Manzano, M.; Martínez, Á.; Domenech, M.; Vallet-Regí, M.; García, P. Auranofin-loaded nanoparticles as a new therapeutic tool to fight streptococcal infections. *Sci. Rep.* **2016**, *6*, 19525. [CrossRef]

nanomaterials

MDPI

Review

Therapeutic Manipulation of Macrophages Using Nanotechnological Approaches for the Treatment of Osteoarthritis

Aldo Ummarino [1,2], Francesco Manlio Gambaro [1], Elizaveta Kon [1,2,*,†] and Fernando Torres Andón [2,3,*,†]

1 Department of Biomedical Sciences, Humanitas University, Via Rita Levi Montalcini 4, 20090 Pieve Emanuele, Milan, Italy; aldo.ummarino@hunimed.eu (A.U.); francescomanlio.gambaro@st.hunimed.eu (F.M.G.)
2 IRCCS Istituto Clinico Humanitas, Via A. Manzoni 56, 20089 Rozzano, Milan, Italy
3 Center for Research in Molecular Medicine & Chronic Diseases (CIMUS), Universidade de Santiago de Compostela, Campus Vida, 15706 Santiago de Compostela, Spain
* Correspondence: elizaveta.kon@humanitas.it (E.K.); Fernando.torres.andon@usc.es (F.T.A.)
† These authors equally contributed to the present review.

Received: 24 June 2020; Accepted: 7 August 2020; Published: 9 August 2020

Abstract: Osteoarthritis (OA) is the most common joint pathology causing severe pain and disability. Macrophages play a central role in the pathogenesis of OA. In the joint microenvironment, macrophages with an M1-like pro-inflammatory phenotype induce chronic inflammation and joint destruction, and they have been correlated with the development and progression of the disease, while the M2-like anti-inflammatory macrophages support the recovery of the disease, promoting tissue repair and the resolution of inflammation. Nowadays, the treatment of OA in the clinic relies on systemic and/or intra-articular administration of anti-inflammatory and pain relief drugs, as well as surgical interventions for the severe cases (i.e., meniscectomy). The disadvantages of the pharmacological therapy are related to the chronic nature of the disease, requiring prolonged treatments, and to the particular location of the pathology in joint tissues, which are separated anatomical compartments with difficult access for the drugs. To overcome these challenges, nanotechnological approaches have been investigated to improve the delivery of drugs toward macrophages into the diseased joint. This strategy may offer advantages by reducing off-target toxicities and improving long-term therapeutic efficacy. In this review, we describe the nanomaterial-based approaches designed so far to directly or indirectly manipulate macrophages for the treatment of osteoarthritis.

Keywords: nanomaterial; macrophage; nanoparticle; drug delivery; immune system; anti-inflammatory; innate immunity; osteoarthritis

1. Introduction

Osteoarthritis (OA) is the most common joint pathology, affecting approximately 33% of the population above 65 years of age with a predilection for the female gender [1]. This disease is able to potentially affect every joint of the human body, but most commonly affecting the knee (85% of the worldwide burden of OA) [2], followed by the hip and the hand joints [3]. The progression of OA pathology results in pain and functional disability, which impact severely on patient's quality of life, making this condition expected to be the 4th leading cause of chronic disability worldwide by the year 2020 [4].

Macrophages are key regulators of OA physiopathology. These innate immune cells trigger the inflammatory response in the joint microenvironment through the secretion of cytokines and other molecular mediators, control the activity of the adaptive immune system, and also influence other cells such as chondrocytes [5]. Macrophages are characterized by a high plasticity dictated by their continuous adaptation and response to specific local stimuli [6]. At the edges of this continuum polarization status of macrophages, two extreme phenotypes can be defined, which have been characterized in terms of gene expression, the pattern of surface molecules, and the production of biological mediators and metabolites [7]. The presence of lipopolysaccharide (LPS), interferon gamma (IFN-γ), and tumor necrosis factor alpha (TNF-α) induces the polarization of macrophages toward an M1-like phenotype, presenting pro-inflammatory functions with the release of interleukin (IL)-1β, IL-6, IL-12, IL-23, and TNF-α [8]. Conversely, their exposure to IL-4 and IL-13 polarizes macrophages toward an M2-like phenotype, which confers to these cells an anti-inflammatory behavior, secreting IL-10 and TGF-β, among others [9]. In OA joints, an imbalance between M1 and M2 macrophages has been observed, with an increase of the first subset that accelerates the onset of the pathology and the related symptoms [10]. Taking into account this knowledge, the reprogramming of M1-like macrophages toward M2-like anti-inflammatory effectors appears to be a reasonable strategy for the treatment of OA-related inflammation.

Most frequently, drugs, such as non-steroidal anti-inflammatory drugs (NSAIDs) or corticosteroids, but also other molecular approaches, for example cytokine-blocking antibodies, anti-inflammatory peptides, or even hyaluronic acid, have been given systemically or locally injected in the joints to ameliorate inflammation [11,12]. Several investigations have studied the pros and cons of different treatments and routes of administration. Systemic (oral) administration is typically used in the clinic, although it is discouraged due to the little amount of drug administered that effectively reaches its target diseased tissue, as well as adverse effects of anti-inflammatory compounds in off-target organs [13]. The intra-articular administration of drugs locally, mainly corticosteroids [14], has been applied in the clinic and also explored in basic research with different methodological approaches [15]. However, this strategy comes also with several obstacles, such as short-term efficacy, in part due to lymphatic and blood drainage of the drug in less than 2 h from the joint [16], and uncomfortable application, typically requiring multiple injections. Specific macrophage targeting has been barely explored, although this strategy may have the advantage to reduce the amount of drug reaching other cells into the joint, such as chondrocytes or fibroblasts.

Nanotechnological approaches offer a wide range of possibilities to overcome these issues, as different nanomaterials can be now engineered to load and deliver therapeutic molecules in a controlled release manner and even help the drug reach specific cell populations, such as macrophages. Indeed, the phagocytic nature of macrophages has been demonstrated to significantly favor the uptake and accumulation of nanostructures, at inflamed sites, inside these immune cells versus other cellular or extracellular compartments [17–19]. In the last decade, numerous types of nanocarriers have been engineered, such as nanoparticles, liposomes, or hybrid nanosystems to improve the delivery of drugs toward macrophages in the diseased joints (Figure 1). Interestingly, also some nanostructures have been designed to prevent macrophage uptake to slow down the drug consumption and prolong the therapeutic effect [20,21]. In this manuscript, we review the nano-based drug delivery strategies aimed to manipulate the immune system in the context of OA, with a particular focus on those designed to specifically target and reprogram macrophages.

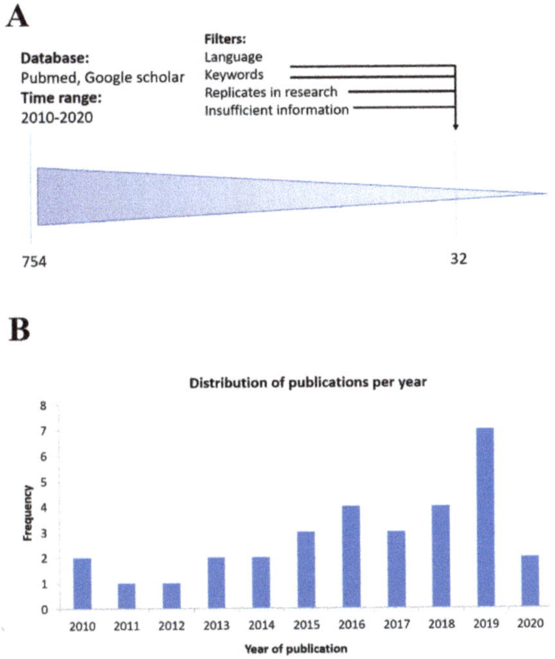

Figure 1. Analysis of nanomaterial-based drug delivery systems in osteoarthritis. (**A**) Procedure used for the literature survey. Studies have been retrieved using the research string "drug delivery AND osteoarthritis AND macrophages OR innate immunity OR inflammation OR immune system OR anti-inflammatory OR nanomaterials OR nanoparticles" on PubMed and Google Scholar, using as a time range the period 2010–2020. With these research criteria, we found 754 studies, and then after excluding the replicates, studies with insufficient information (unclear characteristics of the drug delivery system, missing data about drug dosage or time, uninformative anti-inflammatory readout) and studies not written in English language, we finally selected 32 studies. (**B**) Diagram showing the distribution of the included studies according to the year of publication.

2. Pathophysiology of Osteoarthritis and Role of Macrophages

Osteoarthritis can be classified, according to its leading causes, into primary or secondary based on the underlying etiology. The primary, also known as idiopathic, form of OA presents a complex multifactorial pathophysiology, which can be partially explained by the combination of the following factors: obesity, aging, limbs malalignment, excessive joint loading, and/or genetics. On the other hand, secondary OA is defined by the occurrence of a recognizable causative agent, such as a trauma, joint malformation at birth, rheumatoid arthritis, or surgery (i.e., post-meniscectomy [22]).

In addition to these local triggers of OA, systemic inflammation (as in the case of metabolic syndrome) may play a role in the development of the disease through the establishment of a chronic, systemic low-grade inflammation and the release of circulating adipokines, such as leptin and adiponectin [23]. In particular, leptin in the joints has been shown to increase the expression of inflammatory mediators, such as inducible Nitric oxide synthase (iNOS), cyclooxygenase 2 (COX2), Prostaglandin E2 (PGE2), IL-6, and IL-8 in the cartilage [24]. Meanwhile, adiponectin, presenting lower levels in obesity [25], has a protective role in the articulations by upregulating in chondrocytes the expression of tissue inhibitor metalloproteinase 2 (TIMP2) and IL-10, and preventing cartilage deterioration by the downregulation of matrix metalloproteinase 3 (MMP-3) [26]. In addition, the diagnosis of diabetes mellitus type 2 has emerged as an independent risk predictor of OA severity and arthroplasty requirement [27], possibly owing to a direct detrimental effect of hyperglycemia and chronic low-grade inflammation on cartilage metabolism [28]. Despite the mechanism responsible for the disease progression, OA commonly arises showing similar pathological alterations, as follows: the first joint compartment to be affected is the articular cartilage and then progressively, the disease involves every component of the joint, as the subchondral bone and the synovium, making OA a "whole joint disease" [29].

Increasing basic and clinical experimentations has demonstrated a key role for macrophages in the development and progression of OA [30,31]. The principal involvement of this innate immune cell population has been observed in patients by single-photon emission computed tomography together with conventional tomography (SPECT-CT) in vivo, revealing that 76% of joints affected by OA present activated macrophages and that the number of these cells correlates with radiographic joint disease severity and symptoms [32]. Interestingly, an increased number of activated macrophages is commonly present already at the early stages of OA, suggesting their primary role in the disease development, since the initial phase [33]. The fact that higher macrophage infiltration is observed in early OA, rather than in late OA, further strengthens the concept that these cells are involved from the initial phases of the disease [34]. In addition to their number, the functional polarization of macrophages, i.e., toward an M1-like pro-inflammatory phenotype, plays a fundamental role in the initiation, progression, and resolution of osteoarthritis, also in the knee, as described below.

Physiologically, in the context of the knee, the resident macrophages are present inside the synovial membrane, maintaining their numbers thanks to a pool of locally proliferating mononuclear cells, which are embedded into the synovial tissue and exert a homeostatic function [35]. Whenever these resident monocytic cells detect the presence of exogenous or endogenous pro-inflammatory stimuli, a chain of events known as inflammatory cascade ensues. In the case of OA, acute trauma or chronic overuse of the joint results in tissue injury that is associated with the production of damage-associated molecular patterns (DAMPs), such as fibronectin [36] and oligosaccharides from degraded hyaluronan [37]. These molecules are able to activate resident synovial macrophages toward an M1-like phenotype, by binding to pattern recognition receptors (PRRs) and influencing downstream transcription factors such as the nuclear factor kappa-light-chain-enhancer of activated B cells (NF-κB), which support and boost the pro-inflammatory cascade. Once activated, synovial macrophages exert, directly or indirectly (i.e., stimulating other cells), several actions in the joint microenvironment. Macrophages are responsible for amplification of the inflammatory response, direct tissue injury, and orchestration of other synovial cells. The first action is due to the secretion of signaling molecules, such as pro-inflammatory cytokines (IL-1β, TNF-α, IL-6, IL-12, and IL-23) and chemokines (CCL-2 and CXCL-8) that lead to further leukocyte recruitment, including monocytes. In this way, newly recruited monocytes are differentiated and polarized toward pro-inflammatory macrophages, which join the activated resident macrophages [35]. This accumulation of leukocytes in the OA synovia eventually results in its thickening (a key morphological feature of synovitis) and the perpetration of synovial inflammation. In this context, macrophages can also exert the direct injury of the tissue through the secretion of matrix metalloproteinases (MMP1, MMP3, MMP13), nitric oxide (NO), and reactive oxygen species (ROS) [38,39], leading to the release of more DAMPs and the initiation of a positive feedback loop. Furthermore, the ability of macrophages to orchestrate surrounding cell populations has also been demonstrated. Macrophages can directly inhibit chondrogenesis in mesenchymal stem cells (MSCs), as indicated by decreased expression levels of genes involved in collagen type 2 (COL2) and aggrecan (ACAN) synthesis, which are two fundamental constituents of human cartilage responsible for the resilience of this tissue [40]. The aforementioned actions are exploited mainly by M1-like pro-inflammatory macrophages [41], and their pathological role was confirmed by the selective removal of macrophage-like synovial cells that resulted in the downregulation of pro-inflammatory cytokines and MMP produced by fibroblasts [42].

On the contrary, also in the context of knee OA, it was observed that macrophage polarization toward an M2-like anti-inflammatory phenotype promotes cartilage repair by expressing pro-chondrogenic genes, such as TGF-β and insulin-like growth factor (IGF), resulting in an increased synthesis of collagen type II and glycosaminoglycan, which is accompanied by the inhibition of chondrocytes' apoptosis [43]. These observations are in line with the theoretical classification of M1-classically activated macrophages with a pro-inflammatory behavior versus the M2-alternatively activated cells with anti-inflammatory properties [44] (Figure 2). Furthermore, it was reported that the imbalance between M1 and M2 macrophages in favor of the former is associated with the severity level of osteoarthritis [10].

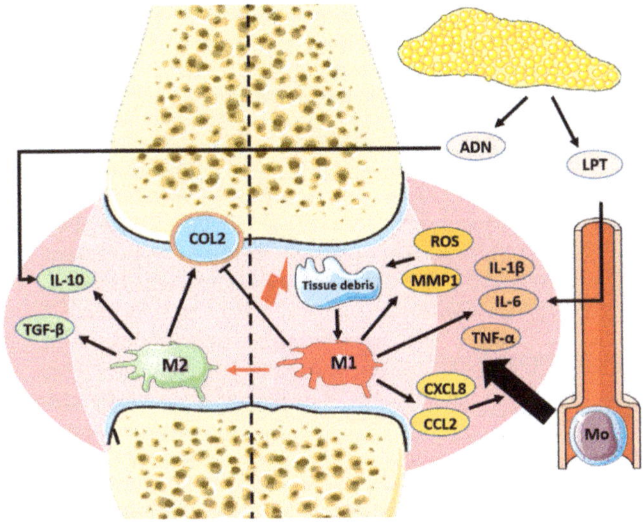

Figure 2. Role of macrophages in the pathophysiology of osteoarthritis. Acute trauma or chronic overuse of the joint results in the activation of resident synovial macrophages toward a harmful pro-inflammatory M1-like phenotype. Once activated, synovial M1-macrophages secrete signaling molecules, such as pro-inflammatory cytokines (interleukin (IL)-1β, tumor necrosis factor alpha (TNF-α), IL-6 and chemokines (CCL-2, CXCL-8) that lead to further leukocyte recruitment, including monocytes (Mo) that infiltrate the joint, become activated toward an M1-like phenotype, and contribute to the thickening of the synovia (a key morphological feature of synovitis). These M1 macrophages also produce matrix metalloproteinases (MMP1) and reactive oxygen species (ROS), which damage directly the joint, worsening the tissue injury and leading to a positive feedback pro-inflammatory loop. Furthermore, M1 macrophages can directly inhibit chondrogenesis through the inhibition of collagen type 2 (COL2) synthesis by mesenchymal stem cells (MSCs) in the joint. Tissue debris and molecules released from the degradation of hyaline cartilage and subchondral bone, which are related to damage of the meniscus, are responsible for the pro-inflammatory properties of the synovial fluid from the early stages of knee OA [45]. In contrast, the polarization of macrophages in the joint toward an M2-like anti-inflammatory phenotype has beneficial effects for the repair of the injury and for the cure of OA disease. It has been demonstrated that M2 macrophages are able to promote cartilage repair through the secretion of TGF-β and IL-10. Once secreted in the synovial fluid, the latter exert their pro-chondrogenic effect by stimulating chondrocytes to secrete type II collagen and proteoglycans. This beneficial action of "alternatively activated" M2 macrophages finds a clinical counterpart in a recent in vivo experiment that correlated the imbalance of M1/M2 ratio as a feature of the severity level of knee OA [10]. In addition to the local triggers of OA, the systemic immune status of the patient is a key responsible for the evolution of the disease. As examples, increased levels of systemic leptin (LPT) increase IL-6 secretion in the joint, supporting deleterious inflammation, while systemic adiponectin (ADN) has shown a protective role by upregulating the secretion of IL-10 in the articulations. Importantly, recent clinical studies have correlated the increased M1/M2 ratio with a higher severity of knee OA disease.

Overall, given the key role played by macrophages in the pathogenesis of OA, it becomes evident that their therapeutic manipulation represents an important target for the treatment of the disease. Some drugs with ability to decrease the M1/M2 macrophage ratio, as desired, for the resolution of knee OA already exist [46–48]. However, the major challenge, still not achieved, consists in the appropriate spatio-temporal manipulation of the immune response in the joint, which may be achieved by a focused therapeutic intervention of macrophages. For this, we believe that the development of new drug delivery approaches is needed, such as administration tools guaranteeing a drug concentration inside the joint at the right dose and for a period of time sufficient to exert a satisfactory long-lasting therapeutic effect. In the next section, we describe recent investigations in the field of nanotechnology aiming to control the delivery of anti-inflammatory drugs toward macrophages in the context of OA.

3. Pharmacological Manipulation of Macrophages for the Actual Treatment of OA

The pharmacological treatment of OA, according to the latest Osteoarthritis Research Society International (OARSI) guidelines [49], is commonly addressed with one or two drugs that are administered either locally (topical or intra-articular) or systemically. To assess the efficacy of the pharmacological treatments, clinicians usually refer to a score established by the OARSI that measures the joint damage in a histopathological manner. This score relies on two parameters: the grade and the stage. The grade is a measure of the vertical extent of the damage of the joint, as this is a reliable indicator of the severity of the disease. On the other hand, the stage is a horizontal measure of the surface/area/volume that is affected by OA. The final OARSI score is obtained by multiplying the grade for the stage, and it allows following the therapeutic activity in a quantitative manner [50].

The drugs currently approved for OA that perform their action at least in part by direct or indirect manipulation of macrophages can be classified into the following main categories: non-selective non-steroidal anti-inflammatory drugs (NSAIDs), NSAIDs inhibiting selectively cyclooxygenase (COX)-2 (coxibs), corticosteroids, and/or hyaluronic acid. Other pharmacological strategies, such as the use of mAbs or nucleic acids are nowadays the object of intensive investigations, but they have not yet entered the clinic [48,51,52].

Non-steroidal anti-inflammatory drugs (NSAIDs), such as aspirin, ibuprofen, diclofenac, or naproxen, exert their anti-inflammatory effect by inhibiting cyclooxygenase (COX) enzymes (both the isoform COX-1 and COX-2) expressed by macrophages [53,54] that metabolize arachidonic acid into thromboxanes and prostaglandins involved in inflammation. Due to their broad effect, non-selective NSAIDs have shown a series of harmful effects on the gastrointestinal tract [55] and kidneys' functions [56]. To overcome these issues, semi-selective NSAIDs (i.e., indomethacin, diclofenac, meloxicam) with a higher affinity for COX-2 versus COX-1, and coxibs (i.e., celecoxib, etoricoxib, parecoxib) specifically targeting COX-2 enzymes have been introduced in the clinical practice. Unfortunately, the systemic administration of COX-2 inhibitors showed also harmful side effects in patients with a known cardiovascular risk [57]. NSAIDs are commonly used, either locally or systemically, for OA. Although the oral administration is always advantageous for the possibility of self-administration, ease of ingestion, and pain avoidance, the local approach is preferred to achieve an intra-articular efficacy and to minimize the adverse events described above.

Corticosteroids are a class of steroid hormones with a powerful anti-inflammatory effect that is mediated by their binding to the glucocorticoid receptor, which is activated and translocated to the nucleus of immune cells, activating the synthesis of lipocortin-1 and gluconeogenesis, among others [58]. Through this mechanism, they modulate a wide range of physiological processes, including stress and immune response. In the clinic, prednisolone, dexamethasone, and others represent well-established treatment options for several rheumatological and orthopaedical pathological conditions, including knee osteoarthritis [59–61]. Their use in OA is usually restricted to intra-articular injections for short periods, as prolonged treatment with corticosteroids can induce extreme immune suppression, which avoids the resolution of the inflammation [62] and/or bone resorption in the joint, by impairment of osteoblasts and osteoclasts recruitment [63].

Although not classified as a drug, the intra-articular administration of hyaluronic acid (HA), a glycosaminoglycan widely distributed throughout the body in several forms related to different molecular weights, has shown relative efficacy in some cases of OA. While low molecular weight HA presents pro-inflammatory effects mainly acting on toll-like receptor-2 (TLR-2) and toll-like receptor-4 (TLR-4) receptors on macrophages [64]; on the contrary, physiologically produced or therapeutically injected high molecular weight hyaluronic acid (HMW-HA) has demonstrated anti-inflammatory effects on macrophages [65] in different settings [66–68]. The local injection of HMW-HA in the knee of patients has demonstrated a significant improvement in OA symptoms [66]. Furthermore, HA is widely applied in dentistry [69], regenerative medicine [70,71], and ophthalmology [72]; and it is gradually becoming a useful therapeutic tool for the intervention of other pathological conditions [73].

Finally, monoclonal antibodies-based therapies are increasingly being used in randomized clinical trials, presenting mixed results in some cases. For example, the weekly subcutaneous injection of adalimumab, an antibody that interferes with TNF-α signaling, which is one of the main pro-inflammatory pathways in macrophages [74], did not result in a positive effect in OA management versus placebo in patients with erosive hand osteoarthritis (HUMOR trial [75]). On the contrary, the injection of 10 mg of the same antibody in the knee joint of patients with moderate/severe knee OA was effective and well tolerated [76]. This finding was also reported in a separate clinical trial for the intra-articular injection of etanercept, which is a fusion protein produced by recombinant DNA used to inhibit the TNF-α receptor [77]. Promising results had been observed by nerve growth factor (NGF) inhibition, which is produced also by macrophages [78], using fasinumab antibodies to prevent OA pain [79]. Subcutaneous injection of fasinumab improved knee/hip OA pain and function [80]. Several ongoing clinical trials are evaluating monoclonal antibodies to inhibit other macrophagic pro-inflammatory pathways such as anti-IL-1β or anti-IL-6 signaling. Lutikizumab, anti-IL-1α/β, resulted in a limited improvement in patients with knee OA [81], while no clear evidence is available for IL-6 blockade, despite its common application in rheumatoid arthritis [82].

Among the pharmacological approaches presented, the systemic or local administration of NSAIDs is given to most of the patients with OA, whilst intra-articular corticosteroids and hyaluronan are conditionally recommended only for the management of particular cases of knee OA. However, the local application of these drugs is able to reduce the inflammation only upon administration, and they are rapidly cleared from the joint by blood and/or lymphatic drainage [83], thus restricting the long-term efficacy of the therapy at the desired target location. For this reason, the oral administration of non-selective NSAIDs or Coxibs, despite their side effects [55,57], is usually prescribed in high doses for extended periods of time to almost all the patients with knee OA. Interestingly, it has been observed that a dose of NSAIDs 100–1000-fold higher than the one used to reduce inflammation could be also beneficial to inhibit the apoptosis of chondrocytes and prevent their dedifferentiation [84]. As it would be dangerous to administer such a dose orally, further efforts to optimize intra-articular delivery are highly desirable. For this, new drug delivery systems are being explored, aiming to implement the local treatment with high and sustained therapeutic efficacy on macrophages in the joint, by controlling the dose and time of release of specific drugs at the right location, while avoiding their systemic biodistribution and consequent adverse effects. The optimal drug delivery approach into the joint must allow a unique implantation, avoiding also adverse effects connected with the practice of multiple injections, such as mild swelling [85] or infection [86] of the joint. In the next section, we present the most relevant nanomaterial-based approaches, which have been investigated so far for this purpose, manipulating macrophage behavior in osteoarthritis.

4. Nanomaterial-Based Approaches for Macrophage Manipulation in OA

The therapeutic manipulation of macrophages using nanotechnology and other drug delivery systems has been usually approached taking into consideration the high ability of these cells to recognize and phagocyte "non-self" or "potentially" dangerous pathogens. The physicochemical properties of nanoparticles (NPs), such as size or surface charge, or even the surface functionalization of nanomaterials can be designed to favor their non-specific [87–89] or specific, receptor-mediated uptake by macrophages [90,91]. The decoration of NPs with specific ligands, such as sugars, lipids, peptides, or even antibodies, has showed improved macrophage targeting [92]. Some of these ligands have been implemented to target macrophages in other pathologies, i.e., cancer, atherosclerosis, or infectious diseases, and they have been reviewed elsewhere [19,90,91,93]. Although out of the scope of this review, these investigations could provide important information for NP–macrophage targeting in OA.

Upon recognition and internalization by macrophages, these NPs are commonly disassembled inside the lysosomes or cytosol of the cells, allowing drug release. As a contrary approach, some biomaterial-based approaches have been designed with non-spherical sizes or enveloped into protective coatings (i.e., PEG or erythrocyte membranes), to avoid or delay macrophage recognition [94,95]. This strategy has been used in the context of intra-articular delivery to achieve a long-lasting release of the drug from the biomaterial, which is not rapidly internalized by macrophages [20,21]. Finally, some nanotechnology-based approaches have been designed to release the drug extracellularly, not inside macrophages, or even using selected ligands to target other cellular components of the joint (i.e., chondrocytes, synoviocytes, fibroblasts), but always aiming to achieve an anti-inflammatory effect.

The majority of the nanomaterial-based approaches designed to inhibit macrophage-induced inflammation for the treatment of OA have used natural or synthetic polymers with a good regulatory profile [96]. Liposomal formulations, made up of a phospholipidic bilayers resembling cellular membranes, are the second most common group of nanosystems applied to improve the delivery of hydrophilic (loaded in the inner core) or lipophilic (trapped in the lipidic bilayer) anti-inflammatory drugs [97]. Furthermore, here we provide some examples of metallic- or carbon-based NPs and nanomaterial-based scaffolds or gels that have been engineered to control the intra-articular release of drugs in the context of OA. In all cases, for the selection of the nanomaterials, their biocompatibility, biodegradability, and safety are major premises that must be tested, in addition to the capability of the nanotechnological approach to improve the therapeutic efficacy of the free pharmacological molecule. A schematic presentation of all the nanomaterial-based approaches presented in this review manuscript is provided in Table 1.

4.1. NSAIDs-Loaded Polymeric Nanoparticles

NSAIDs, as the most used anti-inflammatory and pain relief drugs used worldwide, are commonly given by oral or local administration to patients with knee OA. Several polymeric-NSAID-based approaches have been investigated to improve their local efficacy and reduce their side effects. As an example, Kang et al. developed thermoresponsive polymeric nanospheres containing diclofenac (DCF) and kartogenin (KGN), a pro-chondrogenic compound. They used F127 pluronics and triblock copolymers linked to obtain an amphiphilic final structure and then emulsified with KGN molecules conjugated to the natural polymer chitosan (CS), allowing the binding of KGN/CS molecules on the hydrophilic part of the F127. Subsequently, diclofenac was loaded into the inner hydrophobic core of the NP. These nanospheres showed, in vitro, the individual and sustained drug release of the two drugs, KGN and DCF, which can be accelerated when exposed to cold temperature (4 °C). This spontaneous drug release, subsequent to the cold temperature, is achieved by the enlargement of the F127 segments, generating a loose structure that is more prone to undergo hydrolysis with the consequent release of KGN. In parallel, the increased water permeability occurring at low temperature allows a rapid burst release (12 h) of DCF from the lipidic core.

These nanospheres prevented the secretion of interleukin-6 (IL-6) from LPS-treated U937 cells. Despite these positive results using U937 as an in vitro model of human monocytes from tumoral origin, similar experiments with primary macrophages would be preferred for better mimicking the clinical situation. In rat models of OA induced by anterior cruciate ligament transection (ACLT) and destabilization of the medial meniscus (DMM), these nanospheres showed a satisfactory reduction of the OARSI score [98]. In another study, self-assembling nanosystems made up of Poloxamer 407 (highly hydrophilic) and Tetronic 90R4 (intermediate hydrophilic) were loaded with indomethacin. In addition to these amphiphilic polymers with surfactant properties, also poly (lactic-co-glycolic acid) (PLGA) and articular proteoglycans (collagen, gelatin, and glucosamine HCl) were added in different ratios to achieve a controlled and sustained drug release. The best prototypes, based on their drug-retaining capacity, were investigated in arthritis models consisting of male albino rats injected in their knees with the antigens ovalbumin and complete Freund's adjuvant. After 2 intra-articular injections, the indomethacin nanosystems showed significant therapeutic efficacy in terms of knees' histopathological features and TNF-α concentration in serum. The same dose of the free drug was not effective, which is probably due to its poor solubility in the synovial fluid and is not a problem in the case of the nanosystems [84]. Piroxicam is another NSAID used for the long-term therapy of joints' inflammatory diseases, which has been encapsulated for the intra-articular delivery using NPs with different surface charges [99]. In this case, the NPs composed of PLGA and Eudragit RL, a positive charged polymer intended to interact with negative charged HA, were investigated to reduce the efflux of NPs from the joint. As expected, upon intra-articular injection in healthy rats, the cationic NPs showed a higher retention of piroxicam in the synovial fluid versus the neutral NPs or the free drug, as evaluated by LC-MS/MS. Accordingly, the kinetics of piroxicam in the blood showed a delayed and minor peak for the cationic NPs group in contrast with the rapid increase observed for the free drug, thus reducing the risk of systemic adverse events [99].

Among coxibs, with the ability to inhibit specifically COX2 enzyme, celecoxib (CXB) has shown the safest profile related to the induction of cardiovascular side effects [100]. For OA, Villamagna and colleagues designed CXB-loaded NPs, based on degradable poly(ester amide)s (PEAs), with different monomers intended to modulate their thermal and mechanical behavior, and consequently the drug release. By dialysis membrane, in vitro, a slow release of only 25% of CXB at 40 days, with the drug still present in NPs at day 60, was observed. Using sheep in vivo models of OA, lameness, joint effusion, periarticular swelling, fever, heart rate, synovial fluid, and plasma were evaluated, showing satisfactory anti-inflammatory activity for the CXB NPs, with only a minor increase in white blood cells in synovial fluid and mild synovial intimal hyperplasia [101]. The sheep or equine model represents important added value, in terms of the anatomical and histological similarity of the knee to humans, but also immunological response versus murine models. The evaluation of macroscopic lesions and degrees of damage in mice is more challenging due to their small size [102]. NPs with PLGA and PEG have been also prepared to load etoricoxib, which is a drug with higher therapeutic activity at lower doses but also higher adverse effects than CXB. Sustained drug release was observed for these NPs up to 1 month, by the dialysis membrane, although showing an initial burst of 25% release in the first five days. In rats with OA, induced by the anterior cruciate ligament transection technique, the injection of etoricoxib NPs showed a lower OARSI score, no signs of inflammation, higher expression of type II collagen and aggrecan (mandatories for cartilage integrity), and lower levels of MMP-13 and A disintegrin and metalloproteinase with thrombospondin motifs 5 (ADAMTS-5), which are two proteases produced by macrophages that are responsible for joint destruction [96]. Despite the promising anti-inflammatory activity for these NSAIDs-loaded NPs, their translation to the clinic is delayed by still ongoing pre-clinical experiments and toxicity/safety studies, which must be ideally performed in different animal species i.e., rodents, sheep, and/or equine models.

4.2. Corticosteroid-Loaded Polymeric Nanoparticles

With many corticosteroids currently applied in the clinical practice, dexamethasone (DX) is one of the most popular for encapsulation into NPs, thanks to its powerful anti-inflammatory activity, even at low dose [103]. The first attempts to encapsulate DX in PLGA polymeric NPs suffered from a low drug loading and a fast crystallization [104]. To overcome this impasse, dexamethasone palmitate (DXP), a prodrug of DX characterized by a high hydrophobicity, was encapsulated in poly(ethylene glycol) (PEG)ylated NPs with high efficiency (98% *w/w*) and sustained release in vitro up to 25 h, showing a peak of 60% of DXP release at 5 h. Using LPS-stimulated RAW 264.7 murine macrophages, these DXP NPs versus the free drug showed better inhibition of TNF-α secretion. In this case, primary macrophages may also give a more sensitive indication of the anti-inflammatory efficacy of DXP NPs than the RAW 264.7 cell line. Upon intravenous injection in a murine model of rheumatoid arthritis obtained through the intradermal injection of an emulsion of complete Freund's adjuvant and type II collagen, DXP NPs demonstrated a higher accumulation into the inflamed joints, with lower systemic biodistribution and mild to little adverse reactions. The testing of different doses revealed the necessity of 1 mg/kg of DXP NPs to achieve a significant reduction in inflammatory histological signs [105]. In another report, betamethasone sodium phosphate (BSP) was incorporated into PLGA nanospheres to reduce the inflammation in rabbit models of ovalbumin-induced chronic synovitis. The intra-articular injection of BSP nanospheres, together with the antigen ovalbumin, in one of the two joints of the rabbits was able to reduce joint swelling up to 21 days. This prolonged therapeutic effect, not observed for the free steroid, demonstrated the comparative advantage of the nanosystem [106]. These data demonstrate the feasibility of using nanotechnological approaches for the long-term intra-articular delivery of steroids. However, due to the local harmful effects of these drugs, which are described in Section 3, we would prioritize the development of steroid-based drug delivery systems to facilitate their administration and short-/medium-term release (less than 1 month).

4.3. Polymeric Nanoparticles Loaded with Other Anti-Inflammatory Molecules

As an alternative to conventional anti-inflammatory drugs, another approach has considered the use of anti-inflammatory peptides, with the ability to inhibit inflammatory pathways, and their loading into NPs was explored to improve their efficacy in vivo. The cell-penetrating anti-inflammatory peptide KAFAK was loaded into hollow thermosensitive poly(N-isopropylacrylamide) (pNIPAM) with ability to reduce IL-6 secretion. These NPs present the advantage of undergoing hydrophobic collapse at physiological temperature; thus, the peptide is trapped in the core of the NP upon injection, and its release is prolonged over time [107,108]. The in vitro testing of pNIPAM-NPs showed high uptake by RAW 264.7 macrophages, and a stronger inhibition of IL-6 production than the free anti-inflammatory peptide KAFAK was observed using ex vivo models of OA, which were obtained from bovine cartilage plugs treated in vitro with trypsin to remove aggrecan and induce inflammation [109]. In another report, KAFAK-loaded pNIPAM-NPs were co-polymerized with 2-acrylamido-2-methyl-1-propanesulfonic acid (AMPS), which enhances the interaction between the NPs and the KAFAK peptide, resulting in increased drug loading. These NPs were tested in vitro using LPS pre-stimulated-THP-1 macrophages, and ex vivo using cartilage plugs from bovine knee joints pre-treated with interleukin-1β (IL-1β) to initiate inflammation. In both cases, the KAFAK NPs were able to reduce the inflammation, as determined by TNF-α production by the THP-1 cells and IL-6 secretion in the ex vivo models [110].

The strong pro-inflammatory effect of IL-1β can also be blocked by the IL-1 receptor antagonist (IL-1ra), which is a receptor naturally secreted by polymorphonuclear cells after their stimulation that has been effectively used in the clinic as a recombinant protein (Anakinra®) [111,112]. In the context of OA, IL-1Ra-poly(2-hydroxyethyl methacrylate)-pyridine NPs have been developed and tested in vitro on RAW 264.7 macrophage-like cells and a B-cell precursor acute lymphoblastic leukemia cell line (EU1), showing no toxicity on the former and a significant reduction of NF-κβ activation upon IL-1β stimulation [113]. Another approach consisted of the development of polymeric NPs to target the A2A adenosine receptor, as it has been demonstrated that mice with impaired adenosine signaling within macrophages of the joints develop OA spontaneously [114]. Six types of adenosine functionalized poly(lactic acid)-poly(ethylene glycol) (PLA-PEG) NPs were tested in vitro on IL-1β-stimulated macrophage-like RAW264.7 cells and in vivo in a rat post-traumatic knee OA model, which was induced through anterior cruciate ligament (ACL) rupture with a single load of tibial compression. In vitro, the adenosine PLA-PEG NPs led to a significant reduction of IL-6, MMP-3, and collagen 10 mRNA expression, whilst rats injected with the NPs into the joint showed a significant reduction in knee swelling, cartilage protection, and decreased OARSI score when compared with control rats [115].

Polymeric NPs with the ability to release the drug in response to physicochemical stimuli have been also investigated. Considering the drop of the joint's pH in inflammatory conditions, acid-activable curcumin polymer (ACP) NPs were designed to maximize the release of curcumin in diseased joints. Curcumin is a flavonoid from natural origin with anti-inflammatory and antioxidant properties in vitro and in vivo [116]. Consequently, the ACP–curcumin NPs were tested in mice models of knee OA induced by mono iodoacetic acid, which is a corrosive molecule that destroys joint's components and stimulates an inflammatory response [117]. The injection of ACP–curcumin NPs into the inflamed acid joints led to their fusion to form micelles and curcumin release, resulting in the suppression of TNF-α and IL-1β [118]. Hemoglobin-based PLGA-PEG-conjugated nanogenerators with the ability to produce nitric oxide (NO) upon a photothermal trigger (650 nm light irradiation) were loaded with short interfering RNA (siRNA) to inhibit Notch1. Upon the intra-articular injection of these NPs in the hindlimbs of papain OA murine models and local irradiation, the mice showed a significant reduction in the arthritis score, reduced cartilage erosion, and a lower synovial inflammation, characterized by the immunohistochemical evaluation of TNF-α, IL-1β, IL-6, and Notch-1 [119].

4.4. Hyaluronic Acid-Based Polymeric Nanoparticles

The local injection of HA is commonly used in the clinic, as described in Section 3. Interestingly, the use of hyaluronic acid (HA) as a free polymer, not loaded with pharmacological agents, has presented beneficial effects as a treatment for OA, due to its intrinsic immunomodulatory properties [65]. Thus, in this separate section, we provide a summary of some investigations using HA polymers to prepare NPs and their results.

Mota et al. have prepared PLGA-NPs with oleic acid and HA on their surface, showing a similar anti-inflammatory activity to diclofenac and higher than HA free solution, in rats implanted with cotton pellets subcutaneously to promote granuloma and inflammation [120]. HA and chitosan (HA/CS) NPs have also been developed to deliver into the joints the gene CrmA, cytokine response modifier A, a protease inhibitor that binds and blocks caspase-1 enzyme, which is responsible for the generation of IL-1β in OA. These HA/CS-CrmA-NPs showed a constant release of CrmA up to 70% by day 22. The intra-articular injection of these NPs in rats with knee OA showed attenuation of cartilage lesion, increase in glycosaminoglycans, intact surface, conservation of type II collagen in the joint, reduced inflammatory infiltrate, drop of IL-1β, MMP-3, and MMP-13, and better OARSI score [121]. These investigations provide satisfactory results related to the application of hyaluronic acid-based nano-approaches in OA.

4.5. Liposome-Based Anti-Inflammatory Approaches

Liposomes are nanospherical vesicles made up of a phospholipidic bilayer that resembles the normal cellular membrane. Due to their amphiphilic nature, liposomes can be used to deliver both hydrophilic drugs (localized in the inner core) and lipophilic drugs (trapped in the lipidic bilayer) [97]. Several liposome-based approaches have been explored to deplete synovial macrophages to prevent their detrimental effect on joint's components. As an example, clodronate liposomes were able to ameliorate inflammation in STR/ort mice developing OA in a progressive way comparable to humans [122]. Specifically, STR/ort mice were injected intraperitoneally with clodronate liposomes to induce macrophage apoptosis, and this treatment resulted in a drop of IL-1β and TNF-α RNA expression in the synovial tissue. Interestingly, an increase in the nerve growth factor, related with persistent pain in OA patients, was also observed [78]. Similar findings were also reported in rat models of monoiodoacetate-induced OA [123]. In contrary to these results, a very recent study by Bailey et al. has demonstrated that intra-articular injection of clodronate liposomes in post-traumatic arthritis murine models did not reduce the synovitis, and the M1/M2 ratio was increased in some treated mice, advocating that clodronate liposomes could lead to the depletion not only of the M1 pro-inflammatory macrophages, but also of the M2-like immunomodulator counterparts [124]. Indeed, clodronate liposomes may present high systemic toxicity and poor targeting specificity toward the joint, thus killing macrophages in other organs, which limit the confidence on the experimental observations and also their possibilities for safe translation to the clinic. These evidences encourage higher efforts on strategies to reprogram macrophages versus their depletion.

Liposomes loaded with indomethacin were formulated using different concentrations of phosphatidyl choline, cholesterol, and stearylamine or phosphatidyl glycerol, which are common lipids that are present in the cellular plasmatic membrane. This composition resulted in prolonged and sustained release of the drug in vitro and higher anti-inflammatory activity in both acute and chronic arthritis rat models compared to the free indomethacin, as well as a reduction of gastrointestinal ulcers [125]. Similarly, liposomal formulations containing celecoxib and hyaluronate were intra-articularly injected into the knee joints of rabbits with surgically induced OA. Two weeks after the surgery, animals were sacrificed, and histological specimens from their joints demonstrated a significant alleviation of cartilage degeneration compared to celecoxib or hyaluronate alone [126]. Liposomal dexamethasone reduced the inflammatory response of human macrophages in vitro [127] and reduced local and systemic inflammation in adjuvant arthritis rat models. Liposomal dexamethasone showed prolonged effect (up to 48 h) and higher efficacy at lower doses than free drug [128]. Avnir et al. designed liposomes with a high loading and prolonged release of prednisolone hemisuccinate, an amphipathic weak acid glucocorticoid, by modulating the gradient of calcium ions concentration between the inner core of the liposomes and the medium. Consistently with their in vitro studies, the intravenous injection of the prednisolone liposomes led to a better arthritis score than the free drug in Lewis rats with adjuvant-induced arthritis [129]. Finally, hybrid nanosystems based on the conjugation of calcium phosphate NPs with liposomes decorated with folate were loaded with the immunosuppressive drug methotrexate and siRNA to inhibit NF-kβ activation in joint macrophages. Upon intravenous administration, these folate-targeted liposomes reduced significantly the paw thickness and arthritis score versus similar non-targeted liposomes in murine models of intradermal collagen-induced arthritis. Indeed, a specific macrophage uptake, related to the high expression of folate receptors, was demonstrated in vitro using LPS-activated RAW 264.7 cells [130].

4.6. Other Nanomaterial-Based Anti-Inflammatory Nanoparticles

Other nanomaterials, such as carbon-based NPs or metal-based NPs, have been also investigated to target macrophages in OA. For example, fullerenes are hollow nanospheres consisting of carbon atoms connected by single and double bonds with antioxidant properties [131]. The intra-articular injection of fullerenes alone or in combination with HA in surgically induced rabbit models of knee OA showed a dose-dependent fullerene therapeutic effect and synergistic activity with HA [132]. Similarly, fullerol NPs (a polyhydroxylated form of fullerene [133]) showed anti-inflammatory activity in vitro and the ability to prevent synovial inflammation in rat models of OA induced by the intra-articular injection of monoiodoacetate [134]. Carbon nanotubes or graphene-based nanomaterials have also been investigated for OA treatment [135–139]; however, specific studies to target macrophages are lacking. For example, Liu et al. observed a reduction of MMP-3 in the knee joints of rats following the intra-articular injection of hyaluronic acid reinforced with graphene oxide [139], and it is reasonable to speculate that this effect is secondary to macrophages' modulation. In another report, PEGylated single-walled carbon nanotubes (SWCNTs) loaded with antisense oligomers injected in the knee joint of OA mice showed a prolonged persistence in joint cavity (more than 14 days), without induction of TNF-α or IL-1β. The loading of SWCNTs with oligomers showed the ability to inhibit gene expression in homeostatic and hypertrophic chondrocytes in vivo [137]. To our knowledge, the direct effect of this approach on macrophages was not evaluated; however, we envision the functionalization and optimization of these types of SWCNTs as an interesting strategy to target and reprogram macrophages in the joint.

Table 1. Summary of nanoparticle-based approaches to target macrophages using in vivo pre-clinical models of osteoarthritis (OA).

Type of Nanoparticle	Nanocarrier Composition	Therapeutic Load	Size and Surface Charge (nm/mV)	Route of Administration	Animal Model	Therapeutic Effect	Ref
Polymeric NPs	Pluronic-based Thermoresponsive	*Diclofenac/Kartogenin*	305–650 nm/n.r.	i.a. (knee)	Rats	↓ of OARSI score	[98]
	Self-assembling PLGA-coated	*Indomethacin*	37–255 nm/ (−5.81)–(−9.36) mV #	i.a. (knee)	Rats	↓ of diameter; favorable hystology; ↓ TNF-α in serum	[84]
	PLGA + Eudragit RL	*Piroxicam*	221–243 nm/ (+2.4)–(+11.5) mV #	i.a. (knee)	Rats	Prolonged retention into joint compared to NPs without Eudragit RL	[99]
	PEAs	*Celecoxib*	398–836 nm/n.r. #	i.a. (knee)	Sheeps	↓ joint effusion; ↓ WBC	[101]
	PLGA/PEG	*Etoricoxib*	339 nm (mean value)/ (+1.68 ± 0.85) mV	i.a. (knee)	Rats	Favorable μCT; ↓ MMP-13 and ADAMTS-5; ↑ collagen and aggrecan	[96]
	PEG	*Dexamethasone*	130 ± 3 nm/ (−55 ± 2) mV	i.v.	Mice†	Accumulation in inflamed joints upon administration	[105]
	PLGA	*Betamethasone*	300–490 nm/n.r. #	i.a. (knee)	Rabbits	↓ joint swelling and temperature	[106]
	pNIPAM	*KAFAK*	238–469 nm/ (−5.38)–(−8.48) mV #	ex vivo (knee)	Bovine*	↓ IL-6	[109]
	pNIPAM/AMPS	*KAFAK*	232–358 nm/ (−6.1)–(−22.9) mV #	ex vivo (knee)	Bovine*	↓ IL-6	[110]
	PLA-PEG	*Adenosine*	129–144 nm/n.r. #	i.a. (knee)	Rats	↓ OARSI score	[115]
	Acid-activable PAE	*Curcumin*	170 nm/n.r.	i.a. (knee)	Mice	↓ TNF-α and IL-1β production Favorable histology	[118]
	PLGA-PEG	*NO-Hemoglobin Notch-1 siRNA*	200 nm/0 mV	i.a. (limb)	Mice	↓ TNF-α, IL-6, IL-1β, Notch-1 in immunohistochemistry	[119]
Hyaluronic acid-based NPs	PLGA	*Oleic acid and HA*	4561 ± 3466 nm/ (−0.59)–(−16.65) mV	s.c.	Rats	↓ of inflammation in cotton pellets	[120]
	HA and Chitosan	*CrmA*	100–300 nm/n.r.	i.a. (knee)	Rats	↓ OARSI score; ↓ IL-1β, MMP-3, MMP-13; collagen conserved	[121]
Liposomes	Not specified	*Clodronate*	n.r.	i.p.	Mice‡	↓ IL-1β and TNF-α expression in synovium; ↓ NGF in the joint	[78]
	Clophosome®	*Clodronate*	100–500 nm/ 0 mV	i.v.	Rats	↓ IL-1β and NGF in the joint	[123]
	Phosphatidyl choline; cholesterol; stearylamine; phosphatydil glycerol	*Indomethacin*	50–100 nm/n.r. #	i.p. (knee)	Rats	↓ joint volume	[125]
	SPC and cholesterol + hyaluronan addition	*Celecoxib*	4980 nm/n.r.	i.a. (knee)	Rabbits	Favorable hystology	[126]
	DPPC + DPPG + cholesterol	*Dexamethasone*	283–310 nm/n.r.	i.v.	Rats†	Favorable histology and WBC count	[128]
	NSSLs	*Methyl prednisolone*	80 nm/n.r.	i.v.	Rats†	↓ of the arhtritis score	[129]
	Calcium phosphate NPs in liposomes	*Methotrexate NF-κB siRNA*	170 nm/ (−23.6) mV	i.v.	Mice	↓ limb arhtritis score ↓ paw thickness	[130]

Table 1. *Cont.*

Type of Nanoparticle	Nanocarrier Composition	Therapeutic Load	Size and Surface Charge (nm/mV)	Route of Administration	Animal Model	Therapeutic Effect	Ref
Carbon-based NPs	Fullerene	-	1.1 nm/n.r.	i.a. (knee)	Rabbits	Favorable hystology	[132]
	Fullerol	-	n.r.	i.v. (knee)	Mice	Favorable hystology	[134]
	Graphene oxide	*Hyaluronan conjugation*	n.r.	i.a. (knee)	Rats	↓ MMP-3 concentration in the joint	[139]
	Carbon nanotubes	*Antisense oligomers*	109 ± 49 nm/(−11) mV	i.a. (knee)	Mice	Inhibition of protein synthesis in chondrocytes and reduction of inflammation	[137]
Metal-based NPs	Silica	*Hyaluronan synthase 2*	175 nm/(+12) mV	i.a. (TMJ)	Rats	Favorable hystology	[140]
	Gold	*Fish oil protein, both in DPPC liposomes*	15.3 ± 1.9 nm/(+4.15 ± 3.9) mV	i.a.	Rats	Reduction of inflammation	[141]
	Selenium	*NPs dispersed in coumaric acid*	68,000 ± 10,000 nm/n.r.	i.p.	Rats	Reduction of catalase, COX-2, GPx1	[142]
Other NPs	ZIF-8 (MOF)	*S-methylisothiourea Catalase Anti-CD16/32*	160 nm/(−13)–(+20) mV #	i.a. (knee)	Mice	Favorable histology and X-ray	[143]

Legend: ADAMTS-5: A disintegrin and metalloproteinase with thrombospondin motifs 5; **AMPS:** 2-acrylamido-2-methyl-1-propanesulfonic acid; **COX-2:** cyclooxygenase 2; **CrmA:** cytokine response modifier A; **DPPC:** 1,2-dipalmitoyl-sn-glycero-3-phosphocholine; **DPPG:** 1,2-dipalmitoyl-sn-glycero-3-(phosphor-rac-(1-glycerol))(sodium salt); **GPx1:** Glutathione peroxidase 1; **HA:** hyaluronic acid; **i.a.:** intra-articular; **IL-1β:** interleukin-1β; **IL-6:** interleukin-6; **i.p.:** intraperitoneal; **i.v.:** intravenous; **μCT**: microtomography; **MMP-3:** matrix metalloproteinase 3; **MMP-13:** matrix metalloproteinase 13; **NGF:** nerve growth factor; **n.r.:** not reported; **NSSLs**: sterically stabilized nanoliposomes; **OARSI**: Osteoarthritis Research Society International; **PAE:** poly(β-amino ester); **PEAs:** poly(ester amide)s; **PEG:** poly(ethylene glycol); **PLA:** poly(lactic acid): **PLGA**: poly(lactic-*co*-glycolic acid); **pNIPAM:** poly(N-isopropylacrylamide); **s.c.:** subcutaneous; **SPC:** soybean phosphatidylcholine; **TMJ:** *temporomandibular joint;* **TNF-α:** tumor necrosis factor alpha; **WBC:** white blood cells; **ZIF-8**: zeolitic imidazolate framework-8; * Ex vivo; † Rheumatoid arthritis; **‡** STR/Ort mice that develops spontaneously OA. # NPs with different but defined size and charge within the indicated range were tested.

Silica NPs, characterized by a good biocompatibility and high capacity to load proteins, were used to deliver hyaluronan synthase 2 toward cnidocytes in the temporomandibular joint of OA rat models with the aim to increase HA production and achieve anti-inflammatory effects. The single intra-articular injection of these silica NPs showed histological improvements lasting for more than 3 weeks, thus improving the direct HA supply, which requires multiple painful injections [140]. The encapsulation of gold NPs conjugated with fish oil proteins was also explored for OA. The injection of these hybrid nanosystems in the joint of rat models in which OA was induced using bacterial collagenase showed the ability to reduce inflammation [141]. Selenium NPs dispersed in P-coumaric acid (an anti-inflammatory compound) were applied to reduce inflammation in rats with rheumatoid arthritis, reducing the expression of pro-inflammatory activators, such as COX-2 [142]. Finally, within the group of metal organic frameworks (MOFs), zeolitic imidazolate framework-8 (ZIF-8) NPs were designed to deliver s-methylisothiourea hemisulfate salt and catalase to synovial macrophages, to inhibit iNOS and H_2O_2 activity. These NPs were decorated with adsorbed CD16/32 antibodies to improve their recognition by M1-like macrophages and prolong their retention into the joint [143]. Their intra-articular administration in ACLT-induced OA murine models led to significant histological improvements characterized by the narrowing reversion of joint spaces, decrease of CD16/CD32-positive M1-like macrophages, and increase of CD206-positive M2-like counterparts [143].

5. Conclusions

Here, we have described the pathophysiology of OA, with a particular focus on the inflammation supported by macrophages, a brief summary of the current pharmacological treatment, and a wide range of nanoparticle-based approaches to mitigate the local inflammation and improve the recovery and cure of OA disease (Figure 3). Taking this information into account, we foresee a bright future in the use of nanomedicines for the therapeutic manipulation of macrophages in the context of OA. In the last decade, we have perceived a progressive increase of experimental efforts to implement new nanotechnological strategies to improve the delivery of traditional anti-inflammatory drugs, such as NSAIDs and corticoids, toward diseased joints. Novel molecules not yet approved in the clinical practice are also being intensively investigated, including anti-inflammatory peptides or gene therapies, which will likely need the implementation of nanodrug delivery approaches to avoid their degradation and/or improve their biodistribution profile, thus allowing their effective application in vivo [110,119]. In parallel, in the field of immunology, several investigations have revealed the important role of joint macrophages in OA [144–146]. Macrophage polarization has been recently identified as a possible marker of prognosis [145], influencing also neighbor cells in the joint (i.e., chondrocytes). However, an important challenge to clearly dissect the role of macrophages versus other cellular and molecular components in OA is the availability and relevance of the in vitro and in vivo models commonly used in pre-clinical research. In particular, there is a lack of appropriate in vitro models of chronic inflammation mimicking the joint OA environment. The information related to the specific therapeutic targeting of macrophages in the joints is also limited; thus, if the higher precision in local macrophage targeting could lead to better results remains also to be elucidated. We have found a significant amount of scientific reports testing new anti-inflammatory approaches that resulted in a direct or indirect effect on macrophage phenotype and functions, which was correlated with improved outcomes. Despite these promising scientific observations, the clear discernment of macrophage targeting requires costly in vivo experiments focused on NP and/or drug pharmacokinetics and biodistribution at the tissular and cellular level, which we expect to see in the coming years. Finally, a few clinical trials are investigating anti-inflammatory drugs for OA treatment [31,147,148], although focused efforts examining the role of macrophages and/or the use of nanomaterial-based approaches are lacking.

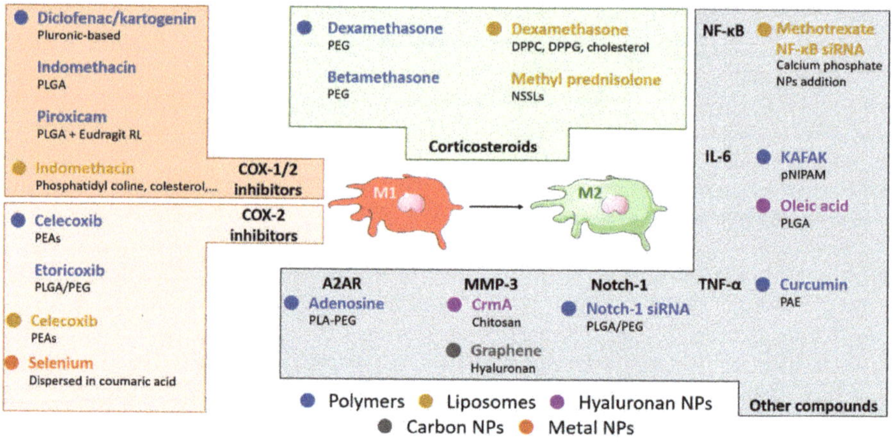

Figure 3. Nanotechnological approaches targeting macrophages in OA. Nanomedicine offers a wide range of drug delivery systems to inhibit the pro-inflammatory activity of M1-like macrophages in OA joints. Polymeric and hyaluronan-based nanoparticles (NPs) and liposomes have been investigated to inhibit inflammation by delivering non-steroidal anti-inflammatory drugs (NSAIDs, i.e., indomethacin, diclofenac, etc.) for COX-1/2 inhibition, COX-2 specific inhibitors (i.e., celecoxib and etoricoxib) or corticosteroids (i.e., dexamethasone, betamethasone, and prednisolone) to block glucocorticoid receptor in OA joints. NPs loaded with other pharmacological molecules have been used to selectively block the release of specific cytokines, such as IL-1β by IL-1Ra or IL-6 by KAFAK peptide. Clodronate-loaded liposomes were also used to deplete macrophages in experimental settings, showing mixed results. Metabolic or genetic manipulation of macrophages was explored using NPs to deliver adenosine and NF-κB or Notch homolog 1, translocation-associated (Notch-1) siRNAs. These approaches have showed promising experimental results related to the reprogramming of macrophages toward the M2 anti-inflammatory phenotype in the joint microenvironment, thus becoming potential candidates to improve the current treatment of OA disease.

In this line of research, we are currently working in the frame of the MEFISTO consortium H2020 project granted to develop a "meniscal functionalized scaffold to prevent knee osteoarthritis onset after meniscectomy". Therefore, we expect that the imminent combination of both fields of research, namely, the better understanding of macrophages' role in OA together with the advances in nanotechnology to control the timely and precise delivery of drugs, will provide important benefits to improve the quality of life of patients with OA.

Author Contributions: A.U. and F.M.G. writing and elaboration of figures; F.T.A. writing and organization of tables; F.T.A. and E.K. writing, review and editing. All authors have read and agreed to the published version of the manuscript.

Funding: This project has received funding from the European Union's Horizon 2020 research and innovation programme under grant agreement No 814444 (MEFISTO).

Acknowledgments: F.T.A. is recipient of a grant by the AECC ("Asociación Española Contra el Cáncer, Spain).

Conflicts of Interest: The authors declare no conflicts of interest. The authors certify that they have no affiliations with or involvement in any organization or entity with any financial interest or non-financial interest in the subject matter or materials discussed in this manuscript.

References

1. Felson, D.T.; Naimark, A.; Anderson, J.; Kazis, L.; Castelli, W.; Meenan, R.F. The prevalence of knee osteoarthritis in the elderly. The framingham osteoarthritis study. *Arthritis Rheum.* **1987**, *30*, 914–918. [CrossRef] [PubMed]

2. Vos, T.; Allen, C.; Arora, M.; Barber, R.M.; Bhutta, Z.A.; Brown, A.; Carter, A.; Casey, D.C.; Charlson, F.J.; Chen, A.Z.; et al. Global, regional, and national incidence, prevalence, and years lived with disability for 310 diseases and injuries, 1990–2015: A systematic analysis for the Global Burden of Disease Study 2015. *Lancet* **2016**, *388*, 1545–1602. [CrossRef]
3. Allen, K.D.; Golightly, Y.M. Epidemiology of osteoarthritis: State of the evidence. *Curr. Opin. Rheumatol.* **2015**, *27*, 276–283. [CrossRef] [PubMed]
4. Woolf, A.D.; Pfleger, B. Burden of major musculoskeletal conditions. *Bull. World Health Organ.* **2003**, *81*, 646–656. [CrossRef] [PubMed]
5. Dreier, R.; Wallace, S.; Fuchs, S.; Bruckner, P.; Grässel, S. Paracrine interactions of chondrocytes and macrophages in cartilage degradation: Articular chondrocytes provide factors that activate macrophage-derived pro-gelatinase B (pro-MMP-9). *J. Cell Sci.* **2001**, *114*, 3813–3822. [PubMed]
6. Mantovani, A.; Sica, A.; Sozzani, S.; Allavena, P.; Vecchi, A.; Locati, M. The chemokine system in diverse forms of macrophage activation and polarization. *Trends Immunol.* **2004**, *25*, 677–686. [CrossRef]
7. Murray, P.J. Macrophage Polarization. *Annu. Rev. Physiol.* **2017**, *79*, 541–566. [CrossRef]
8. Cook, A.D.; Braine, E.L.; Hamilton, J.A. The phenotype of inflammatory macrophages is stimulus dependent: Implications for the nature of the inflammatory response. *J. Immunol.* **2003**, *171*, 4816–4823. [CrossRef]
9. Martinez, F.O.; Helming, L.; Gordon, S. Alternative activation of macrophages: An immunologic functional perspective. *Annu. Rev. Immunol.* **2009**, *27*, 451–483. [CrossRef]
10. Liu, B.; Zhang, M.; Zhao, J.; Zheng, M.; Yang, H. Imbalance of M1/M2 macrophages is linked to severity level of knee osteoarthritis. *Exp. Ther. Med.* **2018**, *16*, 5009–5014. [CrossRef]
11. Ayhan, E.; Kesmezacar, H.; Akgun, I. Intraarticular injections (corticosteroid, hyaluronic acid, platelet rich plasma) for the knee osteoarthritis. *World J. Orthop.* **2014**, *5*, 351–361. [CrossRef] [PubMed]
12. Hunter, D.J.; Bierma-Zeinstra, S. Osteoarthritis. *Lancet* **2019**, *393*, 1745–1759. [CrossRef]
13. Pelletier, J.P.; Martel-Pelletier, J.; Rannou, F.; Cooper, C. Efficacy and safety of oral NSAIDs and analgesics in the management of osteoarthritis: Evidence from real-life setting trials and surveys. *Semin. Arthritis Rheum.* **2016**, *45*, S22–S27. [CrossRef] [PubMed]
14. Wernecke, C.; Braun, H.J.; Dragoo, J.L. The Effect of Intra-articular Corticosteroids on Articular Cartilage. *Orthop. J. Sports Med.* **2015**, 3. [CrossRef] [PubMed]
15. Jüni, P.; Hari, R.; Rutjes, A.W.; Fischer, R.; Silletta, M.G.; Reichenbach, S.; da Costa, B.R. Intra-articular corticosteroid for knee osteoarthritis. *Cochrane Database Syst. Rev.* **2015**. [CrossRef] [PubMed]
16. Holyoak, D.T.; Wheeler, T.A.; van der Meulen, M.C.H.; Singh, A. Injectable mechanical pillows for attenuation of load-induced post-traumatic osteoarthritis. *Regen. Biomater.* **2019**, *6*, 211–219. [CrossRef]
17. Gustafson, H.H.; Holt-Casper, D.; Grainger, D.W.; Ghandehari, H. Nanoparticle Uptake: The Phagocyte Problem. *Nano Today* **2015**, *10*, 487–510. [CrossRef]
18. Jin, K.; Luo, Z.; Zhang, B.; Pang, Z. Biomimetic nanoparticles for inflammation targeting. *Acta Pharm. Sin. B* **2018**, *8*, 23–33. [CrossRef]
19. Hu, G.; Guo, M.; Xu, J.; Wu, F.; Fan, J.; Huang, Q.; Yang, G.; Lv, Z.; Wang, X.; Jin, Y. Nanoparticles Targeting Macrophages as Potential Clinical Therapeutic Agents Against Cancer and Inflammation. *Front. Immunol.* **2019**, 10. [CrossRef]
20. Abou-ElNour, M.; Ishak, R.A.H.; Tiboni, M.; Bonacucina, G.; Cespi, M.; Casettari, L.; Soliman, M.E.; Geneidi, A.S. Triamcinolone acetonide-loaded PLA/PEG-PDL microparticles for effective intra-articular delivery: Synthesis, optimization, in vitro and in vivo evaluation. *J. Control. Release Off. J. Control. Release Soc.* **2019**, *309*, 125–144. [CrossRef]
21. Arunkumar, P.; Indulekha, S.; Vijayalakshmi, S.; Srivastava, R. Poly (caprolactone) microparticles and chitosan thermogels based injectable formulation of etoricoxib for the potential treatment of osteoarthritis. *Mater. Sci. Eng. C Mater. Biol. Appl.* **2016**, *61*, 534–544. [CrossRef] [PubMed]
22. Roos, H.; Laurén, M.; Adalberth, T.; Roos, E.M.; Jonsson, K.; Lohmander, L.S. Knee osteoarthritis after meniscectomy: Prevalence of radiographic changes after twenty-one years, compared with matched controls. *Arthritis Rheum.* **1998**, *41*, 687–693. [CrossRef]
23. Sellam, J.; Berenbaum, F. Is osteoarthritis a metabolic disease? *Jt. Bone Spine* **2013**, *80*, 568–573. [CrossRef] [PubMed]

24. Vuolteenaho, K.; Koskinen, A.; Kukkonen, M.; Nieminen, R.; Päivärinta, U.; Moilanen, T.; Moilanen, E. Leptin enhances synthesis of proinflammatory mediators in human osteoarthritic cartilage—Mediator role of NO in leptin-induced PGE2, IL-6, and IL-8 production. *Mediat. Inflamm.* **2009**, *2009*, 345838. [CrossRef] [PubMed]
25. Nigro, E.; Scudiero, O.; Monaco, M.L.; Palmieri, A.; Mazzarella, G.; Costagliola, C.; Bianco, A.; Daniele, A. New Insight into Adiponectin Role in Obesity and Obesity-Related Diseases. *Biomed. Res. Int.* **2014**. [CrossRef]
26. Chen, T.H.; Chen, L.; Hsieh, M.S.; Chang, C.P.; Chou, D.T.; Tsai, S.H. Evidence for a protective role for adiponectin in osteoarthritis. *Biochim. Biophys. Acta* **2006**, *1762*, 711–718. [CrossRef] [PubMed]
27. Schett, G.; Kleyer, A.; Perricone, C.; Sahinbegovic, E.; Iagnocco, A.; Zwerina, J.; Lorenzini, R.; Aschenbrenner, F.; Berenbaum, F.; D'Agostino, M.A.; et al. Diabetes Is an Independent Predictor for Severe Osteoarthritis. *Diabetes Care* **2013**, *36*, 403–409. [CrossRef]
28. Kluzek, S.; Newton, J.L.; Arden, N.K. Is osteoarthritis a metabolic disorder? *Br. Med. Bull.* **2015**, *115*, 111–121. [CrossRef]
29. Poole, A.R. Osteoarthritis as a whole joint disease. *HSS J.* **2012**, *8*, 4–6. [CrossRef]
30. Han, S.A.; Lee, S.; Seong, S.C.; Lee, M.C. Effects of CD14 macrophages and proinflammatory cytokines on chondrogenesis in osteoarthritic synovium-derived stem cells. *Tissue Eng. Part A* **2014**, *20*, 2680–2691. [CrossRef]
31. Young, L.; Katrib, A.; Cuello, C.; Vollmer-Conna, U.; Bertouch, J.V.; Roberts-Thomson, P.J.; Ahern, M.J.; Smith, M.D.; Youssef, P.P. Effects of intraarticular glucocorticoids on macrophage infiltration and mediators of joint damage in osteoarthritis synovial membranes: Findings in a double-blind, placebo-controlled study. *Arthritis Rheum.* **2001**, *44*, 343–350. [CrossRef]
32. Kraus, V.B.; McDaniel, G.; Huebner, J.L.; Stabler, T.V.; Pieper, C.F.; Shipes, S.W.; Petry, N.A.; Low, P.S.; Shen, J.; McNearney, T.A.; et al. Direct in vivo evidence of activated macrophages in human osteoarthritis. *Osteoarthr. Cartil.* **2016**, *24*, 1613–1621. [CrossRef] [PubMed]
33. Piscaer, T.M.; Müller, C.; Mindt, T.L.; Lubberts, E.; Verhaar, J.A.N.; Krenning, E.P.; Schibli, R.; Jong, M.D.; Weinans, H. Imaging of activated macrophages in experimental osteoarthritis using folate-targeted animal single-photon–emission computed tomography/computed tomography. *Arthritis Rheum.* **2011**, *63*, 1898–1907. [CrossRef] [PubMed]
34. Benito, M.; Veale, D.; FitzGerald, O.; van den Berg, W.B.; Bresnihan, B. Synovial tissue inflammation in early and late osteoarthritis. *Ann. Rheum. Dis.* **2005**, *64*, 1263–1267. [CrossRef] [PubMed]
35. Culemann, S.; Grüneboom, A.; Nicolás-Ávila, J.Á.; Weidner, D.; Lämmle, K.F.; Rothe, T.; Quintana, J.A.; Kirchner, P.; Krljanac, B.; Eberhardt, M.; et al. Locally renewing resident synovial macrophages provide a protective barrier for the joint. *Nature* **2019**, *572*, 670–675. [CrossRef] [PubMed]
36. Okamura, Y.; Watari, M.; Jerud, E.S.; Young, D.W.; Ishizaka, S.T.; Rose, J.; Chow, J.C.; Strauss, J.F. The Extra Domain a of Fibronectin Activates Toll-like Receptor 4. *J. Biol. Chem.* **2001**, *276*, 10229–10233. [CrossRef] [PubMed]
37. Termeer, C.; Benedix, F.; Sleeman, J.; Fieber, C.; Voith, U.; Ahrens, T.; Miyake, K.; Freudenberg, M.; Galanos, C.; Simon, J.C. Oligosaccharides of Hyaluronan Activate Dendritic Cells via Toll-like Receptor 4. *J. Exp. Med.* **2002**, *195*, 99–111. [CrossRef]
38. Haltmayer, E.; Ribitsch, I.; Gabner, S.; Rosser, J.; Gueltekin, S.; Peham, J.; Giese, U.; Dolezal, M.; Egerbacher, M.; Jenner, F. Co-culture of osteochondral explants and synovial membrane as in vitro model for osteoarthritis. *PLoS ONE* **2019**, *14*, e0214709. [CrossRef]
39. Nagai, H.; Kumamoto, H.; Fukuda, M.; Takahashi, T. Inducible nitric oxide synthase and apoptosis-related factors in the synovial tissues of temporomandibular joints with internal derangement and osteoarthritis. *J. Oral Maxillofac. Surg.* **2003**, *61*, 801–807. [CrossRef]
40. Horkay, F.; Basser, P.J.; Hecht, A.M.; Geissler, E. Structure and Properties of Cartilage Proteoglycans. *Macromol. Symp.* **2017**, *372*, 43–50. [CrossRef]
41. Fahy, N.; de Melle, M.L.V.; Lehmann, J.; Wei, W.; Grotenhuis, N.; Farrell, E.; van der Kraan, P.M.; Murphy, J.M.; Bastiaansen-Jenniskens, Y.M.; van Osch, G.J.V.M. Human osteoarthritic synovium impacts chondrogenic differentiation of mesenchymal stem cells via macrophage polarisation state. *Osteoarthr. Cartil.* **2014**, *22*, 1167–1175. [CrossRef] [PubMed]

42. Bondeson, J.; Wainwright, S.D.; Lauder, S.; Amos, N.; Hughes, C.E. The role of synovial macrophages and macrophage-produced cytokines in driving aggrecanases, matrix metalloproteinases, and other destructive and inflammatory responses in osteoarthritis. *Arthritis Res. Ther.* **2006**, *8*, R187. [CrossRef] [PubMed]
43. Dai, M.; Sui, B.; Xue, Y.; Liu, X.; Sun, J. Cartilage repair in degenerative osteoarthritis mediated by squid type II collagen via immunomodulating activation of M2 macrophages, inhibiting apoptosis and hypertrophy of chondrocytes. *Biomaterials* **2018**, *180*, 91–103. [CrossRef] [PubMed]
44. Shapouri-Moghaddam, A.; Mohammadian, S.; Vazini, H.; Taghadosi, M.; Esmaeili, S.A.; Mardani, F.; Seifi, B.; Mohammadi, A.; Afshari, J.T.; Sahebkar, A. Macrophage plasticity, polarization, and function in health and disease. *J. Cell. Physiol.* **2018**, *233*, 6425–6440. [CrossRef]
45. Mathiessen, A.; Conaghan, P.G. Synovitis in osteoarthritis: Current understanding with therapeutic implications. *Arthritis Res. Ther.* **2017**, *19*, 18. [CrossRef]
46. de Girolamo, L.; Kon, E.; Filardo, G.; Marmotti, A.G.; Soler, F.; Peretti, G.M.; Vannini, F.; Madry, H.; Chubinskaya, S. Regenerative approaches for the treatment of early OA. *Knee Surg. Sports Traumatol. Arthrosc.* **2016**, *24*, 1826–1835. [CrossRef]
47. Conaghan, P.G.; Cook, A.D.; Hamilton, J.A.; Tak, P.P. Therapeutic options for targeting inflammatory osteoarthritis pain. *Nat. Rev. Rheumatol.* **2019**, *15*, 355–363. [CrossRef]
48. Ghouri, A.; Conaghan, P.G. Treating osteoarthritis pain: Recent approaches using pharmacological therapies. *Clin. Exp. Rheumatol.* **2019**, *37*, 124–129.
49. Bannuru, R.R.; Osani, M.C.; Vaysbrot, E.E.; Arden, N.K.; Bennell, K.; Bierma-Zeinstra, S.M.A.; Kraus, V.B.; Lohmander, L.S.; Abbott, J.H.; Bhandari, M.; et al. OARSI guidelines for the non-surgical management of knee, hip, and polyarticular osteoarthritis. *Osteoarthr. Cartil.* **2019**, *27*, 1578–1589. [CrossRef]
50. Pritzker, K.P.H.; Gay, S.; Jimenez, S.A.; Ostergaard, K.; Pelletier, J.P.; Revell, P.A.; Salter, D.; van den Berg, W.B. Osteoarthritis cartilage histopathology: Grading and staging. *Osteoarthr. Cartil.* **2006**, *14*, 13–29. [CrossRef]
51. Ji, Q.; Xu, X.; Kang, L.; Xu, Y.; Xiao, J.; Goodman, S.B.; Zhu, X.; Li, W.; Liu, J.; Gao, X.; et al. Hematopoietic PBX-interacting protein mediates cartilage degeneration during the pathogenesis of osteoarthritis. *Nat. Commun.* **2019**, *10*, 313. [CrossRef] [PubMed]
52. Schnitzer, T.J.; Easton, R.; Pang, S.; Levinson, D.J.; Pixton, G.; Viktrup, L.; Davignon, I.; Brown, M.T.; West, C.R.; Verburg, K.M. Effect of Tanezumab on Joint Pain, Physical Function, and Patient Global Assessment of Osteoarthritis Among Patients With Osteoarthritis of the Hip or Knee: A Randomized Clinical Trial. *JAMA* **2019**, *322*, 37–48. [CrossRef] [PubMed]
53. Giroux, M.; Descoteaux, A. Cyclooxygenase-2 Expression in Macrophages: Modulation by Protein Kinase C-α. *J. Immunol.* **2000**, *165*, 3985–3991. [CrossRef] [PubMed]
54. Olszowski, T.; Gutowska, I.; Baranowska-Bosiacka, I.; Piotrowska, K.; Korbecki, J.; Kurzawski, M.; Chlubek, D. The Effect of Cadmium on COX-1 and COX-2 Gene, Protein Expression, and Enzymatic Activity in THP-1 Macrophages. *Biol. Trace Elem. Res.* **2015**, *165*, 135–144. [CrossRef] [PubMed]
55. Lanas, A.; Dumonceau, J.M.; Hunt, R.H.; Fujishiro, M.; Scheiman, J.M.; Gralnek, I.M.; Campbell, H.E.; Rostom, A.; Villanueva, C.; Sung, J.J.Y. Non-variceal upper gastrointestinal bleeding. *Nat. Rev. Dis. Primers* **2018**, *4*, 18020. [CrossRef] [PubMed]
56. Ković, S.V.; Vujović, K.S.; Srebro, D.; Medić, B.; Ilic-Mostic, T. Prevention of Renal Complications Induced by Non- Steroidal Anti-Inflammatory Drugs. *Curr. Med. Chem.* **2016**, *23*, 1953–1964. [CrossRef]
57. Cannon, C.P.; Cannon, P.J. COX-2 Inhibitors and Cardiovascular Risk. *Science* **2012**, *336*, 1386–1387. [CrossRef]
58. Rhen, T.; Cidlowski, J.A. Antiinflammatory action of glucocorticoids–new mechanisms for old drugs. *N. Engl. J. Med.* **2005**, *353*, 1711–1723. [CrossRef]
59. Jevsevar, D.S.; Shores, P.B.; Mullen, K.; Schulte, D.M.; Brown, G.A.; Cummins, D.S. Mixed Treatment Comparisons for Nonsurgical Treatment of Knee Osteoarthritis: A Network Meta-analysis. *J. Am. Acad. Orthop. Surg.* **2018**, *26*, 325–336. [CrossRef]
60. Askari, A.; Gholami, T.; NaghiZadeh, M.M.; Farjam, M.; Kouhpayeh, S.A.; Shahabfard, Z. Hyaluronic acid compared with corticosteroid injections for the treatment of osteoarthritis of the knee: A randomized control trail. *Springerplus* **2016**, 5. [CrossRef]
61. DeRogatis, M.; Anis, H.K.; Sodhi, N.; Ehiorobo, J.O.; Chughtai, M.; Bhave, A.; Mont, M.A. Non-operative treatment options for knee osteoarthritis. *Ann. Transl. Med.* **2019**, *7*, S245. [CrossRef] [PubMed]
62. Flynn, J.K.; Dankers, W.; Morand, E.F. Could GILZ Be the Answer to Glucocorticoid Toxicity in Lupus? *Front. Immunol.* **2019**, *10*, 1684. [CrossRef] [PubMed]

63. Azetsu, Y.; Chatani, M.; Dodo, Y.; Karakawa, A.; Sakai, N.; Negishi-Koga, T.; Takami, M. Treatment with synthetic glucocorticoid impairs bone metabolism, as revealed by in vivo imaging of osteoblasts and osteoclasts in medaka fish. *Biomed. Pharmacother.* **2019**, *118*, 109101. [CrossRef]
64. Litwiniuk, M.; Krejner, A.; Speyrer, M.S.; Gauto, A.R.; Grzela, T. Hyaluronic Acid in Inflammation and Tissue Regeneration. *Wounds* **2016**, *28*, 78–88. [PubMed]
65. Rayahin, J.E.; Buhrman, J.S.; Zhang, Y.; Koh, T.J.; Gemeinhart, R.A. High and low molecular weight hyaluronic acid differentially influence macrophage activation. *ACS Biomater. Sci. Eng.* **2015**, *1*, 481–493. [CrossRef] [PubMed]
66. Shi, Q.; Zhao, L.; Xu, C.; Zhang, L.; Zhao, H. High Molecular Weight Hyaluronan Suppresses Macrophage M1 Polarization and Enhances IL-10 Production in PM2.5-Induced Lung Inflammation. *Molecules* **2019**, *24*, 1766. [CrossRef] [PubMed]
67. Liu, M.; Tolg, C.; Turley, E. Dissecting the Dual Nature of Hyaluronan in the Tumor Microenvironment. *Front. Immunol.* **2019**, *10*, 947. [CrossRef]
68. Kim, Y.; Eom, S.; Park, D.; Kim, H.; Jeoung, D. The Hyaluronic Acid-HDAC3-miRNA Network in Allergic Inflammation. *Front. Immunol.* **2015**, *6*, 210. [CrossRef]
69. Casale, M.; Moffa, A.; Vella, P.; Sabatino, L.; Capuano, F.; Salvinelli, B.; Lopez, M.A.; Carinci, F.; Salvinelli, F. Hyaluronic acid: Perspectives in dentistry. A systematic review. *Int. J. Immunopathol. Pharmcol.* **2016**, *29*, 572–582. [CrossRef]
70. Stellavato, A.; La Noce, M.; Corsuto, L.; Pirozzi, A.V.A.; De Rosa, M.; Papaccio, G.; Schiraldi, C.; Tirino, V. Hybrid Complexes of High and Low Molecular Weight Hyaluronans Highly Enhance HASCs Differentiation: Implication for Facial Bioremodelling. *Cell. Physiol. Biochem.* **2017**, *44*, 1078–1092. [CrossRef]
71. Chen, K.L.; Yeh, Y.Y.; Lung, J.; Yang, Y.C.; Yuan, K. Mineralization Effect of Hyaluronan on Dental Pulp Cells via CD44. *J. Endod.* **2016**, *42*, 711–716. [CrossRef] [PubMed]
72. La Gatta, A.; Corsuto, L.; Salzillo, R.; D'Agostino, A.; De Rosa, M.; Bracco, A.; Schiraldi, C. In Vitro Evaluation of Hybrid Cooperative Complexes of Hyaluronic Acid as a Potential New Ophthalmic Treatment. *J. Ocul. Pharmcol. Ther.* **2018**, *34*, 677–684. [CrossRef] [PubMed]
73. Mowbray, C.A.; Shams, S.; Chung, G.; Stanton, A.; Aldridge, P.; Suchenko, A.; Pickard, R.S.; Ali, A.S.; Hall, J. High molecular weight hyaluronic acid: A two-pronged protectant against infection of the urogenital tract? *Clin. Transl. Immunol.* **2018**, *7*, e1021. [CrossRef] [PubMed]
74. Parameswaran, N.; Patial, S. Tumor Necrosis Factor-α Signaling in Macrophages. *Crit. Rev. Eukaryot. Gene Exp.* **2010**, *20*, 87–103. [CrossRef]
75. Aitken, D.; Laslett, L.L.; Pan, F.; Haugen, I.K.; Otahal, P.; Bellamy, N.; Bird, P.; Jones, G. A randomised double-blind placebo-controlled crossover trial of HUMira (adalimumab) for erosive hand OsteoaRthritis—The HUMOR trial. *Osteoarthr. Cartil.* **2018**, *26*, 880–887. [CrossRef]
76. Wang, J. Efficacy and safety of adalimumab by intra-articular injection for moderate to severe knee osteoarthritis: An open-label randomized controlled trial. *J. Int. Med. Res.* **2018**, *46*, 326–334. [CrossRef]
77. Ohtori, S.; Orita, S.; Yamauchi, K.; Eguchi, Y.; Ochiai, N.; Kishida, S.; Kuniyoshi, K.; Aoki, Y.; Nakamura, J.; Ishikawa, T.; et al. Efficacy of Direct Injection of Etanercept into Knee Joints for Pain in Moderate and Severe Knee Osteoarthritis. *Yonsei Med. J.* **2015**, *56*, 1379–1383. [CrossRef]
78. Takano, S.; Uchida, K.; Inoue, G.; Miyagi, M.; Aikawa, J.; Iwase, D.; Iwabuchi, K.; Matsumoto, T.; Satoh, M.; Mukai, M.; et al. Nerve growth factor regulation and production by macrophages in osteoarthritic synovium. *Clin. Exp. Immunol.* **2017**, *190*, 235–243. [CrossRef]
79. Denk, F.; Bennett, D.L.; McMahon, S.B. Nerve Growth Factor and Pain Mechanisms. *Annu. Rev. Neurosci.* **2017**, *40*, 307–325. [CrossRef]
80. Dakin, P.; DiMartino, S.J.; Gao, H.; Maloney, J.; Kivitz, A.J.; Schnitzer, T.J.; Stahl, N.; Yancopoulos, G.D.; Geba, G.P. The Efficacy, Tolerability, and Joint Safety of Fasinumab in Osteoarthritis Pain: A Phase IIb/III Double-Blind, Placebo-Controlled, Randomized Clinical Trial. *Arthritis Rheumatol.* **2019**, *71*, 1824–1834. [CrossRef]
81. Fleischmann, R.M.; Bliddal, H.; Blanco, F.J.; Schnitzer, T.J.; Peterfy, C.; Chen, S.; Wang, L.; Feng, S.; Conaghan, P.G.; Berenbaum, F.; et al. A Phase II Trial of Lutikizumab, an Anti-Interleukin-1α/β Dual Variable Domain Immunoglobulin, in Knee Osteoarthritis Patients with Synovitis. *Arthritis Rheumatol.* **2019**, *71*, 1056–1069. [CrossRef] [PubMed]

82. Yoshida, Y.; Tanaka, T. Interleukin 6 and Rheumatoid Arthritis. *Biomed. Res. Int.* **2014**, *2014*, 698313. [CrossRef] [PubMed]
83. Stefani, R.M.; Lee, A.J.; Tan, A.R.; Halder, S.S.; Hu, Y.; Guo, X.E.; Stoker, A.M.; Ateshian, G.A.; Marra, K.G.; Cook, J.L.; et al. Sustained low-dose dexamethasone delivery via a PLGA microsphere-embedded agarose implant for enhanced osteochondral repair. *Acta Biomater.* **2020**, *102*, 326–340. [CrossRef] [PubMed]
84. Kamel, R.; Salama, A.H.; Mahmoud, A.A. Development and optimization of self-assembling nanosystem for intra-articular delivery of indomethacin. *Int. J. Pharm.* **2016**. [CrossRef] [PubMed]
85. Chen, A.L.; Desai, P.; Adler, E.M.; Di Cesare, P.E. Granulomatous inflammation after Hylan G-F 20 viscosupplementation of the knee: A report of six cases. *J. Bone Jt. Surg. Am.* **2002**, *84*, 1142–1147. [CrossRef]
86. Charalambous, C.P.; Tryfonidis, M.; Sadiq, S.; Hirst, P.; Paul, A. Septic arthritis following intra-articular steroid injection of the knee—A survey of current practice regarding antiseptic technique used during intra-articular steroid injection of the knee. *Clin. Rheumatol.* **2003**, *22*, 386–390. [CrossRef]
87. Andón, F.T.; Fadeel, B. Programmed cell death: Molecular mechanisms and implications for safety assessment of nanomaterials. *Acc. Chem. Res.* **2013**, *46*, 733–742. [CrossRef]
88. Boraschi, D.; Italiani, P.; Palomba, R.; Decuzzi, P.; Duschl, A.; Fadeel, B.; Moghimi, S.M. Nanoparticles and innate immunity: New perspectives on host defence. *Semin. Immunol.* **2017**, *34*, 33–51. [CrossRef]
89. Wilhelm, S.; Tavares, A.J.; Dai, Q.; Ohta, S.; Audet, J.; Dvorak, H.F.; Chan, W.C.W. Analysis of nanoparticle delivery to tumours. *Nat. Rev. Mater.* **2016**, *1*, 16014. [CrossRef]
90. Andón, F.T.; Digifico, E.; Maeda, A.; Erreni, M.; Mantovani, A.; Alonso, M.J.; Allavena, P. Targeting tumor associated macrophages: The new challenge for nanomedicine. *Semin. Immunol.* **2017**, *34*, 103–113. [CrossRef]
91. Mosaiab, T.; Farr, D.C.; Kiefel, M.J.; Houston, T.A. Carbohydrate-based nanocarriers and their application to target macrophages and deliver antimicrobial agents. *Adv. Drug Deliv. Rev.* **2019**, *151*, 94–129. [CrossRef] [PubMed]
92. Gaspar, N.; Zambito, G.; Löwik, C.M.W.G.; Mezzanotte, L. Active Nano-targeting of Macrophages. *Curr. Pharm. Des.* **2019**, *25*, 1951–1961. [CrossRef] [PubMed]
93. Zhang, J.; Zu, Y.; Dhanasekara, C.S.; Li, J.; Wu, D.; Fan, Z.; Wang, S. Detection and treatment of atherosclerosis using nanoparticles. *Wiley Interdiscip. Rev. Nanomed. Nanobiotechnol.* **2017**, 9. [CrossRef] [PubMed]
94. Wibroe, P.P.; Anselmo, A.C.; Nilsson, P.H.; Sarode, A.; Gupta, V.; Urbanics, R.; Szebeni, J.; Hunter, A.C.; Mitragotri, S.; Mollnes, T.E.; et al. Bypassing adverse injection reactions to nanoparticles through shape modification and attachment to erythrocytes. *Nat. Nanotechnol.* **2017**, *12*, 589–594. [CrossRef]
95. Moghimi, S.M.; Simberg, D.; Skotland, T.; Yaghmur, A.; Hunter, A.C. The Interplay between Blood Proteins, Complement, and Macrophages on Nanomedicine Performance and Responses. *J. Pharmacol. Exp. Ther.* **2019**, *370*, 581–592. [CrossRef]
96. Liu, P.; Gu, L.; Ren, L.; Chen, J.; Li, T.; Wang, X.; Yang, J.; Chen, C.; Sun, L. Intra-articular injection of etoricoxib-loaded PLGA-PEG-PLGA triblock copolymeric nanoparticles attenuates osteoarthritis progression. *Am. J. Transl. Res.* **2019**, *11*, 6775–6789.
97. Malam, Y.; Loizidou, M.; Seifalian, A.M. Liposomes and nanoparticles: Nanosized vehicles for drug delivery in cancer. *Trends Pharmcol. Sci.* **2009**, *30*, 592–599. [CrossRef]
98. Kang, M.L.; Kim, J.E.; Im, G.I. Thermoresponsive nanospheres with independent dual drug release profiles for the treatment of osteoarthritis. *Acta Biomater.* **2016**, *39*, 65–78. [CrossRef]
99. Kim, S.R.; Ho, M.J.; Kim, S.H.; Cho, H.R.; Kim, H.S.; Choi, Y.S.; Choi, Y.W.; Kang, M.J. Increased localized delivery of piroxicam by cationic nanoparticles after intra-articular injection. *Drug Des. Devel. Ther.* **2016**, *10*, 3779–3787. [CrossRef]
100. Sooriakumaran, P. COX-2 inhibitors and the heart: Are all coxibs the same? *Postgrad. Med. J.* **2006**, *82*, 242–245. [CrossRef]
101. Villamagna, I.J.; Gordon, T.N.; Hurtig, M.B.; Beier, F.; Gillies, E.R. Poly(ester amide) particles for controlled delivery of celecoxib. *J. Biomed. Mater. Res. A* **2019**, *107*, 1235–1243. [CrossRef] [PubMed]
102. Cope, P.J.; Ourradi, K.; Li, Y.; Sharif, M. Models of osteoarthritis: The good, the bad and the promising. *Osteoarthr. Cartil.* **2019**, *27*, 230–239. [CrossRef] [PubMed]
103. Nicolaides, N.C.; Pavlaki, A.N.; Maria Alexandra, M.A.; Chrousos, G.P. Glucocorticoid Therapy and Adrenal Suppression. In *Endotext*; Feingold, K.R., Anawalt, B., Boyce, A., Chrousos, G., Dungan, K., Grossman, A., Hershman, J.M., Kaltsas, G., Koch, C., Kopp, P., et al., Eds.; MDText.com, Inc.: South Dartmouth, MA, USA, 2000.

104. Gómez-Gaete, C.; Tsapis, N.; Besnard, M.; Bochot, A.; Fattal, E. Encapsulation of dexamethasone into biodegradable polymeric nanoparticles. *Int. J. Pharm.* **2007**, *331*, 153–159. [CrossRef] [PubMed]
105. Lorscheider, M.; Tsapis, N.; Ur-Rehman, M.; Gaudin, F.; Stolfa, I.; Abreu, S.; Mura, S.; Chaminade, P.; Espeli, M.; Fattal, E. Dexamethasone palmitate nanoparticles: An efficient treatment for rheumatoid arthritis. *J. Control. Release Off. J. Control. Release Soc.* **2019**, *296*, 179–189. [CrossRef]
106. Horisawa, E.; Hirota, T.; Kawazoe, S.; Yamada, J.; Yamamoto, H.; Takeuchi, H.; Kawashima, Y. Prolonged anti-inflammatory action of DL-lactide/glycolide copolymer nanospheres containing betamethasone sodium phosphate for an intra-articular delivery system in antigen-induced arthritic rabbit. *Pharm. Res.* **2002**, *19*, 403–410. [CrossRef] [PubMed]
107. Gan, D.; Lyon, L.A. Tunable swelling kinetics in core–shell hydrogel nanoparticles. *J. Am. Chem. Soc.* **2001**, *123*, 7511–7517. [CrossRef]
108. Bartlett, R.L.; Medow, M.R.; Panitch, A.; Seal, B. Hemocompatible poly(NIPAm-MBA-AMPS) colloidal nanoparticles as carriers of anti-inflammatory cell penetrating peptides. *Biomacromolecules* **2012**, *13*, 1204–1211. [CrossRef]
109. McMasters, J.; Poh, S.; Lin, J.B.; Panitch, A. Delivery of anti-inflammatory peptides from hollow PEGylated poly(NIPAM) nanoparticles reduces inflammation in an ex vivo osteoarthritis model. *J. Control Release* **2017**, *258*, 161–170. [CrossRef]
110. Bartlett, R.L.; Sharma, S.; Panitch, A. Cell-penetrating peptides released from thermosensitive nanoparticles suppress pro-inflammatory cytokine response by specifically targeting inflamed cartilage explants. *Nanomedicine* **2013**, *9*, 419–427. [CrossRef]
111. Re, F.; Mengozzi, M.; Muzio, M.; Dinarello, C.A.; Mantovani, A.; Colotta, F. Expression of interleukin-1 receptor antagonist (IL-1ra) by human circulating polymorphonuclear cells. *Eur. J. Immunol.* **1993**, *23*, 570–573. [CrossRef]
112. Clements, A.E.B.; Murphy, W.L. Injectable biomaterials for delivery of interleukin-1 receptor antagonist: Toward improving its therapeutic effect. *Acta Biomater.* **2019**, *93*, 123–134. [CrossRef] [PubMed]
113. Agarwal, R.; Volkmer, T.M.; Wang, P.; Lee, L.A.; Wang, Q.; García, A.J. Synthesis of self-assembled IL-1Ra-presenting nanoparticles for the treatment of osteoarthritis. *J. Biomed. Mater. Res. A* **2016**, *104*, 595–599. [CrossRef] [PubMed]
114. Corciulo, C.; Lendhey, M.; Wilder, T.; Schoen, H.; Cornelissen, A.S.; Chang, G.; Kennedy, O.D.; Cronstein, B.N. Endogenous adenosine maintains cartilage homeostasis and exogenous adenosine inhibits osteoarthritis progression. *Nat. Commun.* **2017**, *8*, 15019. [CrossRef] [PubMed]
115. Liu, X.; Corciulo, C.; Arabagian, S.; Ulman, A.; Cronstein, B.N. Adenosine-Functionalized Biodegradable PLA-b-PEG Nanoparticles Ameliorate Osteoarthritis in Rats. *Sci. Rep.* **2019**, *9*, 7430. [CrossRef] [PubMed]
116. Aggarwal, B.B.; Harikumar, K.B. Potential therapeutic effects of curcumin, the anti-inflammatory agent, against neurodegenerative, cardiovascular, pulmonary, metabolic, autoimmune and neoplastic diseases. *Int. J. Biochem. Cell Biol.* **2009**, *41*, 40–59. [CrossRef] [PubMed]
117. Udo, M.; Muneta, T.; Tsuji, K.; Ozeki, N.; Nakagawa, Y.; Ohara, T.; Saito, R.; Yanagisawa, K.; Koga, H.; Sekiya, I. Monoiodoacetic acid induces arthritis and synovitis in rats in a dose- and time-dependent manner: Proposed model-specific scoring systems. *Osteoarthr. Cartil.* **2016**, *24*, 1284–1291. [CrossRef]
118. Kang, C.; Jung, E.; Hyeon, H.; Seon, S.; Lee, D. Acid-activatable polymeric curcumin nanoparticles as therapeutic agents for osteoarthritis. *Nanomedicine* **2020**, *23*, 102104. [CrossRef]
119. Chen, X.; Liu, Y.; Wen, Y.; Yu, Q.; Liu, J.; Zhao, Y.; Liu, J.; Ye, G. A photothermal-triggered nitric oxide nanogenerator combined with siRNA for precise therapy of osteoarthritis by suppressing macrophage inflammation. *Nanoscale* **2019**, *11*, 6693–6709. [CrossRef]
120. Mota, A.H.; Direito, R.; Carrasco, M.P.; Rijo, P.; Ascensão, L.; Viana, A.S.; Rocha, J.; Eduardo-Figueira, M.; Rodrigues, M.J.; Custódio, L.; et al. Combination of hyaluronic acid and PLGA particles as hybrid systems for viscosupplementation in osteoarthritis. *Int. J. Pharm.* **2019**, *559*, 13–22. [CrossRef]
121. Zhou, P.H.; Qiu, B.; Deng, R.H.; Li, H.J.; Xu, X.F.; Shang, X.F. Chondroprotective Effects of Hyaluronic Acid-Chitosan Nanoparticles Containing Plasmid DNA Encoding Cytokine Response Modifier A in a Rat Knee Osteoarthritis Model. *Cell. Physiol. Biochem.* **2018**, *47*, 1207–1216. [CrossRef]
122. Staines, K.A.; Poulet, B.; Wentworth, D.N.; Pitsillides, A.A. The STR/ort mouse model of spontaneous osteoarthritis—An update. *Osteoarthr. Cartil.* **2017**, *25*, 802–808. [CrossRef] [PubMed]

123. Sakurai, Y.; Fujita, M.; Kawasaki, S.; Sanaki, T.; Yoshioka, T.; Higashino, K.; Tofukuji, S.; Yoneda, S.; Takahashi, T.; Koda, K.; et al. Contribution of synovial macrophages to rat advanced osteoarthritis pain resistant to cyclooxygenase inhibitors. *Pain* **2019**, *160*, 895–907. [CrossRef] [PubMed]
124. Bailey, K.N.; Furman, B.D.; Zeitlin, J.; Kimmerling, K.A.; Wu, C.L.; Guilak, F.; Olson, S.A. Intra-articular depletion of macrophages increases acute synovitis and alters macrophage polarity in the injured mouse knee. *Osteoarthr. Cartil.* **2020**. [CrossRef] [PubMed]
125. Srinath, P.; Vyas, S.P.; Diwan, P.V. Preparation and pharmacodynamic evaluation of liposomes of indomethacin. *Drug Dev. Ind. Pharm.* **2000**, *26*, 313–321. [CrossRef] [PubMed]
126. Dong, J.; Jiang, D.; Wang, Z.; Wu, G.; Miao, L.; Huang, L. Intra-articular delivery of liposomal celecoxib-hyaluronate combination for the treatment of osteoarthritis in rabbit model. *Int. J. Pharm.* **2013**, *441*, 285–290. [CrossRef] [PubMed]
127. Bartneck, M.; Peters, F.M.; Warzecha, K.T.; Bienert, M.; van Bloois, L.; Trautwein, C.; Lammers, T.; Tacke, F. Liposomal encapsulation of dexamethasone modulates cytotoxicity, inflammatory cytokine response, and migratory properties of primary human macrophages. *Nanomedicine* **2014**, *10*, 1209–1220. [CrossRef]
128. Anderson, R.; Franch, A.; Castell, M.; Perez-Cano, F.J.; Bräuer, R.; Pohlers, D.; Gajda, M.; Siskos, A.P.; Katsila, T.; Tamvakopoulos, C.; et al. Liposomal encapsulation enhances and prolongs the anti-inflammatory effects of water-soluble dexamethasone phosphate in experimental adjuvant arthritis. *Arthritis Res. Ther.* **2010**, *12*, R147. [CrossRef]
129. Avnir, Y.; Ulmansky, R.; Wasserman, V.; Even-Chen, S.; Broyer, M.; Barenholz, Y.; Naparstek, Y. Amphipathic weak acid glucocorticoid prodrugs remote-loaded into sterically stabilized nanoliposomes evaluated in arthritic rats and in a Beagle dog: A novel approach to treating autoimmune arthritis. *Arthritis Rheum.* **2008**, *58*, 119–129. [CrossRef]
130. Duan, W.; Li, H. Combination of NF-kB targeted siRNA and methotrexate in a hybrid nanocarrier towards the effective treatment in rheumatoid arthritis. *J. Nanobiotechnol.* **2018**, *16*, 58. [CrossRef]
131. Sergeeva, V.; Kraevaya, O.; Ershova, E.; Kameneva, L.; Malinovskaya, E.; Dolgikh, O.; Konkova, M.; Voronov, I.; Zhilenkov, A.; Veiko, N.; et al. Antioxidant Properties of Fullerene Derivatives Depend on Their Chemical Structure: A Study of Two Fullerene Derivatives on HELFs. *Oxid. Med. Cell. Longev.* **2019**, *2019*, 4398695. [CrossRef]
132. Yudoh, K.; Shishido, K.; Murayama, H.; Yano, M.; Matsubayashi, K.; Takada, H.; Nakamura, H.; Masuko, K.; Kato, T.; Nishioka, K. Water-soluble C60 fullerene prevents degeneration of articular cartilage in osteoarthritis via down-regulation of chondrocyte catabolic activity and inhibition of cartilage degeneration during disease development. *Arthritis Rheum.* **2007**, *56*, 3307–3318. [CrossRef] [PubMed]
133. Yang, X.; Ebrahimi, A.; Li, J.; Cui, Q. Fullerene-biomolecule conjugates and their biomedicinal applications. *Int. J. Nanomed.* **2014**, *9*, 77–92. [CrossRef] [PubMed]
134. Pei, Y.; Cui, F.; Du, X.; Shang, G.; Xiao, W.; Yang, X.; Cui, Q. Antioxidative nanofullerol inhibits macrophage activation and development of osteoarthritis in rats. *Int. J. Nanomed.* **2019**, *14*, 4145–4155. [CrossRef] [PubMed]
135. Yu, Y.; Shen, X.; Luo, Z.; Hu, Y.; Li, M.; Ma, P.; Ran, Q.; Dai, L.; He, Y.; Cai, K. Osteogenesis potential of different titania nanotubes in oxidative stress microenvironment. *Biomaterials* **2018**, *167*, 44–57. [CrossRef]
136. Mohammadinejad, R.; Ashrafizadeh, M.; Pardakhty, A.; Uzieliene, I.; Denkovskij, J.; Bernotiene, E.; Janssen, L.; Lorite, G.S.; Saarakkala, S.; Mobasheri, A. Nanotechnological Strategies for Osteoarthritis Diagnosis, Monitoring, Clinical Management, and Regenerative Medicine: Recent Advances and Future Opportunities. *Curr. Rheumatol. Rep.* **2020**, *22*, 12. [CrossRef]
137. Sacchetti, C.; Liu-Bryan, R.; Magrini, A.; Rosato, N.; Bottini, N.; Bottini, M. Polyethylene-glycol-modified single-walled carbon nanotubes for intra-articular delivery to chondrocytes. *ACS Nano* **2014**, *8*, 12280–12291. [CrossRef]
138. Lee, Y.K.; Kim, S.W.; Park, J.Y.; Kang, W.C.; Kang, Y.J.; Khang, D. Suppression of human arthritis synovial fibroblasts inflammation using dexamethasone-carbon nanotubes via increasing caveolin-dependent endocytosis and recovering mitochondrial membrane potential. *Int. J. Nanomed.* **2017**, *12*, 5761–5779. [CrossRef]
139. Liu, A.; Wang, P.; Zhang, J.; Ye, W.; Wei, Q. Restoration Effect and Tribological Behavior of Hyaluronic Acid Reinforced with Graphene Oxide in Osteoarthritis. *J. Nanosci. Nanotechnol.* **2019**, *19*, 91–97. [CrossRef]

140. Li, H.; Guo, H.; Lei, C.; Liu, L.; Xu, L.; Feng, Y.; Ke, J.; Fang, W.; Song, H.; Xu, C.; et al. Nanotherapy in Joints: Increasing Endogenous Hyaluronan Production by Delivering Hyaluronan Synthase 2. *Adv. Mater.* **2019**, *31*, e1904535. [CrossRef]
141. Sarkar, A.; Carvalho, E.; D'souza, A.A.; Banerjee, R. Liposome-encapsulated fish oil protein-tagged gold nanoparticles for intra-articular therapy in osteoarthritis. *Nanomedicine* **2019**, *14*, 871–887. [CrossRef]
142. Ren, S.X.; Zhan, B.; Lin, Y.; Ma, D.S.; Yan, H. Selenium Nanoparticles Dispersed in Phytochemical Exert Anti-Inflammatory Activity by Modulating Catalase, GPx1, and COX-2 Gene Expression in a Rheumatoid Arthritis Rat Model. *Med. Sci. Monit.* **2019**, *25*, 991–1000. [CrossRef] [PubMed]
143. Zhou, F.; Mei, J.; Yang, S.; Han, X.; Li, H.; Yu, Z.; Qiao, H.; Tang, T. Modified ZIF-8 Nanoparticles Attenuate Osteoarthritis by Reprogramming the Metabolic Pathway of Synovial Macrophages. *ACS Appl. Mater. Interfaces* **2020**, *12*, 2009–2022. [CrossRef] [PubMed]
144. Griffin, T.M.; Scanzello, C.R. Innate inflammation and synovial macrophages in osteoarthritis pathophysiology. *Clin. Exp. Rheumatol.* **2019**, *37*, 57–63. [PubMed]
145. Xie, J.; Huang, Z.; Yu, X.; Zhou, L.; Pei, F. Clinical implications of macrophage dysfunction in the development of osteoarthritis of the knee. *Cytokine Growth Factor Rev.* **2019**, *46*, 36–44. [CrossRef]
146. Wu, C.L.; Harasymowicz, N.S.; Klimak, M.A.; Collins, K.H.; Guilak, F. The role of macrophages in osteoarthritis and cartilage repair. *Osteoarthr. Cartil.* **2020**, *28*, 544–554. [CrossRef]
147. Alvarez-Soria, M.A.; Largo, R.; Santillana, J.; Sánchez-Pernaute, O.; Calvo, E.; Hernández, M.; Egido, J.; Herrero-Beaumont, G. Long term NSAID treatment inhibits COX-2 synthesis in the knee synovial membrane of patients with osteoarthritis: Differential proinflammatory cytokine profile between celecoxib and aceclofenac. *Ann. Rheum. Dis.* **2006**, *65*, 998–1005. [CrossRef]
148. Pasquali Ronchetti, I.; Guerra, D.; Taparelli, F.; Boraldi, F.; Bergamini, G.; Mori, G.; Zizzi, F.; Frizziero, L. Morphological analysis of knee synovial membrane biopsies from a randomized controlled clinical study comparing the effects of sodium hyaluronate (Hyalgan) and methylprednisolone acetate (Depomedrol) in osteoarthritis. *Rheumatology* **2001**, *40*, 158–169. [CrossRef]

MDPI
St. Alban-Anlage 66
4052 Basel
Switzerland
Tel. +41 61 683 77 34
Fax +41 61 302 89 18
www.mdpi.com

Nanomaterials Editorial Office
E-mail: nanomaterials@mdpi.com
www.mdpi.com/journal/nanomaterials

www.ingramcontent.com/pod-product-compliance
Lightning Source LLC
LaVergne TN
LVHW070734100526
838202LV00013B/1231